COVID-19 AND IMMUNOMODULATION WITH SPECIAL EMPHASIS ON NUTRACEUTICAL AND HERBAL FORMULATION

COVID-19 AND IMMUNOMODULATION WITH SPECIAL EMPHASIS ON NUTRACEUTICAL AND HERBAL FORMULATION

Edited by

Rajesh K. Kesharwani

Raj K. Keservani

AAP | APPLE ACADEMIC PRESS

First edition published 2024

Apple Academic Press Inc.
1265 Goldenrod Circle, NE,
Palm Bay, FL 32905 USA

760 Laurentian Drive, Unit 19,
Burlington, ON L7N 0A4, CANADA

CRC Press
2385 NW Executive Center Drive,
Suite 320, Boca Raton FL 33431

4 Park Square, Milton Park,
Abingdon, Oxon, OX14 4RN UK

Library and Archives Canada Cataloguing in Publication

Title: COVID-19 and immunomodulation with special emphasis on nutraceutical and herbal formulation / edited by Rajesh K. Kesharwani, Raj K. Keservani.
Names: Kesharwani, Rajesh K., 1978- editor. | Keservani, Raj K., 1981- editor.
Description: First edition. | Includes bibliographical references and index.
Identifiers: Canadiana (print) 20230450466 | Canadiana (ebook) 20230450539 | ISBN 9781774913178 (hardcover) | ISBN 9781774913185 (softcover) | ISBN 9781003347804 (ebook)
Subjects: LCSH: COVID-19 (Disease)—Treatment. | LCSH: COVID-19 (Disease)—Immunotherapy. | LCSH: Functional foods. | LCSH: Herbs—Therapeutic use. | LCSH: Immune response—Regulation.
Classification: LCC RA644.C67 C68 2024 | DDC 614.5/92414406—dc23

Library of Congress Cataloging-in-Publication Data

CIP data on file with US Library of Congress

ISBN: 978-1-77491-317-8 (hbk)
ISBN: 978-1-77491-318-5 (pbk)
ISBN: 978-1-00334-780-4 (ebk)

About the Editors

Rajesh K. Kesharwani, PhD, MTech

Rajesh K. Kesharwani, PhD, MTech, has more than 10 years of research and eight years of teaching experience at various institutes of India, imparting bioinformatics and biotechnology education. He has received several awards, including the NASI-Swarna Jayanti Puruskar by The National Academy of Sciences of India. He has supervised PhD, postgraduate, and undergraduate students in their research work and has authored over 40 peer-reviewed articles, 20 book chapters, and 11 edited books with international publishers. He has been a member of many scientific communities as well as a reviewer for many international journals. He has presented many papers in various national and international conferences. Dr. Kesharwani received his PhD from the Indian Institute of Information Technology, Allahabad, India, and has worked at NIT Warangal. He has been a recipient of the Ministry of Human Resource Development (India) Fellowship and Senior Research Fellowship from the Indian Council of Medical Research, India. His research fields of interest are medical informatics, protein structure and function prediction, computer-aided drug designing, structural biology, drug delivery, cancer biology, nanobiotechnology, and biomedical sciences.

Raj K. Keservani, MPharm

Raj K. Keservani, MPharm, is a Faculty of B. Pharmacy, CSM Group of Institutions, Allahabad, India. He has more than 12 years of academic (teaching) experience from various institutes of India in pharmaceutical education. He has published 31 peer-reviewed papers in the field of pharmaceutical sciences in national and international journals, 43 book chapters, 3 coauthored books, and 18 edited books. He is also active as a reviewer for several international scientific journals. Mr. Keservani graduated with a degree in pharmacy from the Department of Pharmacy,

Kumaun University, Nainital, Uttarakhand, India. He received his MPharm degree (specialization in pharmaceutics) from the School of Pharmaceutical Sciences, Rajiv Gandhi Proudyogiki Vishwavidyalaya, Bhopal, India. Mr. Keservani is a life member of Society of Pharmaceutical Education and Research (SPER). His research interests include nutraceutical and functional foods, novel drug delivery systems (NDDS), transdermal drug delivery/drug delivery, health science, cancer biology, and neurobiology.

Contents

Contributors

Anamika
Department of Kaumarbhritya, State Ayurvedic College and Hospital, Lucknow, Uttar Pradesh, India

Eknath D. Ahire
Department of Pharmaceutics, SSS's Divine College of Pharmacy, Satana, Maharashtra, India

Anamika Basu
Department of Biochemistry, Gurudas College, Narkeldanga, Kolkata, India

Mounika Bharat
Department of Pharmaceutics, Shri D. D. Vispute College of Pharmacy & Research Center, Panvel, Dist Raigad, Maharashtra, India

Umesh Dhakad
Department of Pharmacy, Ravishankar College of Pharmacy, Bhopal, Madhya Pradesh, India

Ashish S. Jain
Department of Pharmaceutics, Shri D. D. Vispute College of Pharmacy & Research Center, Panvel, Maharashtra, India

Urmila Jarouliya
School of Studies in Biochemistry, Jiwaji University, Gwalior, Madhya Pradesh, India

Khushwinder Kaur
Department of Chemistry and Centre of Advanced Studies in Chemistry, Panjab University, Chandigarh, Punjab, India

Raj K. Keservani
Faculty of B. Pharmacy, CSM Group of Institutions, Prayagraj, Uttar Pradesh, India

Ravi Kesharwani
Department of Pharmacy, Ravishankar College of Pharmacy, Bhopal, Madhya Pradesh, India

Kapil Khatri
Department of Pharmacy, Ravishankar College of Pharmacy, Bhopal, Madhya Pradesh, India

Sanjay J. Kshirsagar
Department of Pharmaceutics, MET's Institute of Pharmacy, Bhujbal Knowledge City, Nashik, Maharashtra, India

Umesh D. Laddha
Department of Pharmaceutics, MET's Institute of Pharmacy, Bhujbal Knowledge City, Nashik, Maharashtra, India

Rajkumari Lodhi
Department of Pharmacy, Ravishankar College of Pharmacy, Bhopal, Madhya Pradesh, India

Shanti Bhushan Mishra
Department of Pharmacognosy, United Institute of Pharmacy, Prayagraj, Uttar Pradesh, India

Bhushan R. Rane
Department of Pharmaceutics, Shri D. D. Vispute College of Pharmacy & Research Center, Panvel, Maharashtra, India

Satish Shilpi
Department of Pharmacy, Ravishankar College of Pharmacy, Bhopal, Madhya Pradesh, India

Amit Kumar Singh
Department of Pharmaceutics, United Institute of Pharmacy, Prayagraj, Uttar Pradesh, India

Anil Kumar Singh
Department of Pharmaceutics, United Institute of Pharmacy, Prayagraj, Uttar Pradesh, India

Shradhanjali Singh
Department of Pharmaceutical Chemistry, United Institute of Pharmacy, Prayagraj, Uttar Pradesh, India

Vijayraj N. Sonawane
Department of Pharmaceutics, SSS's Divine College of Pharmacy, Satana, Maharashtra, India

Anupam Srivastava
Department of Kayachikitsa, Chandra Shekhar Singh Ayurved Sansthan, Kaushambi, Uttar Pradesh, India

Khemchand R. Surana
Department of Pharmaceutics, SSS's Divine College of Pharmacy, Satana, Maharashtra, India

Tejas S. Telange
Department of Pharmaceutics, Shri D. D. Vispute College of Pharmacy & Research Center, Panvel, Maharashtra, India

Gokul S. Talele
Department of Pharmaceutics, Matoshri College of Pharmacy, Eklahare, Nashik, Maharashtra, India

Swati G. Talele
Department of Pharmaceutics, Sandip Institute of Pharmaceutical Sciences, Nashik, Maharashtra, India

Ritesh Tiwari
Department of Pharmaceutical Chemistry, Chandra Shekhar Singh College of Pharmacy, Kaushambi, Uttar Pradesh, India

Pranit S. Waghchaure
Department of Pharmaceutics, Shri D. D. Vispute College of Pharmacy & Research Center, Panvel, Maharashtra, India

V. Wiwanitkit
Dr DY Patil University, Pimpri-Chinchwad, Maharashtra, India
Hainan Medical University, China

S. Yasri
KMT Primary Care Center, Bangkok, Thailand

Abbreviations

ACE2	angiotensin-converting enzyme 2
AGTR2	angiotensin II receptor type 2
ARDS	acute respiration distress syndrome
ATP	adenosine triphosphate
BCG	Bacillus Calmette–Guérin
BCRs	B-cell receptors
BoHV-1	antibovine herpes virus type 1
CARDS	COVID-19-induced ARDS
CBD	cannabidiol
CCL20	C–C motif chemokine ligand 20
CD154	receptors on the cell surface
CM	Chinese medicine
CoV	coronavirus
COVID-19	coronavirus disease
COX-2	cyclooxygenase-2
CSF	colony-stimulating factor
CT	computed tomography
CTD	comparative toxicogenomics database
CTL	cytotoxic T lymphocyte
CTM	Chinese traditional medicine
CYP450	cytochrome p 450
DC	dendritic cells
DPP4	dipeptidyl peptidase-4
ECMO	extracorporeal membrane oxygenation
EGCG	epigallocatechin gallate
EGR1	early growth response 1
ER	endoplasmic reticulum
ERK1/2	extracellular signal–regulated protein kinase
FGF-2	fibroblast growth factor 2
G-CSF	granulocyte colony-stimulating factor
GG	ground or ground glass
GM-CSF	granulocyte-macrophage colony-stimulating factor

GRNs	gene regulatory networks
HCV	hepatitis C virus
HIV	human immunodeficiency virus
HLH	hemophagocytic lymphohistiocytosis
HNF4G	hepatocyte nuclear factor 4 gamma
HPV	human papillomavirus
HRCT	high-resolution computed tomography
ICTV	International Committee on Taxonomy of Viruses
ICU	intensive care unit
IFN	interferon
IL-1	interleukin-1
IL-6	interleukin-6
IL-8	interleukin-8
IP	inducible protein-10
ISGs	IFN-stimulated genes
ISM	Indian systems of medicine
ISRE	IFN-stimulated response element
IVIg	intravenous immunoglobulin
LAMP	loop-mediated isothermal amplification
LDH	lactate dehydrogenase
MAPK	mitogen-activated protein kinase
MAS	macrophage activation syndrome
MCP-1	monocyte chemo attractant protein-1
MERS-CoV	Middle East Respiratory Syndrome coronavirus
MeV	measles virus
MHC	major histocompatibility complex
MIP-1a	macrophage inflammatory protein-1a
MMR	measles, mumps, and rubella
MWM	modern western medicine
nCoV	novel coronavirus
NF-κB	nuclear factor-kappa B
NHS	National Health Service
NK	natural killer
NLP	neem leaf
NLR	neutrophil-to-lymphocyte relative count
NSPs	nonstructural proteins
ORA	overrepresentation analysis
OSSO	*Ocimum tenuiflorum,* L. seed oil

PAI-1	plasminogen activator inhibitor-1
PAMPs	pathogen-associated molecular patterns
PF	pulmonary fibrosis
PGs	prostaglandins
PLpro	papain-like protease
PPIs	protein–protein interactions
PUI	persons beneath analysis
RDB	receptor-binding domain
RDRP	RNA-dependent RNA polymerase
RNA	ribonucleic acid
ROS	reactive oxygen species
RTC	replication–transcription complex
RT-PCR	reversal polymerase chain reaction
RT-qPCR	reverse transcription quantitative polymerase chain reaction
SAC	S-allyl cysteine
SARI	severe acute respiratory illness
SARS-CoV-2	severe acute respiratory syndrome coronavirus-2
SEC	S-ethyl cysteine
sHLH	second hemophagocytic lymphohistiocytosis
SIR1	silent information regulator 1
SPC	S-propyl cysteine
SRBC	anti-sheep crimson blood cells
ssRNA	single-stranded RNA
STAT	signal transducer and activator of transcription
T cells	thymus
TC	T cytotoxic
TCRs	T-cell receptors
TGF-β1	transforming growth factor beta 1
TH1	T-helper-1
TMPRSS2	transmembrane protease serine precursor-2
TNF-a	tumor necrosis factor-a
TPP	target product profile
TSM	traditional systems of medicine
USA	United States of America
VSN	variance stabilizing normalization
WHO	World Health Organization
3CLpro	3 chymotrypsin-like protease

Preface

Covid (CoV) is a lethal coronavirus strain that causes respiratory infections ranging from the common cold to more serious illnesses. More noteworthy discoveries concerning this novel COVID virus (nCoV) have not been recently found in humans.

The overall well-being of humans is being undermined due to a continuous outbreak of the coronavirus. A breathing illness is brought about by the unusual coronavirus SARS-CoV-2, which was first identified in December 2019 in Wuhan, China. Coronavirus is infectious and causes signs or symptoms with the manifestations of fever, pneumonia, thrombocytopenia, hacking, dyspnea, myalgia, and asthenia in patients.

The discovery of anti-infection agents derived from home-grown medicinal plants in the form of herbal preparations play a fundamental role in curing diseases. The purified compounds and the standardized extracts from medicinal plants offer favorable mixtures of bioactive compounds for the improvement of novel antiviral medications.

Healthy verdures had been used in providing good health and well-being along with traditional medicines to combat illnesses. Herbal products offer an ancillary way to release one-of-a-kind mysteries to fight illnesses. With this knowledge base, this book describes the use of selected nutraceuticals and herbal medicines that might be helpful as pharmacological remedies in preventing COVID-19-associated complications in infected patients.

The book, *COVID-19 and Immunomodulation with Special Emphasis on Nutraceutical and Herbal Formulation,* contains 10 chapters that deal with recent advances, management, prevention, future prospects, and applications of nutraceuticals and herbs for COVID-19. This book demonstrates proper nutrition and use of medication for a disease-free life. This book covers nutraceuticals, spices, polyphenols, customary (traditional) medications, natural products, ayurveda, antioxidants, trace elements, vitamins, and vaccines.

Numerous food additives have an immunomodulatory effect on immune function, and adequate dietary ingredients are required for the immune system to function properly.

Chapter 1, *Role of Immunomodulators in SARS-Cov-2 Treatment: An In-Silico Study Using Network Biology*, written by Anamika Basu, discusses the immunomodulatory properties of natural products.

Herbal immunomodulators provide an inherent benefit over prescribed/artificial drugs because they have fewer side effects side effects, as discussed in Chapter 2, *COVID-19: Role of Polyphenols as Immunomodulators*, written by Khushwinder Kaur. It also gives a standard concept of flavonoids function in immune boosting.

Chapter 3, *Herbal formulation and COVID-19,* written by Rajkumari Lodhi et al., discusses the role of ayurvedic medicines in the control and prevention of COVID-19 disease.

Rane and his associates summarize the most current discoveries and have covered key factors of SARS-CoV-2 genetics, pathophysiology, and the host immune response in Chapter 4, *COVID-19 Pandemic: Role of Ayurveda for Prevention and Treatment.*

Chapter 5, *Developing Vaccine against COVID-19 and Immune Response*, written by Jarouliya and associates, describes the functions of the immune system and the antiviral effect it has on vaccines against COVID-19 infection and also gives information about the different available vaccines against COVID-19.

Mishra et al. illustrate how medicinal vegetation might be used to prevent or treat viruses. It also discusses some yoga protocols to improve respiratory and cardiac efficiency and to strengthen immunity, as described in Chapter 6, *Traditional System of Medicine and Lifestyle for the Management, Prevention, and Treatment of COVID-19.*

Chapter 7, *Role of Synthetic Medicines as Immunomodulators for Cure of COVID–19,* written by Ahire et al., explains the pharmacological results alongside precise immunomodulator agents such as immunostimulators and immunosuppressant, and additionally conveys instances of immunity and distinctive immunomodulator sellers.

Chapter 8, *Immunomodulators for New Emerging Virus Infections (Zika virus infection, MERS, and COVID-19)*, written by Yasri and Wiwanitkit, provides information about three important new emerging viral infections: Zika virus infection, MERS, and COVID-19. In addition, this chapter discusses new effective and safe immunomodulatory agents for the treatment of COVID-19.

Rane et al. discuss the nature of coronavirus and how it resulted in fast-expending pandemic and how the world has managed its containment in Chapter 9, *COVID-19 Infection and Recent Investigations and Future Prospects*.

Chapter 10, *Advances of Traditional System of Medicine for COVID-19*, written by Srivastava et al., discusses recent advances in the traditional system of medicine for the control of COVID-19 disease.

CHAPTER 1

Role of Immunomodulators in SARS-CoV-2 Treatment: An In-Silico Study Using Network Biology

ANAMIKA BASU

Department of Biochemistry, Gurudas College, Kolkata, West Bengal, India

ABSTRACT

Severe acute respiratory tract infection caused by the novel coronavirus (SARSCoV2) sources as one of the most deliberate infectious diseases in the world. During virus–host interactions, different classes of biomolecules are accountable for invasion of virus particle and replication of these viruses inside the host cells. Understanding the response of the human host against this virus is very important to develop new therapies for the treatment of SARS-CoV-2. In systems' pharmacology approach, the consequence of the complex network of interactions of a drug is considered compared to the conventional approach with a single drug–molecule interaction. In this study, an integrative antiviral drug discovery procedure is presented here, which combines a gene network from microarray dataset of coronavirus disease (COVID-19)-infected patients via virus–host interactome generation. It finally creates a system pharmacology-based network that identifies drug to treat SARS-CoV-2. Viral-infected epithelial cells of respiratory tract are a major resource of immunoglobulin molecules such as beta and lambda interferons. These infected cells can initiate innate immune response in the lungs that is principally intermediated by

COVID-19 and Immunomodulation with Special Emphasis on Nutraceutical and Herbal Formulation. Rajesh K. Kesharwani & Raj K. Keservani (Eds)

pro-inflammatory macrophages and granulocytes. Levels of inflammatory cytokines (interleukin 1 [IL-1], tumor necrosis factor [TNF]) have been reported to be elevated in the lungs of COVID-19 patients. The innate immune response to several tissue damage caused by the virus could result in acute respiratory distress syndrome. Pro-inflammatory cytokines are produced excessively in presence of the SARS-CoV-2 virus which leads to cytokine storm. During this immune response, immune cells are continuously activated to produce a vast number of cytokines from lymphocytes and macrophages. The anti-inflammatory immunotherapy has become mandatory to control the cytokine response in SARS-CoV-2 treatment. Increased levels of pro-inflammatory cytokines (IL-1 and IFN) and chemokines (CXCL10 and CCL2) are strongly related with the activation of T-helper-1 cells during SARS-CoV-2 infection. Immunomodulators can control the immune system response by either increasing (known as immunostimulators) or decreasing (known as immunosuppressors) the production of biomolecule related to our immune system. Microarray data from a single sample in a single experiment has become a strong tool for studying genes involved in a specific disease. We can find medications to cure this disease by analyzing these genes of interest in terms of their biological roles and cellular pathways, such as metabolic, signaling, and so on. A gene network can be built by comparing differentially expressed genes in different cell lines such as human lung, heart, liver, kidney, and jejunum cells from both normal and COVID-19 patients. Two datasets, namely, GSE150316_RawCounts_Final.txt.gz and GSE150316_Log2DE-NormCounts.txt.gz, are analyzed with NetworkAnalyst web tools, and the basic expression profiling such as differential expression analysis of genes, volcano plot, heatmap clustering are performed. For meta-data, significant gene analysis is done with various graphical methods, namely, network visual analysis, ORA (overrepresentation analysis), ORA heatmap clustering, Venn diagram, and Chord diagram. Significant gene analysis contains network visual analytics study with 84 genes. In total, 84 genes are identified as significant genes from the meta-analysis study. The significant gene analysis is done with various graphical methods. Protein–protein interactions network reveals that early growth response 1 protein and hepatocyte nuclear factor 4 gamma proteins can produce inflammatory cytokine proteins. The gene regulatory networks confirm that the transcription factor EGR1 interaction with various genes results in the activation of pro-inflammatory cytokine molecules such as IL-1 and TNF, and the expression of some pro-inflammatory genes including cytokines, chemokines, and so on. Drug–gene interaction network shows that sumatriptan exercises anti-inflammatory and immunomodulatory properties by decreasing mRNA levels of TNF-, IL-1 can interact with 5-hydroxytryptamine receptor 1F gene. This can act as immunomodulator drug in SARS-CoV-2 therapeutics. Gene–chemical interaction network with 13 differentially expressed genes from the IL-17-signaling pathway concludes that baicalein can be used as anti-inflammatory agent in this SARS-CoV-2 infection. This natural product can act as nonspecific immunomodulator due to its low toxicity and high bioavailability in food to combat this viral infection.

1.1 INTRODUCTION—SARS-COV-2 INFECTION AND THE IMMUNE SYSTEM

Severe acute respiratory infection caused by a novel coronavirus (SARS-CoV2) characterizes one of the most deliberate infectious diseases in the world. Host–immune response to novel coronavirus is very complex in nature and involves both innate and adaptive immunity of the human body.

Between the airways and the internal system of the lungs, the bronchial epithelium acts as a barrier against allergens, viruses, bacteria, and pollutants, causing an inflammatory response as part of innate immunity. The expression of cytokines, growth factors, and adhesion molecules in bronchial epithelial cells can be linked to their immunomodulatory role. Leucocyte recruitment from the circulation rises during this inflammatory response, and inflammatory cell survival is boosted within the bronchi via changing cell apoptosis (Chanez and Bourdin, 2008). Activated epithelial cells also secrete leukotrienes, prostaglandins, and extracellular matrix components in addition to cytokines. Infections (viral, bacterial, and fungal), allergies, and air pollutants, all trigger an adaptive immune response in epithelial cells. This is the first step in the antigen neutralization and elimination process. For their attachment to host cells, all viruses use different ways. Different groups of biomolecules are responsible for virus invasion and reproduction inside host cells during virus–host interactions (Maginnis, 2018).

According to World Health Organization, till date, there are no specific medicines or vaccines for coronavirus disease (COVID-19). Different approaches are used to identify effective drugs for the prevention and treatment of this lethal COVID-19, which is produced by novel SARS-CoV-2

(Sarkar and Maulik, 2020). Repurposing of approved and investigational medicines and designing of various antiviral vaccines are at present, hot topics in medical science to combat COVID-19 around the world.

Understanding the response of the human host against this virus is very important to develop new therapies for the treatment of SARS-CoV-2. Similar to that of other coronaviruses, this SARS-CoV-2 also causes mild to severe respiratory tract infection with very high global mortality rate (https://coronavirus.jhu.edu/data/mortality).

In systems' pharmacology approach, the consequence of the complex network of interactions of a drug is considered compared to the conventional approach with a single drug–molecule interaction. Computational strategies based on this system pharmacology approach can integrate gene expression data related to pharmaceuticals and disease states (Ferguson et al., 2018). In study, gene expression profiling with microarray dataset for both COVID-19-infected patients and for normal individuals (Desai et al., 2020) to identify drug for COVID-19 treatment is exploited. Several functional drug–gene network and bioinformatics analyses for different antiviral drug discovery are performed for Zika virus infection (Cheng et al., 2016), Ebola virus infection (Johansen et al., 2013), and Middle East respiratory syndrome coronavirus infection (Dyall et al., 2014).

In this study, an integrative antiviral drug identification method is presented here, which combines a gene network from microarray dataset of COVID-19-infected patients via virus–host interactome generation and finally a systems pharmacology-based network that identifies drug to treat SARS-CoV-2.

The immune system plays a decisive role in the response to SARS-CoV-2 with significant changes among severe and nonsevere patients (Shi et al., 2020). When a defensive immune response is weakened in human body, virus will propagate and massive damage of the affected tissue and organs will happen, especially in organs that have high angiotensin-converting enzyme 2 (ACE2) gene expression, such as intestine and kidney. ACE2 (EC:3.4.17.23), which is a transmembrane protein of human cell membrane, is considered as receptor for spike protein binding of novel coronavirus (SARS-CoV-2). During first stage of infection, that is, asymptomatic state (initial 12 days of virus infection), the inhaled virus particle binds to epithelial cells through ACE2 receptor in surface of the nasal cavity area and the replication process starts (Mason, 2020) with a limited innate immune response from host cell. In the second stage (in next few days), the virus propagates through upper airway, and strong innate immunological response is activated. Viral-infected epithelial cells of respiratory tract are a major source of beta and lambda interferons. In the final stage of infection, the particular virus reaches alveolus, which is the gas exchange unit of the lung. Here, the viral infection starts in alveolar type II cells. The infected cells induce innate inflammatory response in the lungs that is principally intermediated by pro-inflammatory macrophages and granulocytes. It has been reported that the levels of inflammatory cytokines (IL-1, TNF) are raised in the lungs of virus-infected patients. The inflammation in the lung is the main symptom of life-threatening respiratory disorders in its severe stage. The innate immune response leading to tissue damage results in acute respiratory distress syndrome (ARDS). During ARDS, the respiratory failure is caused by the rapid onset of inflammatory reactions in the lungs and following fatality. The mortality rate of severe COVID-19 patients has been informed as high as 49% showed by a recent epidemiological survey in China (Mason, 2020).

Mateus et al. (2020) have found that elevated serum cytokines in some COVID-19 patients stimulate the T cells to provoke cytokines and chemokines for activating and recruiting myeloid cells (Chen and Wherry, 2020). Pro-inflammatory cytokines are produced excessively in presence of the SARS-CoV-2 virus which leads to cytokine storm (Moore and June, 2020). The cytokine storm is caused by an unexpected increase of interleukins, such as interleukin 1 (IL1), IL-7, IL-8, IL-9, IL-10, fibroblast growth factor (FGF), G-CSF (colony-stimulating factor), GM-CSF, IFN (interferon), IP10, TNF (tumor necrosis factor), VEGF (Ragab et al., 2020). The increase in pro-inflammatory cytokine leads to various biological events, namely, destabilization of endothelial cells, vascular barrier, capillary damage, and lung injury. Cytokine storm is an uncontrolled immune response of host cell against this virus. During this immune response, immune cells are continuously activated to produce vast number of cytokines from lymphocytes and macrophages. This type of inflammatory response is also observed earlier in influenza (H5N1, H1N1) and SARS-CoV and MERS-CoV viral infections. This uncontrolled immune response leads to severe acute respiratory illness which results in acute lung damage, subsequently multi-organ failure and ultimately death. Thus, antiviral therapeutics are not sufficient for COVID-19 patient treatment. The anti-inflammatory therapy is also required to control the cytokine response in SARS-CoV-2 treatment. Increased levels of pro-inflammatory cytokines (IL-1 and IFN) and chemokines (CXCL10 and CCL2) are strongly related to the activation of T-helper-1 (TH1) cell during SARS-CoV-2 infection (Coperchini et al., 2020). In this infection, levels of IL-4 and IL-10 also increase due to TH2-oriented activation.

Immunomodulators are chemical compounds which are used to regulate or alter the functions of the immune system. These compounds can be considered as drugs to treat many diseases where immune system plays a major role such as rheumatic diseases (Sakkas et al., 2018), cancers (Mahoney et al., 2015), and AIDS (Suwannarach et al., 2020). Immunomodulators can control the immune system response by either increasing (known as immunostimulators) or decreasing (known as immunosuppressors) the production of biomolecule related to our immune system. During infections, for example, viruses (Naik, 2018), bacteria (Zapater et al., 2015), and fungus (Sam et al., 2018), immunostimulators are used. In case of cancer treatment and immunodeficiency syndromes, they are also prescribed as drugs.

Microarray data from a sample in a single experiment have become a powerful tool for analyzing genes, responsible for a particular disease. The findings of that particular microarray experiment are finally compiled into a list of genes of interest. In both normal and pathological states, these genes are expressed differentially (Rapaport et al., 2007). Analysis of these genes of interest in terms of their biological functions and cellular pathways, for example, metabolic, signaling, and so on, helps us to identify drugs to treat this specific disease. In the context of any disease, a gene network is a graph with genes as vertices and edges that describe relationships between genes based on their biological roles.

1.2 METHODOLOGY

Network-based approach is used to identify molecular signature genes and therapeutic agents in different diseases such as Alzheimer's disease (Rahman et al., 2019a) and colorectal cancer (Rahman et al., 2019b). There are several web-based tools that are available for meta-analysis of gene expression data, for example, INMEX (Xia et al., 2013), NetworkAnalyst 3.0 (Xia et al., 2015), and so on.

For 17 different species, NetworkAnalyst 3.0 (Xia et al., 2015) tool is used. This tool is a visual analytics platform that executes extensive gene expression profiling, at the time meta-analysis, and ultimately network in biology. By using this tool not only protein–protein interaction (PPI) network, but also gene regulatory network, gene coexpression network, toxicogenomics, and pharmacogenomics network (Xia et al., 2014; Zhou et al., 2019) can be constructed. Meta-analysis is a cluster of statistical techniques that assemble data from more than one study into a combined dataset and analyze the new dataset. Workflow for meta-analysis using NetworkAnalyst 3.0 is shown in Figure 1.1.

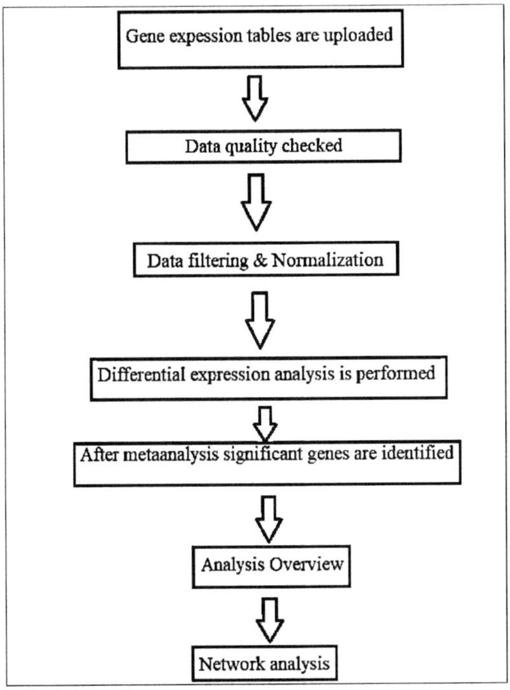

FIGURE 1.1 Workflow for meta-analysis using Network Analyst 3.0.

1.3 STEPS FOR META-ANALYSIS NETWORKANALYST 3.0 WEBTOOLS

1.3.1 UPLOADATION OF GENE EXPRESSION TABLES

Comparing differentially expressed genes in different cell lines such as human lung, liver, heart, jejunum, and kidney cells from both normal and

COVID-19 patients (Desai et al., 2020), a gene network can be constructed. Desai et al. (2020) used in-situ hybridization to visualize viral RNA and immunohistochemistry and total RNA sequencing to analyze the immune infiltration in five COVID-19-positive patients. The interferon signature genes are overrepresented in patients with high amounts of viral RNA. The study highlights the immune response in patients with severe COVID-19 infection. Two datasets, namely, GSE150316_RawCounts_Final.txt.gz and GSE150316_Log2DENormCounts.txt.gz, are analyzed with NetworkAnalyst web tools and the basic expression profiling such as differential analysis, heatmap clustering, and volcano plot are performed.

1.3.2 DATA QUALITY CHECKING

The uploaded samples are checked and results are summarized in Table 1.1, together with several graphical outputs. These graphical outputs, for example, boxplot, count sum, MSD plots, and PCA plot are commonly used for quality check.

TABLE 1.1 Results for Data Quality Checking.

	GSE150316_ RawCounts	**For GSE150316_ Log2RPM**	**Individual datasets: GSE150316_ Log2RPMNormCounts_final.txt; GSE150316_RawCounts.txt**
Data type	Microarray gene expression	Microarray gene expression	Gene expression meta-analysis
Total feature number	19,582	19,582	
Matched gene number	19,582	16,018	32,943
Unmatched gene number	0	3564	
Percent matched	100	81.8	
Sample number	37	38	74
Number of experimental factors	1	1	
Group names	Case; control	Case; control	Case; control

Graphical outputs are shown in Figures 1.2–1.4.

Boxplots for two datasets are shown in Figure 1.2.

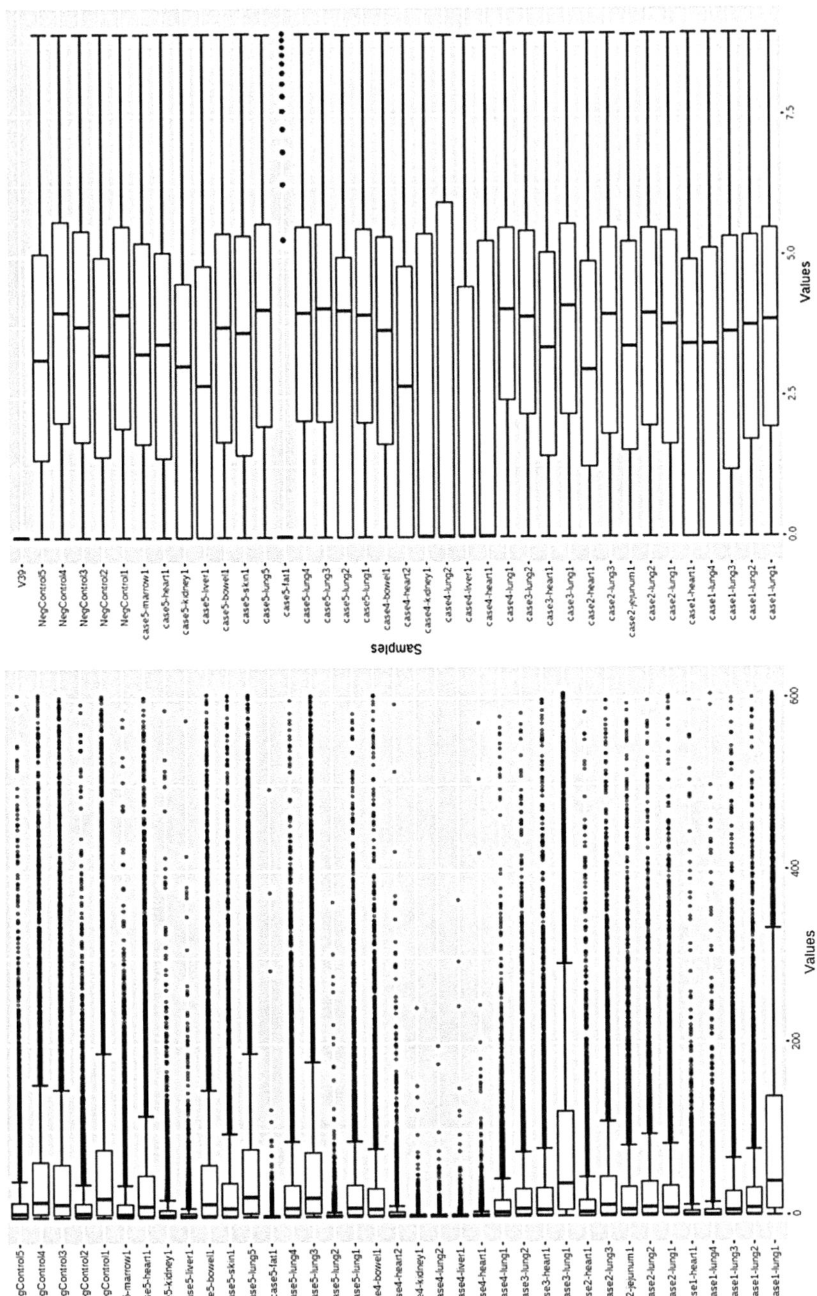

FIGURE 1.2 Boxplots for two datasets.

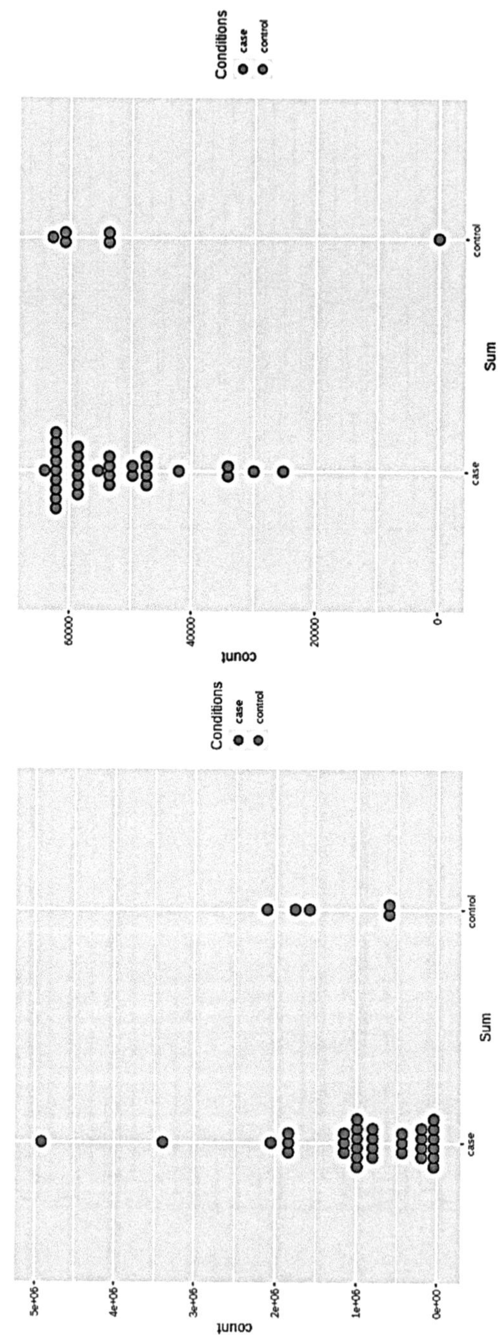

FIGURE 1.3 Count sum graphs for both datasets.

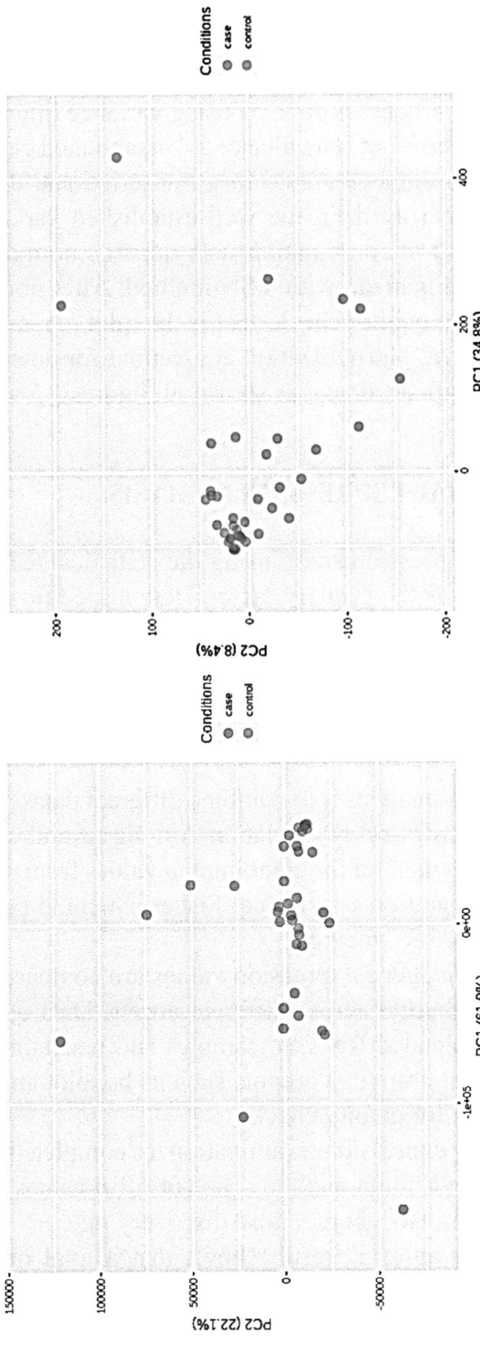

FIGURE 1.4 PCA plots for two datasets.

1.4 DATA FILTERING AND NORMALIZATION

Filtering serves to remove data that are unlikely to be informative or simply erroneous. Filtering process is done by using variance filter with a value of 15 and low abundance is set at a value of 5. Unannotated genes are filtered. Normalization is essential for detecting transcriptional differences with accuracy. For microarray data, the well-established variance stabilizing normalization (VSN) in combination with quantile normalization can be used. Normalization is made with VSN method. After normalization, the graphical outputs for quality check, that is, boxplot, count sum. PCA and MSD plots are drawn. Normalization is essential for detecting transcriptional differences with accuracy, as shown in Figures 1.5 and 1.6.

1.5 DIFFERENTIAL EXPRESSION ANALYSIS

Differential gene expression study using the statistical technique is used, considering "class" as the primary factor. Here a specific comparison has been made with case versus control data as shown in Table 1.2.

1.6 META-ANALYSIS WITH THE TWO DATASETS

The purpose of meta-analysis is to combine different datasets for increased statistical power or cross-study validation. Among several well-established approaches, Fisher's method for combining p values from multiple studies for information integration is selected. Fisher's method ($-2*\sum \text{Log}(p)$) is known as a "weight-free" method.

For meta-analysis, gene expression values are compared at log scales with identical distribution across different arrays. Data quality checking is done with the uploaded RNAseq samples and results are summarized in Table 1.1. Several graphical outputs such as boxplot and PCA plot are shown in Figure 1.7 for quality check.

The differential expression examination is completed on individual dataset based on the Limma method. The cut-off p values are adjusted at 0.05 using Benjamini Hochberg's false discovery rate.

Gene-level meta-analysis result shows that a total of 1021 gene is found in the differential gene expression analysis. Among them, 500 genes

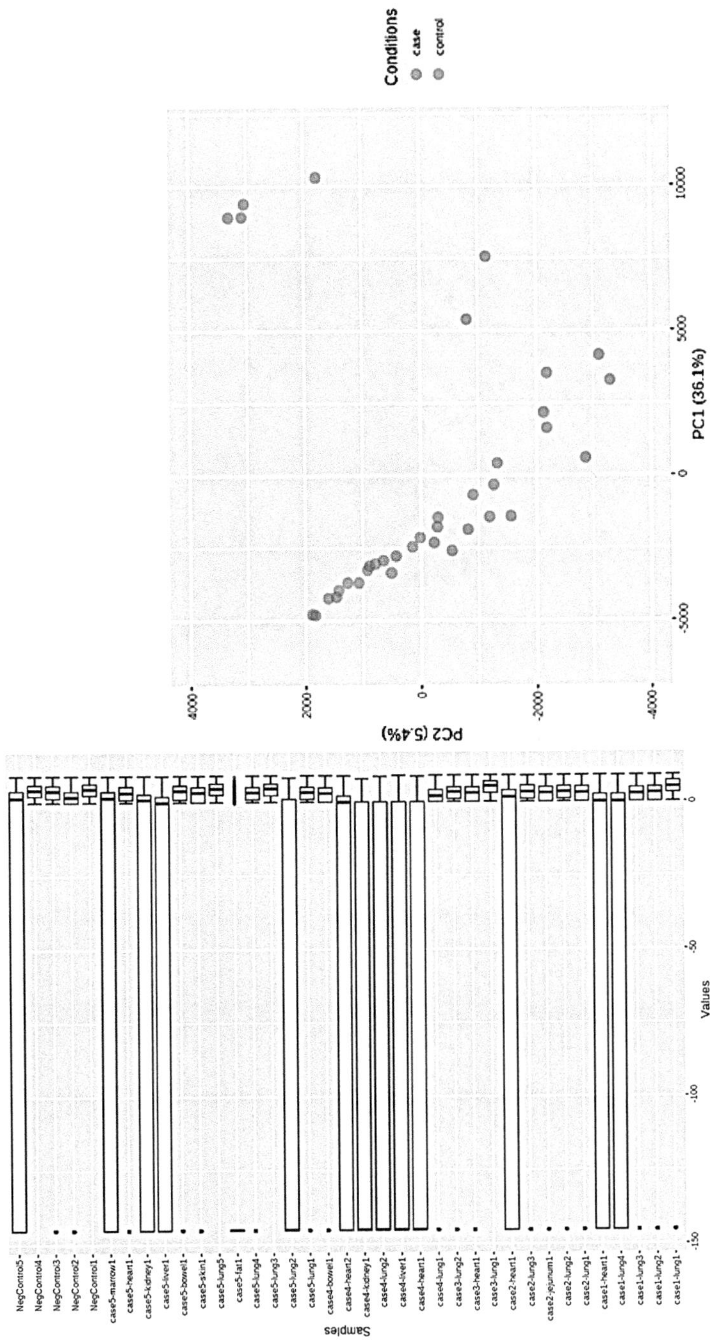

FIGURE 1.5 Box plot and PCA plot after normalization.

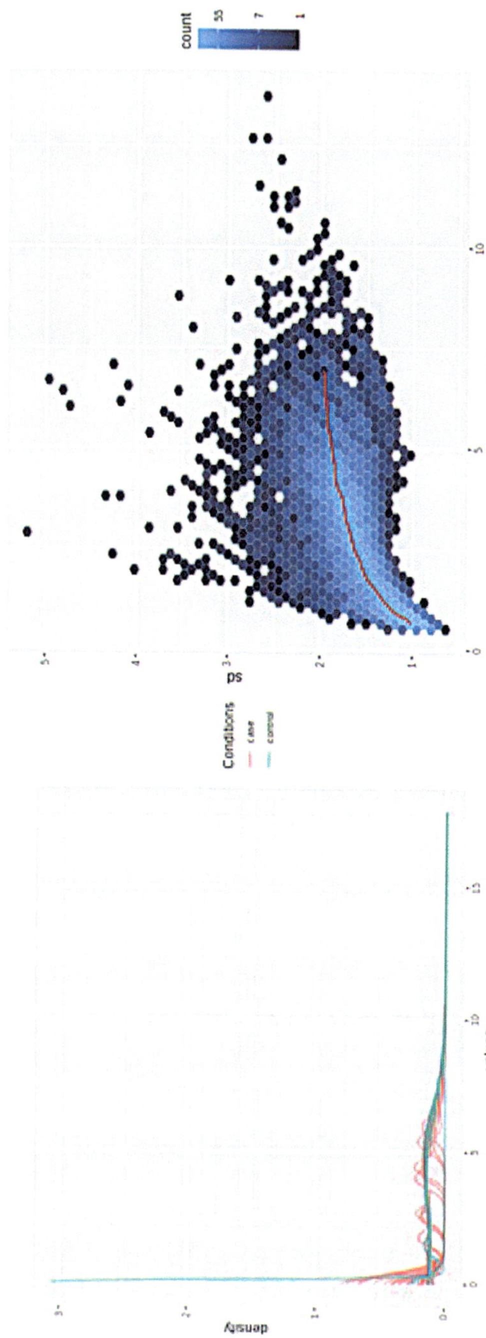

FIGURE 1.6 Density plot and MSD plot after normalization.

TABLE 1.2 Cases and Controls.

Case	Control
case1–lung1 case2–lung1 case3–lung1 case4–liver1 case5–lung1 case5–lung5 case5–heart1	NegControl1
case1–lung2 case2–lung2 case3–heart1 case4–lung2 case5–lung2 case5–skin1 case5–marrow1	NegControl2
case1–lung3 case2–jejunum1 case3–lung2 case4–kidney1 case5–lung3 case5–bowel1	NegControl3
case1–lung4 case2–lung3 case4–lung1 case4–heart2 case5–lung4 case5–liver1	NegControl4
case1–heart1 case2–heart1 case4–heart1 case4–bowel1 case5–fat1 case5–kidney1	NegControl5

according to their p values are nominated for further network analysis. Total 84 genes are identified as significant genes from meta-analysis study.

1.7 ANALYSIS OVERVIEW

1.7.1 NETWORK ANALYSIS

Visual analytics technology from NetworkAnalyst 3.0 aims to participate in interactive visualization of gene network with statistical analysis and will help to navigate complex omics data analysis. For metadata, significant gene analysis is done with various graphical methods, namely, network visual analysis, ORA (overrepresentation analysis), ORA heatmap clustering, Venn diagram, and Chord diagram.

Significant gene analysis contains network visual analytics study with 84 genes. In PPIs network, STRING interactome with a 900 confidence score (Szklarczyk et al., 2015) with experimental evidence is selected as the PPI database. The significant genes (seeds) from the previous analysis are mapped to the corresponding molecular interaction database. The procedure typically produces one big subnetwork ("continent") with several smaller ones ("islands"). Subnetworks with at least three nodes are listed in Table 1.3. Two big subnetworks and five smaller subnetworks are displayed in Figure 1.9.

EGR1 (early growth response 1) protein is a zinc-finger transcription factors (TFs), which can control the expression of around 300 target genes, including TNF-α, ICAM-1, MCP-1, MIP-1, IL-1, IL-6, TGF-α, CD44,

TABLE 1.2 Cases and Controls.

Case	Control
case1–lung1 case2–lung1 case3–lung1 case4–liver1 case5–lung1 case5–lung5 case5–heart1	NegControl1
case1–lung2 case2–lung2 case3–heart1 case4–lung2 case5–lung2 case5–skin1 case5–marrow1	NegControl2
case1–lung3 case2–jejunum1 case3–lung2 case4–kidney1 case5–lung3 case5–bowel1	NegControl3
case1–lung4 case2–lung3 case4–lung1 case4–heart2 case5–lung4 case5–liver1	NegControl4
case1–heart1 case2–heart1 case4–heart1 case4–bowel1 case5–fat1 case5–kidney1	NegControl5

according to their p values are nominated for further network analysis. Total 84 genes are identified as significant genes from meta-analysis study.

1.7 ANALYSIS OVERVIEW

1.7.1 NETWORK ANALYSIS

Visual analytics technology from NetworkAnalyst 3.0 aims to participate in interactive visualization of gene network with statistical analysis and will help to navigate complex omics data analysis. For metadata, significant gene analysis is done with various graphical methods, namely, network visual analysis, ORA (overrepresentation analysis), ORA heatmap clustering, Venn diagram, and Chord diagram.

Significant gene analysis contains network visual analytics study with 84 genes. In PPIs network, STRING interactome with a 900 confidence score (Szklarczyk et al., 2015) with experimental evidence is selected as the PPI database. The significant genes (seeds) from the previous analysis are mapped to the corresponding molecular interaction database. The procedure typically produces one big subnetwork ("continent") with several smaller ones ("islands"). Subnetworks with at least three nodes are listed in Table 1.3. Two big subnetworks and five smaller subnetworks are displayed in Figure 1.9.

EGR1 (early growth response 1) protein is a zinc-finger transcription factors (TFs), which can control the expression of around 300 target genes, including TNF-α, ICAM-1, MCP-1, MIP-1, IL-1, IL-6, TGF-α, CD44,

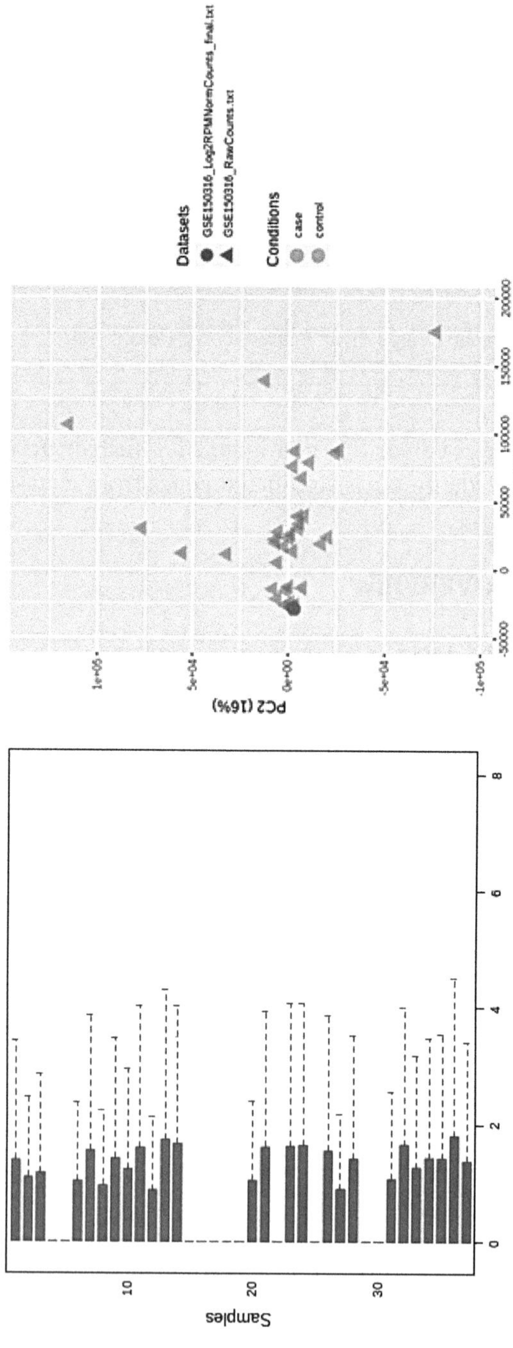

FIGURE 1.7 Box plot and PCA plot for meta-analysis.

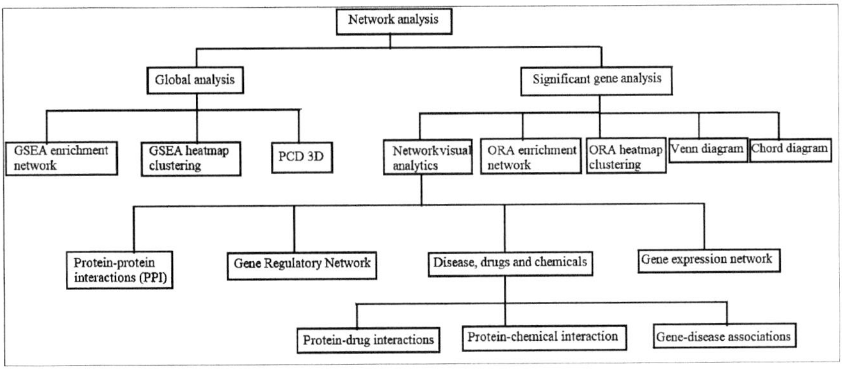

FIGURE 1.8 Schematic representation of network analysis.

PAI-1, and tissue factor (Schmidt et al., 2008). It can act as pleiotropic inflammatory transactivator in molecular inflammatory responses. Among the target genes, TNF-, IL-1, and IL-6 genes produce inflammatory cytokine proteins.

Hepatocyte nuclear factor 4 gamma (HNF4G) protein is a member of the HNF4 (NR2A) TFs. In subnetwork 2, HNF4G interacts with two early growth response proteins such as EGR1 and EGR2 (Fig. 1.2). Thus, this protein indirectly produces TNF-α, IL-1β, and IL-6 inflammatory cytokine proteins.

Importin 4 (IPO4) imports protein in nucleus.

5-Hydroxytryptamine (5-HT) is commonly known as serotonin. 5-HT-mediated cell functions are regulated by expression of different classes of G-protein-coupled serotoninergic receptors (5HTR). Among two types of 5-HTR receptors, the first class consists of five 5-hydroxytryptamine receptor (5-HTR1A, 5-HTR1B, 5-HTR1D, 5-HTR1E, and 5-HTR1F) receptors. Inflammation involves the migration of monocytes into damaged tissues, and in innate immune response, monocytes macrophages eliminate invasive microorganisms (such as viruses) by activating cytokines such as IL-1b, IL-6, IL-8/CXCL8, IL-10, IL-12p40, IL-18, and TNF-a (Dürk et al., 2005).

Fibroblast growth factors (FGFs), such as FGF17, are growth factors and oncogenes that play important roles in embryonic development, cell growth, morphogenesis, tissue repair, inflammation, angiogenesis, and tumor growth and invasion (Hoshikawa et al., 1998).

TABLE 1.3 Different Subnetworks in Protein–Protein Interactions (PPIs) Network.

Networks	Nodes	Edges	Seeds	Gene symbol of seed gene
subnetwork1	38	37	1	EGR1
subnetwork2	25	24	1	HNF4G
subnetwork3	8	7	1	IPO4
subnetwork4	5	4	1	HTR1F
subnetwork5	5	4	1	FGF17
subnetwork6	4	3	1	DLGAP1
subnetwork7	3	2	1	PPEF1

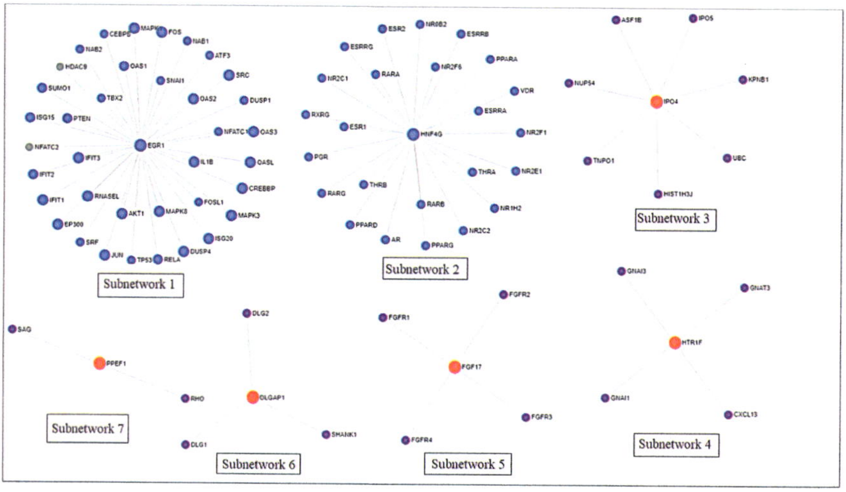

FIGURE 1.9 Different subnetworks in PPI network.

As generic PPI network, a tissue-specific PPI is constructed considering lung as the specific tissue type. This tissue-specific PPI data is collected from the DifferentialNet database. It shows differential PPIs across human tissues using a filter 15.0. The 84 significant genes considered as seeds are mapped to the DifferentialNet database. The procedure produces one big subnetwork ("continent") with seven smaller ones ("islands"). Subnetworks with at least three nodes are listed in Table 1.4 and explored using Cytoscape. In subnetwork1, EGR1 is present as seed gene in lung tissue.

TABLE 1.4 Features of Tissue-Specific Protein–Protein Interaction Networks.

Networks	Nodes	Edges	Seeds
subnetwork1	68	67	4
subnetwork2	14	13	1
subnetwork3	9	8	1
subnetwork4	6	5	1
subnetwork5	4	3	1
subnetwork6	4	3	1
subnetwork7	3	2	1
subnetwork8	3	2	1

Gene regulatory networks (GRNs) are constructed using TF–gene interactions, where TF and their target genes are matched from the JASPAR, a TF-binding site profile database (Bryne et al., 2008). With the help of Cytoscape, a subnetwork is formed containing 89 nodes, 211 edges, and 32 seeds (Fig. 1.11). TF EGR1 interacts with STAT (signal transducer and activator of transcription), POU (POU homeodomain proteins), NFKB, JUN, FOX, and ATF genes. The activation of pro-inflammatory cytokines such as interleukin 1 (IL-1) and TNF, as well as the production of several pro-inflammatory genes, play an important role in inflammation and innate immunity by the NF-B family of TFs (Lawrence, 2009). Inflammatory cytokines enhance collagenases (MMP) gene expression through the mitogen-activated protein kinase (MAPK), a cell signaling pathway, by increasing the levels and phosphorylating different AP-1 components, such as JUN and FOXs (Guma and Firestein, 2012).

In network biology diseases, drugs and chemicals are correlated with the significant genes and the types of interactions. In protein–drug interaction network, the protein and drug target information is collected from the DrugBank database (Version 5.0) (Wishart et al., 2018) for human data. Two subnetworks are visualized (Fig. 1.12) using Cytoscape (Kohl et al., 2011). The features of these two networks are enlisted in Table 1.5.

5-Hydroxytryptamine receptor 1F protein from HTR1F gene is a G-protein coupled receptor for 5-hydroxytryptamine (serotonin). This protein acts as a receptor for several ligands such as different psychoactive substances and alkaloids. The binding of ligand causes a conformation change in the protein that triggers signaling via guanine nucleotide-binding proteins (G proteins) and modulates the activity of downstream effectors, such as adenylate cyclase. Adenylate cyclase activity is also

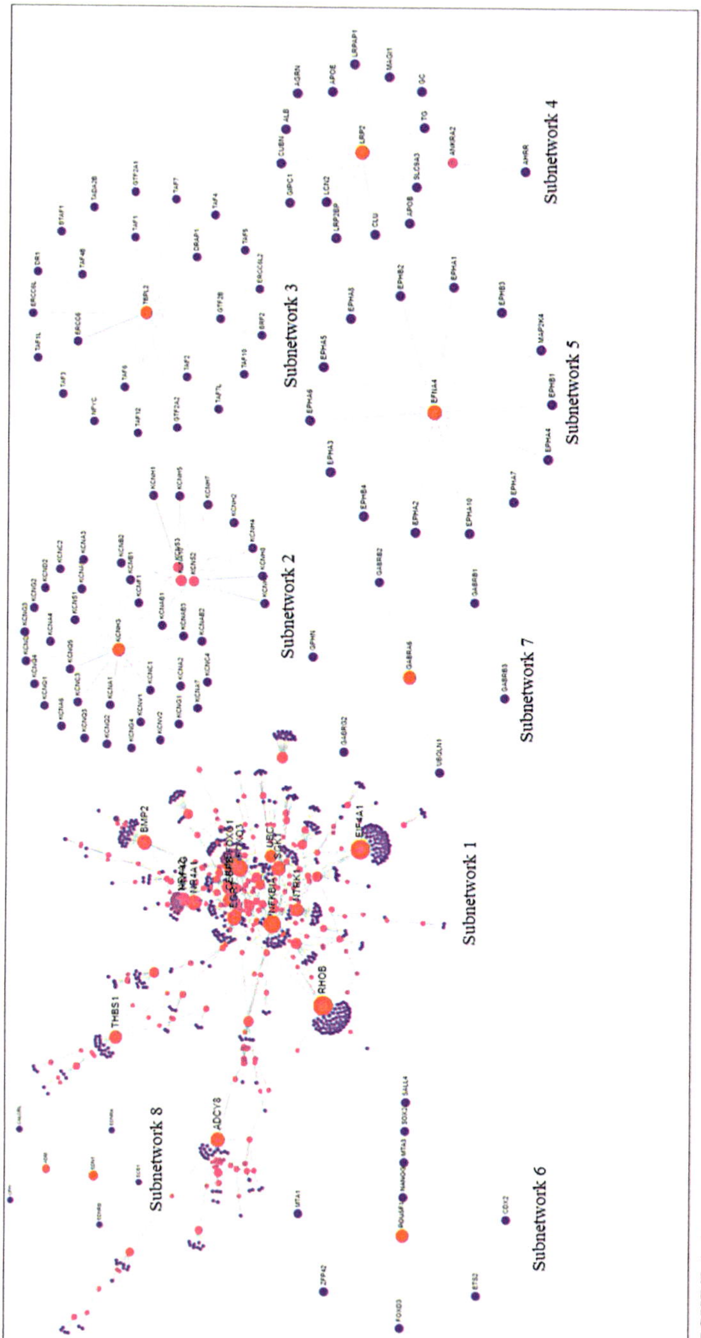

FIGURE 1.10 Different subnetworks in tissue-specific protein–protein interaction networks.

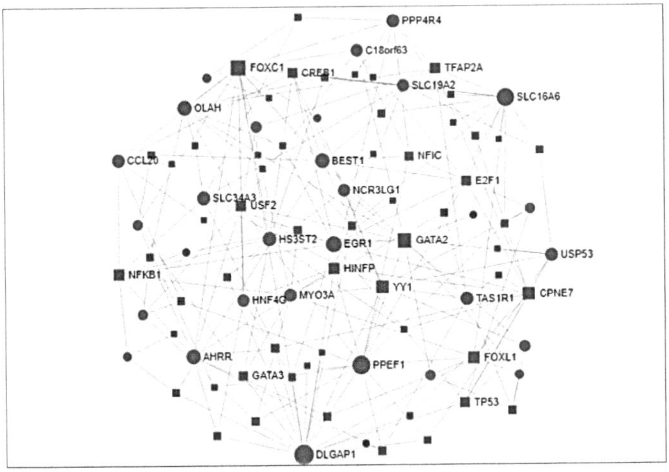

FIGURE 1.11 Gene regulatory networks (GRN) using significant genes.

inhibited by the signaling pathway. In subnetwork1, among 2 networks with protein–drug interactions, HTR1F protein is illustrated as a seed gene having interactions with 10 drugs (Fig. 1.12).

Methysergide is a serotonin antagonist that operates on the central nervous system, stimulating the smooth muscle directly. Mianserin is a tetracyclic antidepressant with antihistaminic, hypnosedative, and anti-histaminic properties. Triptans are a kind of medication that includes Zolmitriptan. It has an effect on a natural molecule called serotonin, which causes blood vessels in the brain to constrict. Sumatriptan, an anti-migraine medication, is a 5-hydroxytryptamine 1B, 1D (5HT1B, 1D) receptor agonist. Studies of other researchers have shown that sumatriptan exercises anti-inflammatory and immunomodulatory properties by decreasing mRNA levels of TNF-, IL-1 (Khalilzadeh et al., 2018). Ergotamine is a vasoconstrictor and alpha-adrenoreceptor antagonist. Eletriptan is a triptan, which is a kind of medication. It has an effect on a natural molecule called serotonin, which causes blood vessels in the brain to constrict. Naratriptan and Rizatriptan belong to a class of medications that is called as selective serotonin receptor agonists.

TABLE 1.5 Subnetworks in Drug–Gene Interaction Network.

Networks	Nodes	Edges	Seeds
subnetwork1	11	10	1
subnetwork2	3	2	1

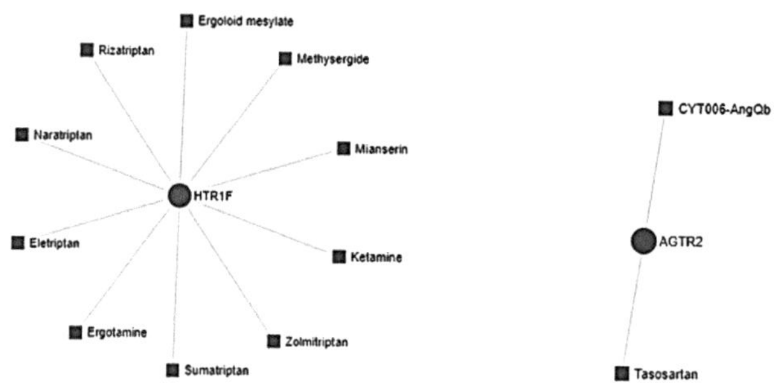

FIGURE 1.12 Subnetworks in drug–gene interaction network.

The AT2 receptor, also known as the angiotensin II (AngII) receptor type 2 (AGTR2), is a protein that is produced by the AGTR2 gene in humans. This protein can function as a receptor for AngII. Since ACE2 (EC:3.4.17.23) is announced as receptor for spike protein binding of novel coronavirus (SARS-CoV-2), tasosartan and CYT006-AngQb are considered as important drugs for this disease. Tasosartan is an AngII receptor blocker with a prolonged half-life. The therapeutic vaccination CYT006-AngQb is being developed for the treatment of hypertension. Its goal is to get the patient's immune system to make antibodies against AngII, a tiny peptide that causes blood vessels to constrict and raises blood pressure (Wishart et al., 2018).

Protein–chemical interactions are displayed in the following network (Fig. 1.13) with 356 nodes, 649 edges, and 30 seeds. The data in network is based on data from the Comparative Toxicogenomics Database (CTD) (downloaded on November 2016) (Davis et al., 2019). Due huge number of nodes and edges are found in this network, further analysis is made with fewer number of genes in the following section.

Gene–disease associations are constructed by using the literature curated for gene–disease association information which is collected from the DisGeNET database for human data (Fig. 1.14) (Piñero et al., 2019). CCL20 (C–C motif chemokine ligand 20) gene is related with several diseases such as pneumonia, diabetes mellitus, and so on.

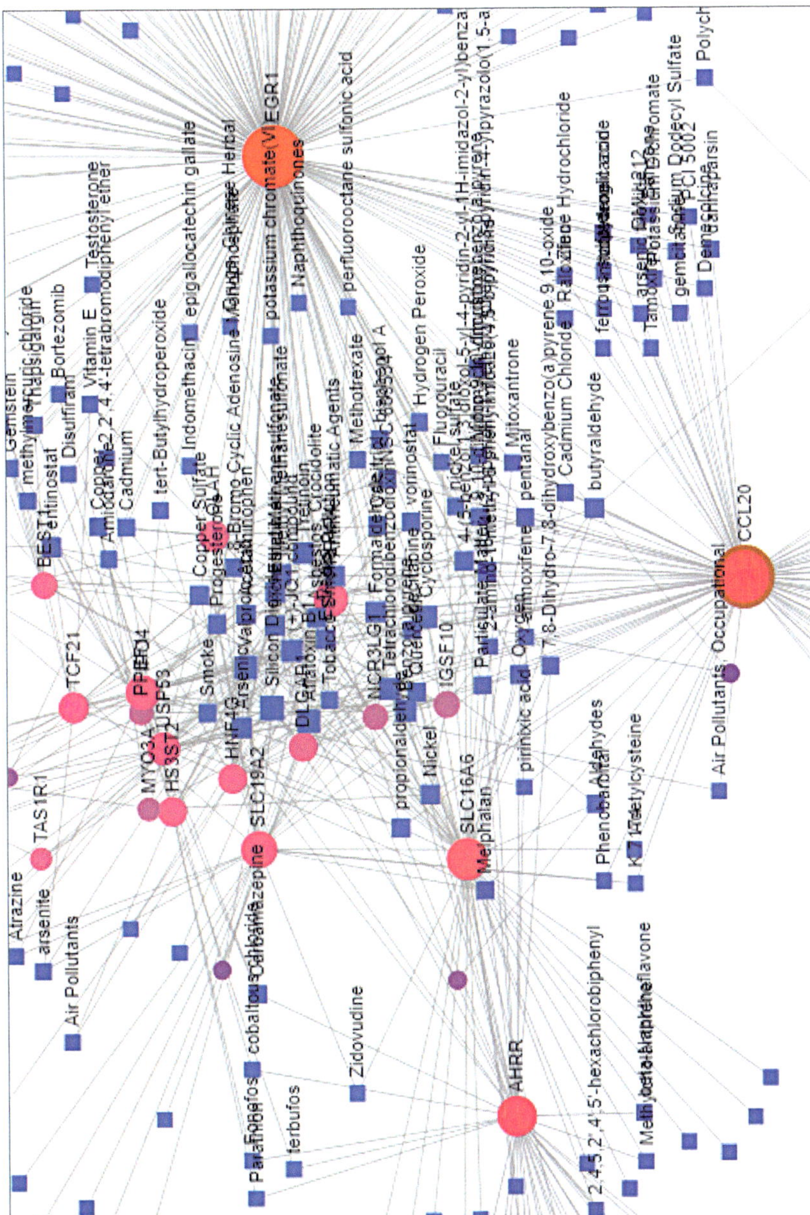

FIGURE 1.13 Protein–chemical interactions.

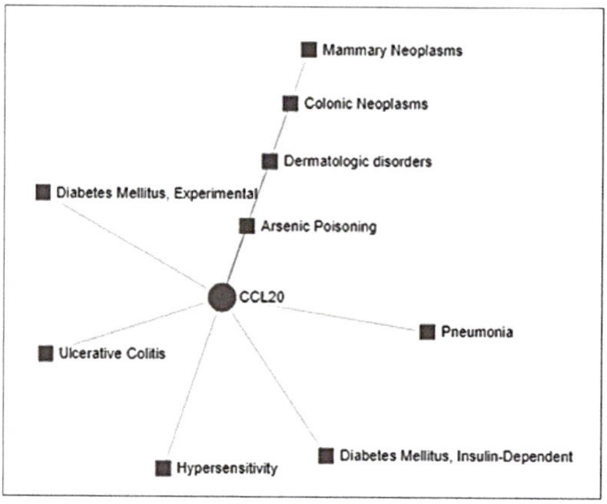

FIGURE 1.14 Gene–disease associations.

ORA heatmap clustering for the metadata is shown in Figure 1.15. This heatmap shows that various genes, namely, CCL20, RNU6-16P (RNA, U6 small nuclear 16, pseudogene), RNA5SP498 (RNA, 5S ribosomal pseudogene 498), and SLC34A3 (solute carrier family 34 member 3).

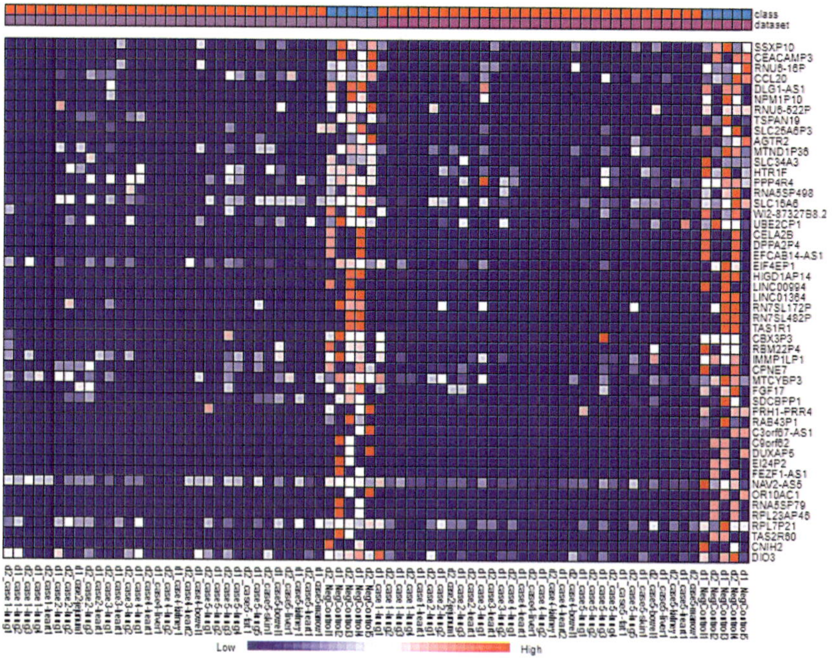

FIGURE 1.15 ORA heatmap clustering for the metadata.

Venn diagram and Chord diagram combining two data, for example, GSE150316_RawCounts.txt and GSE150316_Log2RPMNormCounts_final.txt, are shown in Figure 1.16.

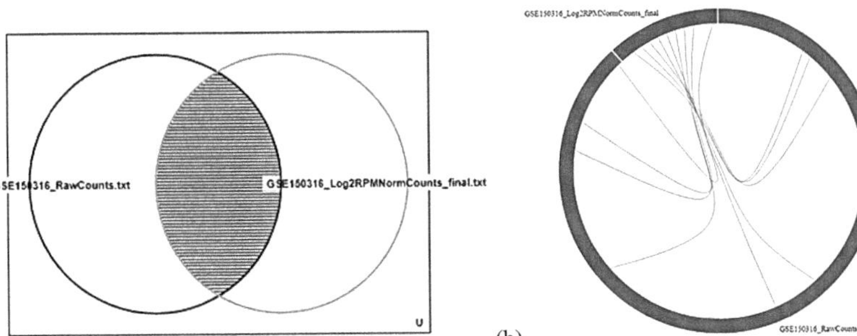

(a) (b)

FIGURE 1.16 (a) Venn diagram and (b) Chord diagram.

In Venn diagrams, different regions in the Venn diagram represent all possible comparisons among the datasets. The enrichment analysis is performed on gene list containing nine genes. These genes are SSXP10, RNU6-16P, CEACAMP3, DLG1-AS1, NPM1P10, MTND1P36, SLC34A3, CCL20, and WI2-87327B8.2.

With data list containing 1022 genes, generated from metadata, gene enrichment analysis with KEGG pathway is performed and results are shown in Table 1.6 and Figure 1.17.

TABLE 1.6 Gene Enrichment Analysis with KEGG Pathway.

Name	Hits	*p* Value	Adj. *p*
Cytokine–cytokine receptor interaction	24/294	1.25e–7	3.97e–5
IL-17-signaling pathway	13/93	2.85e–7	4.52e–5
TNF-signaling pathway	12/110	1.18e–5	0.00125
Taste transduction	10/83	2.69e–5	0.00214
MAPK-signaling pathway	18/295	2.47e–4	0.0141
p53-signaling pathway	8/72	3.08e–4	0.0141
PI3K–Akt-signaling pathway	20/354	0.00031	0.0141
Neuroactive ligand–receptor interaction	18/338	0.00124	0.0493
Transcriptional misregulation in cancer	12/186	0.0017	0.0601
Pathways in cancer	24/530	0.0019	0.0603
NF-kappa B-signaling pathway	8/100	0.00271	0.0783
Renin secretion	6/69	0.00609	0.151

TABLE 1.6 *(Continued)*

Name	Hits	*p* Value	Adj. *p*
Malaria	5/49	0.00616	0.151
Melanoma	6/72	0.00748	0.17
Hematopoietic cell lineage	7/97	0.00863	0.172
Circadian entrainment	7/97	0.00863	0.172
Legionellosis	5/55	0.01	0.179
AGE–RAGE-signaling pathway in diabetic complications	7/100	0.0101	0.179
Vascular smooth muscle contraction	8/132	0.014	0.235
Cellular senescence	9/160	0.0148	0.236
Renin–angiotensin system	3/23	0.017	0.257
Glutamatergic synapse	7/114	0.0197	0.285
Olfactory transduction	18/448	0.0219	0.291
Rheumatoid arthritis	6/91	0.022	0.291
Ras-signaling pathway	11/232	0.024	0.305
Phospholipase D–signaling pathway	8/148	0.026	0.319
cAMP-signaling pathway	10/212	0.0316	0.372
Chagas disease (American trypanosomiasis)	6/103	0.0374	0.406
Toll-like receptor–signaling pathway	6/104	0.0389	0.406
Chemokine-signaling pathway	9/190	0.0394	0.406
FoxO-signaling pathway	7/132	0.0396	0.406
Measles	7/138	0.0484	0.481

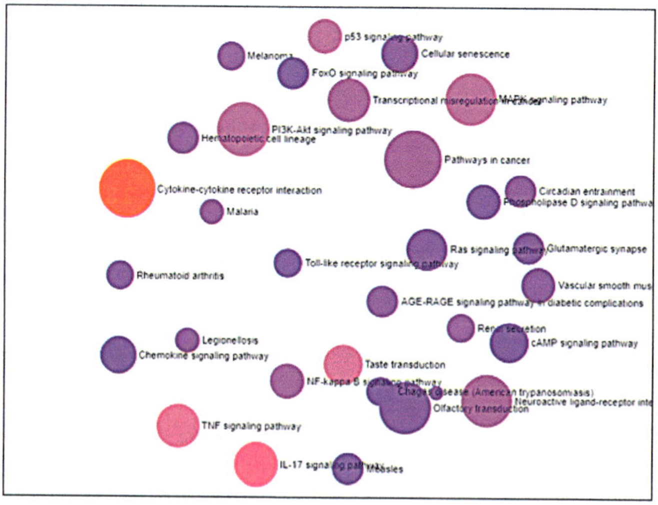

FIGURE 1.17 Gene enrichment analysis with KEGG pathway.

Cytokine–cytokine receptor interaction, TNF-signaling pathway, IL-17-signaling pathway, taste transduction, MAPK-signaling pathway, PI3K-Akt-signaling pathway, and neuroactive ligand–receptor interaction are the KEGG pathways which are related to immunology. Gene lists for those pathways are shown in Table 1.7. These pathways are discussed briefly.

TABLE 1.7 Gene Lists for Functional Annotation of Genes Present in Network (Related to Immune System).

Cytokine–cytokine receptor interaction	IL-17-signaling pathway	TNF-signaling pathway	Taste transduction	MAPK-signaling pathway	PI3K-Akt-signaling pathway	Neuroactive ligand–receptor interaction
CCL20	CCL20	CCL20	HTR1F	IL1B	IFNA5	EDN1
CXCL5	CXCL5	CXCL5	TAS1R1	FGF17	CSF3	HTR1F
GDF5	CXCL2	CXCL2	TAS2R60	CACNG6	CSF3R	GABRA6
BMP2	CSF3	IL1B	TAS2R50	GADD45A	OSM	GABBR2
BMP8A	CXCL8	LIF	ADCY8	PLA2G4B	GNG13	AGTR2
IL24	IL1B	IL18R1	GABRA6	DUSP6	FGF17	EDN2
CCL3L3	CEBPB	CEBPB	GNG13	CACNA1D	FGF8	GLRA2
GDF15	NFKBIA	NFKBIA	TAS2R38	FGF8	NTRK1	GRIA1
CXCL2	TNFAIP3	TNFAIP3	GABBR2	GADD45B	NR4A1	MTNR1A
EDA2R	FOSL1	PTGS2	TAS2R4	NTRK1	FLT3	RXFP3
IFNA5	MAPK15	EDN1		NR4A1	FGFR4	TRHR
IL1R2	MAPK6	JUNB		DUSP5	EFNA4	S1PR2
CSF3	PTGS2			FLT3	PDGFA	ADORA3
IL18RAP				FGFR4	KITLG	C5AR1
TNFSF4				EFNA4	THBS1	ADM
CXCL8				PDGFA	MDM2	AGTR1
RELT				RRAS2	SGK1	GRIK1
IL1RL1				KITLG	TLR2	PTGER2
CSF3R					FOXO3	
IL1B					COL6A6	
LIF						
IL18R1						
OSM						
GDF10						

1.7.2 CYTOKINE–CYTOKINE RECEPTOR INTERACTION—HOMO SAPIENS (HUMAN) (KEGG ID HSA04060)

Cytokines are soluble extracellular proteins or glycoproteins that act as intercellular regulators and mobilizers of cells involved in innate and adaptive immune responses, cell proliferation, differentiation, cell death, angiogenesis, development, and repair during homeostasis restoration. Cytokines are generated by a variety of cells throughout the body in response to a triggering event, and they elicit responses by attaching to particular receptors on target cells' cell surfaces. Cytokines and their receptors can be classified into several groups based on their structure.

1.7.3 IL-17-SIGNALING PATHWAY—HOMO SAPIENS (HUMAN)

In both acute and chronic inflammatory reactions, the interleukin 17 (IL-17) family plays a critical role. This subgroup of cytokines, IL-17A-F, belongs to the interleukin family of proteins. IL-17A, the signature cytokine of the recently characterized T-helper-17 cell subset, is involved in protecting the host against external pathogens while also promoting the inflammatory pathway in autoimmune diseases, and IL-17F is involved in mucosal host defense mechanisms. TH2-immune responses are amplified by IL-17E (IL-25). The biological actions of IL-17C are comparable to those of IL-17A. The IL-17 family stimulates downstream pathways such as NF-kappaB, MAPKs, and C/EBPs (CCAAT-enhancer-binding proteins) to promote the synthesis of antimicrobial peptides, cytokines, and chemokines through signaling through their respective receptors. The primary mediator in IL-17A signaling has been identified as the receptor proximal adaptor Act1 (an NF-kappaB activator 1). Thirteen genes present in metadata, related to IL-17-signaling pathway, along with their pro-inflammatory activities, are shown in Figure 1.18.

ToppGene Suite (http://toppgene.cchmc.org) is executed for gene list functional enrichment. From ToppGene analysis (Chen et al., 2009) with the abovementioned 13 genes, the gene names and IDs are shown in Table 1.8.

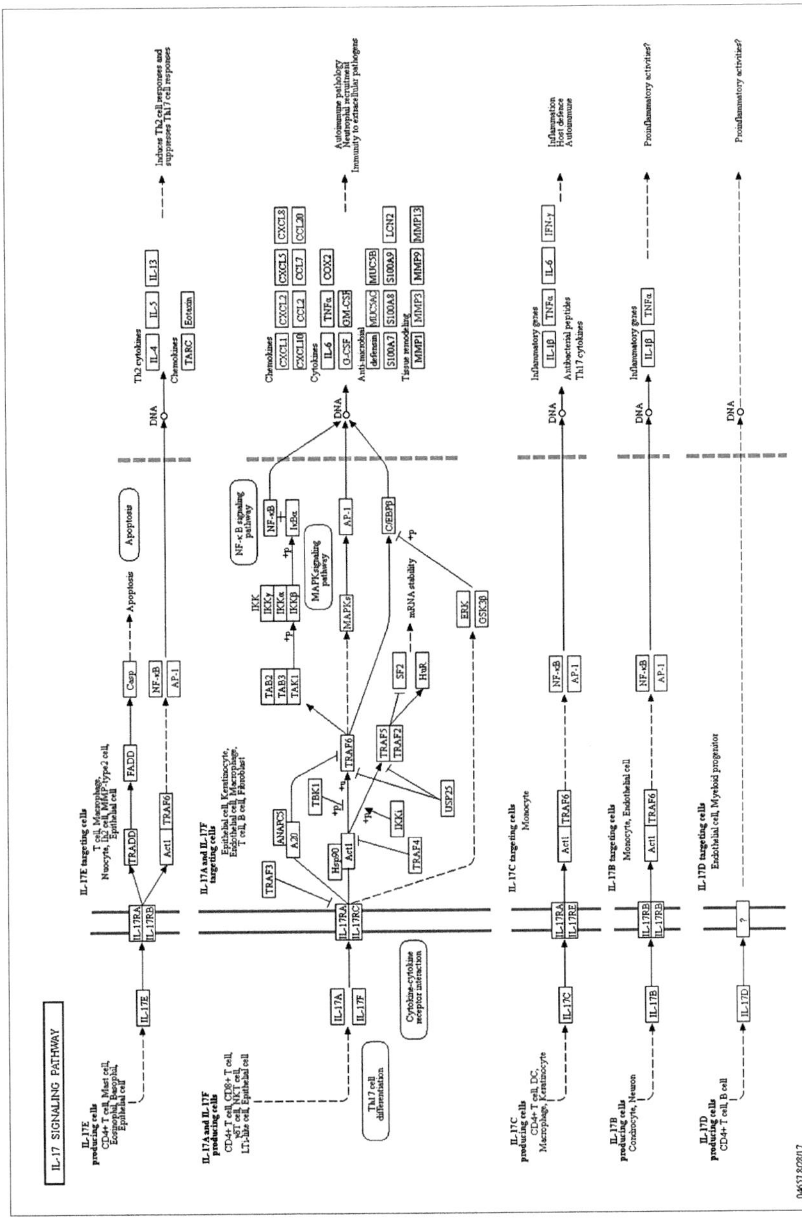

FIGURE 1.18 Thirteen genes of metadata present in the IL-17-signaling pathway.

TABLE 1.8 Name of 13 Genes Present in Metadata Related to the IL-17-Signaling Pathway.

Gene symbol	Gene name	Gene ID
CCL20	CCL20 (C–C motif chemokine ligand 20)	6364
CXCL5	CXCL5 (C–X–C motif chemokine ligand 5)	6374
CXCL2	CXCL2 (C–X–C motif chemokine ligand 2)	2920
CSF3	CSF3 (colony-stimulating factor 3)	1440
CXCL8	CXCL8 (C–X–C motif chemokine ligand 8)	3576
IL-1B	IL-1B (interleukin 1 beta)	3553
CEBPB	CEBPB (CCAAT enhancer binding protein beta)	1051
NFKBIA	NFKBIA (NFKB inhibitor alpha)	4792
TNFAIP3	TNFAIP3 (TNF-alpha induced protein 3)	7128
FOSL1	FOSL1 (FOS like 1, AP-1 transcription factor subunit)	8061
MAPK15	MAPK15 (mitogen-activated protein kinase 15)	225689
MAPK6	MAPK6 (mitogen-activated protein kinase 6)	5597
PTGS2	PTGS2 (prostaglandin-endoperoxide synthase 2)	5743

1.7.4 GENE–CHEMICAL INTERACTION NETWORK

Gene–chemical interaction network for 13 genes present in IL-17-signaling pathway is carried out with ToppGene Suite, webtools (Chen et al., 2009), and a detailed analysis is shown in Table 1.9.

Considering their biological functions, six drugs which are connected by immunological response are analyzed in detail in Table 1.10.

Baicalein can be used as anti-inflammatory agent in several virus infection such as H1N1 (Hour et al., 2013), H5N1 (Sithisarn et al., 2012), Chikungunya (Lee et al., 2014), and Zika virus infection (Oo et al., 2019). This phytochemical interferes with the H5N1 virus-induced production of cytokines, for example, IL-6, IP10, and TNFα.

TABLE 1.9 Chemicals Interacting with 13 Input Genes.

	ID	Name	Source	*p* Value	Genes from input	Biological activity of chemical
1	1791 UP	Azaguanine-8 [134-58-7]; Up 200; 26.2 μM; PC3; HT HG-U133A	Broad Institute CMAP Up	2.018E−17	9	A purine analog with potential antineoplastic activity
2	CID000002750	Ciglitazone	Stitch	3.750E−17	9	Antidiabetic agents with antihyperglycemic activity
3	ctd:C003898	2-Anisidine	CTD	1.183E−16	8	Used in the manufacture of dyes, possible human carcinogen
4	CID000200878	P-38	Stitch	3.554E−16	11	No predicted properties
5	ctd:D004137	Dinitrochlorobenzene	CTD	4.073E−16	10	Induces a type IV hypersensitivity reaction
6	CID000001444	AC1L1BHQ	Stitch	6.304E−16	9	Potent inhibitor of TRPA1 (transient receptor potential cation channel subfamily A member 1)
7	ctd:D004391	Dust	CTD	8.286E−16	9	No predicted properties
8	ctd:D017632	Asbestos, serpentine	CTD	2.222E−15	10	No predicted properties
9	ctd:C433788	Lipopolysaccharide, *E. coli* O26-B6	CTD	2.577E−15	8	No predicted properties
10	ctd:C056507	Gemcitabine	CTD	2.716E−15	9	DNA synthesis inhibitor and an immunosuppressive agent
11	CID000176155	SB203580	Stitch	4.518E−15	11	Inhibitor of mitogen-activated protein kinase and a neuroprotective agent
12	1626 UP	Etoposide [33419-42-0]; Up 200; 6.8 μM; HL60; HG-U133A	Broad Institute CMAP Up	8.631E−15	8	Inhibits topoisomerase II

TABLE 1.9 *(Continued)*

	ID	Name	Source	*p* Value	Genes from input	Biological activity of chemical
13	CID000065351	APDC	Stitch	1.200E−14	9	An anticonvulsant, a neuroprotective agent, a radical scavenger, an antineoplastic agent, and a NF-kappaB inhibitor
14	1230 UP	Thioridazine hydrochloride; Up 200; 10 μM; PC3; HT HG-U133A	Broad Institute CMAP Up	1.450E−14	8	A dopamine antagonist with antipsychotic property
15	1343 UP	Primaquine diphosphate [63-45-6]; Up 200; 8.8 μM; HL60; HT HG-U133A	Broad Institute CMAP Up	1.816E−14	8	Binds to and alters the properties of protozoal DNA
16	CID000003003	Betamethasone-d5	Stitch	1.996E−14	12	A glucocorticoid applied topically in the management of various disorders
17	CID000002900	Isocycloheximide	Stitch	2.594E−14	11	Immunotoxin, inhibition of TNFα-signaling pathway
18	ctd:D013656	Taurocholic acid	CTD	3.626E−14	7	Induces bile flow, inhibitor of cholesterol biosynthesis
19	ctd:D010457	Peptidoglycan	CTD	4.535E−14	6	No predicted properties
20	CID003081257	Peptide 78	Stitch	5.956E−14	7	No predicted properties
21	ctd:C020748	Ferrous sulfate	CTD	6.375E−14	7	Used in iron deficiency anemia
22	ctd:C038459	Curdlan	CTD	7.789E−14	7	Used in fluid and nutrient replacement
23	ctd:D014302	Trinitrobenzenesulfonic acid	CTD	8.148E−14	9	No predicted properties
24	ctd:C032668	1-Nitropyrene	CTD	2.196E−13	8	Carcinogenic agent
25	CID000001287	AC1L1B55	Stitch	2.994E−13	9	Inhibitors of human apurinic/apyrimidinic endonuclease

TABLE 1.9 *(Continued)*

	ID	Name	Source	*p* Value	Genes from input	Biological activity of chemical
26	CID000025500	Nickel hydroxide	Stitch	3.016E−13	8	Increased risk of developing lung and nasal cancers
27	CID005353940	SB202190	Stitch	3.411E−13	7	Purine nucleoside as anti-apoptotic agent
28	CID000004553	NS-398	Stitch	3.518E−13	8	COX-2 inhibitor used in the study of the function of cyclooxygenase
29	CID000004364	NSC350593	Stitch	4.092E−13	8	Chemotactic peptide
30	ctd:C022838	Nickel chloride	CTD	4.674E−13	11	Carcinogen
31	ctd:D052638	Particulate matter	CTD	4.700E−13	12	No predicted properties
32	ctd:D003840	Deoxycholic acid	CTD	4.904E−13	7	Hepatotoxin, metabotoxin, and an oncometabolite
33	ctd:C007262	Deoxynivalenol	CTD	5.036E−13	9	Acute toxic chemical warfare agent
34	ctd:D003035	Cobalt	CTD	5.181E−13	8	No predicted properties
35	ctd:D002211	Capsaicin	CTD	5.735E−13	9	Causes carcinogenesis
36	2338 UP	Mebendazole [31431-39-7]; Up 200; 13.6 µM; HL60; HT HG-U133A	Broad Institute CMAP Up	1.102E−12	7	Anthelmintic agent
37	ctd:D015112	4-Nitroquinoline-1-oxide	CTD	1.125E−12	6	Carcinogenic agent
38	2192 UP	Helveticoside [630-64-8]; Up 200; 7.4 µM; HL60; HT HG-U133A	Broad Institute CMAP Up	1.152E−12	7	No predicted properties
39	ctd:D005944	Glucosamine	CTD	1.314E−12	8	Nutritional supplement
40	ctd:C442865	Lipopolysaccharide, *Helicobacter pylori*	CTD	1.315E−12	5	Upregulates the secretion of superoxide anion resulting in activation of pro-inflammatory cytokine gene expression

TABLE 1.9 *(Continued)*

	ID	Name	Source	*p* Value	Genes from input	Biological activity of chemical
41	CID005281605	Baicalein	Stitch	1.316E−12	7	Antioxidant, prostaglandin antagonist, and anti-inflammatory agent
42	2439 UP	Menadione [58-27-5]; Up 200; 23.2 μM; HL60; HT HG-U133A	Broad Institute CMAP Up	1.498E−12	7	Anticoagulant protein
43	2525 UP	Strophanthidin [66-28-4]; Up 200; 9.8 μM; HL60; HT HG-U133A	Broad Institute CMAP Up	1.564E−12	7	Cardioactive agent
44	CID000000581	*N*-acetylcysteine	Stitch	1.574E−12	9	Inhibits viral stimulation by reactive oxygen intermediates
45	ctd:C040527	Lipoxin A4	CTD	1.628E−12	5	Regulates cellular responses in inflammation
46	CID000005083	Ro 31-8220	Stitch	1.694E−12	8	Inhibits protein kinase C and induces apoptosis
47	2456 UP	Ciclopirox ethanolamine [41621-49-2]; Up 200; 15 μM; HL60; HT HG-U133A	Broad Institute CMAP Up	2.183E−12	7	Anti-inflammatory activity by inhibiting 5-lipoxygenase and cyclooxygenase
48	6697 UP	Ethopropazine hydrochloride [1094-08-2]; Up 200; 11.4 μM; PC3; HT HG-U133A	Broad Institute CMAP Up	4.069E−12	7	A muscarinic antagonist, used as an anti-Parkinson drug
49	ctd:C029728	4-Phenylenediamine	CTD	4.314E−12	6	Antioxidant causing dermatitis, asthma
50	ctd:D014118	Toxins, biological	CTD	5.924E−12	9	No predicted properties

TABLE 1.10 Six Drugs Related to Immunological Response.

	Name of drug related to immunological response	Molecular formula	3D structure	Biological functions	Interacting genes
1	Ciglitazone	$C_{18}H_{23}NO_3S$	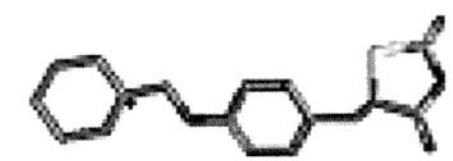	Exerts anti-inflammatory activity through the modulation of nuclear factor-kappaB-mediated pathways (PubChem)	IL-1B CXCL5 CXCL2 PTGS2 CXCL8 NFKBIA TNFAIP3 MAPK15 MAPK6
2	15-Deoxy-delta-12,14-prostaglandin J2 (AC1L1BHQ)	$C_{20}H_{28}O_3$	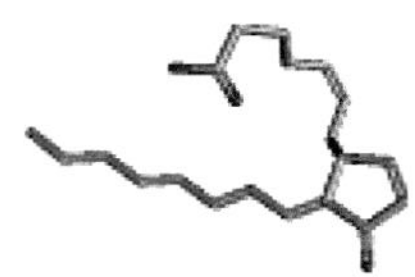	Potent inhibitor of TRPA1 (transient receptor potential cation channel subfamily A member 1) (Superpain database) The transient receptor potential cation channel subfamily A member 1 (TRPA1) plays a key role in chemical sensing in inflammatory pain pathway TRPA1 is permeable to calcium ions and blocked by ruthenium red, which is known to antagonize bronchoconstriction	IL-1B CXCL5 CXCL2 PTGS2 CXCL8 NFKBIA TNFAIP3 MAPK15 MAPK6
3	Gemcitabine	$C_9H_{11}F_2N_3O_4$	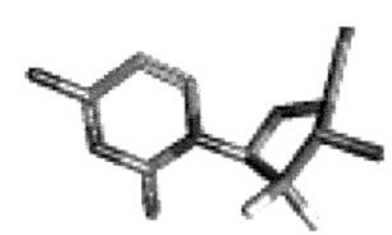	It functions as a photosensitizer, a DNA synthesis inhibitor, a prodrug, an EC 1.17.4.1 (ribonucleoside-diphosphate reductase) inhibitor, an environmental pollutant, a xenobiotic, a radiosensitizer, an antimetabolite, an antiviral drug, and an immunosuppressive agent (PubChem)	CSF3 IL-1B CXCL2 PTGS2 CXCL8 NFKBIA TNFAIP3 CEBPB CCL20

TABLE 1.10 *(Continued)*

	Name of drug related to immunological response	Molecular formula	3D structure	Biological functions	Interacting genes
4	Baicalein	$C_{15}H_{10}O_5$	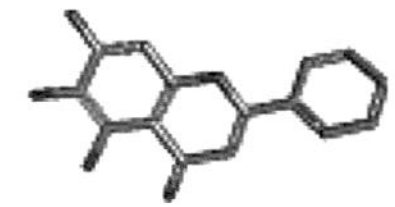	It is used as anti-inflammatory agent in several virus infections. The virus-induced production of cytokines, for example, IL-6, IP10, and TNFα interferes and it imparts anti-inflammatory response by inhibiting NO, cytokines, chemokines, and growth factors via the endoplasmic reticulum stress–CHOP/STAT pathway (Kim et al., 2018)	IL-1B PTGS2 CXCL8 NFKBIA TNFAIP3 MAPK15 MAPK6
5	Lipoxin A4	C20H32O5	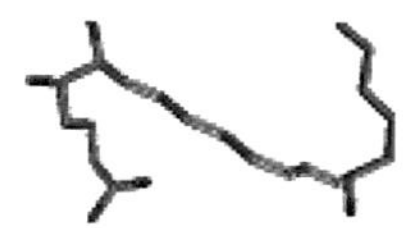	Lipoxin A4 (LXA4) is a 5-lipoxygenase interaction product of activated leukocytes. It is aneicosanoid chemical mediator that displays a potent anti-inflammatory activity. It can act at specific GPCRs as agonists to regulate cellular responses of interest in inflammation (PubChem)	IL-1B CXCL2 PTGS2 CXCL8 NFKBIA
6	Ciclopirox ethanolamine	C14H24N2O3	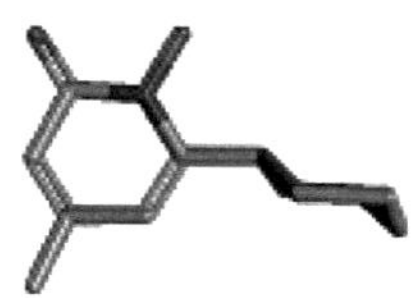	It is a broad-spectrum antifungal that also has antibacterial and anti-inflammatory activities against a variety of Gram-positive and Gram-negative bacteria. It exerts its anti-inflammatory activity by inhibiting 5-lipoxygenase and cyclooxygenase (COX) (PubChem)	IL-1B CXCL2 PTGS2 CXCL8 NFKBIA TNFAIP3 FOSL1

1.8 CONCLUSION

The immune system plays a decisive role in the response to SARS-CoV-2 with substantial changes in gene expression of cytokine genes related to inflammation cytokines (IL-1, TNF). The elevated levels of serum cytokines, known as cytokine storm, results in abrupt increase of interleukins such as IL-1, IL-7, IL-8, IL-9, IL-10, colony-stimulating factors, IFN, and TNF. The anti-inflammatory therapy is required to control the cytokine response in SARS-CoV-2 treatment. Therefore, immunomodulators can be used to regulate or alter the functions of the immune system during COVID-19 pandemic situation. According to the mode of action, the immunomodulator scan be classified as specific and nonspecific. With the help of systems' pharmacology approach, several complex networks of interactions are derived from the gene expression profiling with microarray dataset for both COVID-19-infected patients and for normal individuals. Gene-level meta-analysis result shows that a total 1021 gene is found in the differential gene expression analysis. Among them, 500 genes based on their p values are selected for further network analysis. In total, 84 genes are identified as significant genes from meta-analysis study. The significant gene analysis is done with various graphical methods. PPI network, reveals that EGR1 and HNF4G proteins can produce inflammatory cytokine proteins. The GRNs confirm that the TFs. The interaction of EGRI with multiple genes causes the activation of pro-inflammatory cytokines like interleukin 1 (IL-1) and TNF, as well as the production of pro-inflammatory genes like cytokines and chemokines.

Serotonin (5HT) induces metabolic effects on leukocytes in a concentration-dependent manner by 5HT-induced immunomodulation method, because 5HT can alter diverse activities such as leukocyte activation, proliferation, and at the same time cytokine secretion (Arreola et al., 2015). Serotonin receptors (5HTR), also known as 7-transmembrane receptors, present on immune cells can influence cytokine production (Müller et al., 2009). Drug–gene interaction network shows that sumatriptan exerts anti-inflammatory and immunomodulatory properties by decreasing mRNA levels of TNF and IL-1 that can interact with HTR1F gene. This can act as immunomodulator drug in SARS-CoV-2 therapeutics.

Gene enrichment analysis with KEGG pathway illustrates that cytokine–cytokine receptor interaction, IL-17-signaling pathway, TNF-signaling pathway are related with immunology, which are the biological functions of significant genes of metadata. Thirteen genes present in metadata, related with IL-17-signaling pathway, have their pro-inflammatory activities in immune response. Gene–chemical interaction network for 13 genes present in IL-17-signaling pathway concludes that baicalein can be used as anti-inflammatory agent in this SARS-CoV-2 infection. This natural product can act as a nonspecific immunomodulator, due to its low toxicity and high bioavailability in food, to combat this viral infection.

KEYWORDS

- **gene network**
- **microarray datasets**
- **cytokine storm**
- **immune response**
- **immunomodulators**
- **network visual analysis**
- **pro-inflammatory cytokines**

REFERENCES

Arreola, R.; Becerril-Villanueva, E.; Cruz-Fuentes, C.; Velasco-Velázquez, M. A.; Garcés-Alvarez, M. E.; Hurtado-Alvarado, G.; Quintero-Fabian, S.; Pavón, L. Immunomodulatory Effects Mediated by Serotonin. *J. Immunol. Res.* **2015,** *2015*, 354957.

Bryne, J. C.; Valen, E.; Tang, M. H. E.; Marstrand, T.; Winther, O.; da Piedade, I.; Krogh, A.; Lenhard, B.; Sandelin, A. JASPAR, the Open Access Database of Transcription Factor-Binding Profiles: New Content and Tools in the 2008 Update. *Nucl. Acids Res.* **2007,** *36* (suppl_1), D102–D106.

Chanez, P.; Bourdin, A. Pathophysiology of Asthma. In *Clinical Asthma, Mosby*; Castro, M., Kraft, M., Eds.; 2008; Chapter 3, pp 23–34. ISBN 9780323042895. https://doi.org/10.1016/B978-032304289-5.10003-7. (http://www.sciencedirect.com/science/article/pii/B9780323042895100037).

Chen, Z.; Wherry, E. J. T Cell Responses in Patients with COVID-19. *Nat. Rev. Immunol.* **2020,** *20*, 529–536.

Chen, J.; Bardes, E. E.; Aronow, B. J.; Jegga, A. G. ToppGene Suite for Gene List Enrichment Analysis and Candidate Gene Prioritization. *Nucl. Acids Res.* **2009,** *37* (suppl_2), W305–W311.

Cheng, F.; Murray, J. L.; Rubin, D. H. Drug Repurposing: New Treatments for Zika Virus Infection? *Trends Mol. Med.* **2016,** *22*, 919–921.

Coperchini, F.; Chiovato, L.; Croce, L.; Magri, F.; Rotondi, M. The Cytokine Storm in COVID-19: An Overview of the Involvement of the Chemokine/Chemokine-Receptor System. *Cytokine Growth Factor Rev.* **2020,** *53,* 25–32.

Davis, A. P.; Grondin, C. J.; Johnson, R. J.; Sciaky, D.; McMorran, R.; Wiegers, J.; Wiegers, T. C.; Mattingly, C. J. The Comparative Toxicogenomics Database: Update 2019. *Nucl. Acids Res.* **2019,** *47* (D1), D948–D954.

Desai, N.; Neyaz, A.; Szabolcs, A.; Shih, A. R.; Chen, J. H.; Thapar, V.; Nieman, L. T.; Solovyov, A.; Mehta, A.; Lieb, D. J.; Kulkarni, A. S.; Jaicks, C.; Pinto, C. J.; Juric, D.; Chebib, I.; Colvin, R. B.; Kim, A. Y.; Monroe, R.; Warren, S. E.; Danaher, P.; et al. Temporal and Spatial Heterogeneity of Host Response to SARS-CoV-2 Pulmonary Infection. *medRxiv* **2020**. 2020.07.30.20165241. https://doi.org/10.1101/2020.07.30.20165241

Dürk, T.; Panther, E.; Müller, T.; Sorichter, S.; Ferrari, D.; Pizzirani, C.; Di Virgilio, F.; Myrtek, D.; Norgauer, J.; Idzko, M. 5-Hydroxytryptamine Modulates Cytokine and Chemokine Production in LPS-Primed Human Monocytes Via Stimulation of Different 5-HTR Subtypes. *International Immunology* **2005,** *17* (5), 599–606.

Dyall, J.; et al. Repurposing of Clinically Developed Drugs for Treatment of Middle East Respiratory Syndrome Coronavirus Infection. *Antimicrob. Agents Chemother.* **2014,** *58,* 4885–4893.

Ferguson, L. B.; Harris, R. A.; Mayfield, R. D. From Gene Networks to Drugs: Systems Pharmacology Approaches for AUD. *Psychopharmacology* **2018,** *235* (6), 1635–1662.

Flockerzi, V. TRP Channels. In *Encyclopedia of Molecular Pharmacology*; Offermanns, S., Rosenthal, W., Eds.; Springer: Berlin, Heidelberg, 2008.

Guma, M.; Firestein, G. S. Suppl. 2: c-Jun N-Terminal Kinase in Inflammation and Rheumatic Diseases. *Open Rheumatol. J.* **2012,** *6,* 220.

Hoshikawa, M.; Ohbayashi, N.; Yonamine, A.; Konishi, M.; Ozaki, K.; Fukui, S.; Itoh, N. Structure and Expression of a Novel Fibroblast Growth Factor, FGF-17, Preferentially Expressed in the Embryonic Brain. *Biochem. Biophys. Res. Commun.* **1998,** *244,* 187–191.

Hour, M. J.; Huang, S. H.; Chang, C. Y.; Lin, Y. K.; Wang, C. Y.; Chang, Y. S.; Lin, C. W. Baicalein, Ethyl Acetate, and Chloroform Extracts of *Scutellaria baicalensis* Inhibit the Neuraminidase Activity of Pandemic 2009 H1N1 and Seasonal Influenza A Viruses. *Evid.-Based Complement. Altern. Med.* **2013,** *2013.* https://coronavirus.jhu.edu/data/mortality

Johansen, L. M.; et al. FDA-Approved Selective Estrogen Receptor Modulators Inhibit Ebola Virus Infection. *Sci. Transl. Med.* **2013,** *5,* 190ra179.

Khalilzadeh, M.; Panahi, G.; Rashidian, A.; Hadian, M. R.; Abdollahi, A.; Afshari, K.; Shakiba, S.; Norouzi-Javidan, A.; Rahimi, N.; Momeny, M.; Dehpour, A. R. The Protective Effects of Sumatriptan on Vincristine-Induced Peripheral Neuropathy in a Rat Model. *Neurotoxicology* **2018,** *67,* 279–286.

Kim, Y. J.; Kim, H. J.; Lee, J. Y.; Kim, D. H.; Kang, M. S.; Park, W. Anti-inflammatory Effect of Baicalein on Polyinosinic–Polycytidylic Acid-Induced RAW 264.7 Mouse Macrophages. *Viruses* **2018,** *10* (5), 224.

Kohl, M.; Wiese, S.; Warscheid, B. Cytoscape: Software for Visualization and Analysis of Biological Networks. In *Data Mining in Proteomics*; Humana Press: Totowa, NJ, 2011; pp 291–303.

Lawrence, T. The Nuclear Factor NF-κB Pathway in Inflammation. *Cold Spring Harbor Perspect. Biol.* **2009,** *1* (6), a001651.

Lee, W.; Ku, S.-K.; Bae, J.-S. Anti-inflammatory Effects of Baicalin, Baicalein, and Wogonin In Vitro and In Vivo. *Inflammation*, **2014,** *38*. doi:10.1007/s10753-014-0013-0.

Maginnis, M. S. Virus–Receptor Interactions: The Key to Cellular Invasion. *J. Mol. Biol.* **2018,** *430* (17), 2590–2611.

Mahoney, K. M.; Rennert, P. D.; Freeman, G. J. Combination Cancer Immunotherapy and New Immunomodulatory Targets. *Nat. Rev. Drug Discov.* **2015,** *14* (8), 561–584.

Mason, R. J. Pathogenesis of COVID-19 from a Cell Biologic Perspective. *Eur. Respir. J.* **2020,** *55* (4), 2000607.

Mateus, J.; Grifoni, A.; Tarke, A.; Sidney, J.; Ramirez, S. I.; Dan, J. M.; Burger, Z. C.; Rawlings, S. A.; Smith, D. M.; Phillips, E.; Mallal, S. Selective and Cross-Reactive SARS-CoV-2 T-Cell Epitopes in Unexposed Humans. *Science* **2020,** *370* (6512), 89–94.

Moore, J. B.; June, C. H. Cytokine Release Syndrome in Severe COVID-19. *Science* **2020,** *368*, 473–474. doi:10.1126/science.abb8925pmid:32303591.

Müller, T.; Dürk, T.; Blumenthal, B.; Grimm, M.; Cicko, S.; Panther, E.; Sorichter, S.; Herouy, Y.; Di Virgilio, F.; Ferrari, D.; Norgauer, J. 5-Hydroxytryptamine Modulates Migration, Cytokine and Chemokine Release and T-Cell Priming Capacity of Dendritic Cells In Vitro and In Vivo. *PLoS ONE* **2009,** *4* (7), e6453.

Naik, D. G. Immunomodulation in Viral Infections. *Res. Rev.: J. Immunol.* **2018,** *7* (2), 5–8.

Oo, A.; Teoh, B. T.; Sam, S. S.; Bakar, S. A.; Zandi, K. Baicalein and Baicalin as Zika Virus Inhibitors. *Arch. Virol.* **2019,** *164* (2), 585–593.

Piñero, J.; Ramírez-Anguita, J. M.; Saüch-Pitarch, J.; Ronzano, F.; Centeno, E.; Sanz, F.; Furlong, L. I. The DisGeNET Knowledge Platform for Disease Genomics: 2019 Update. *Nucl. Acids Res.* **2020,** *48* (D1), D845–D855.

Ragab, D.; Salah Eldin, H.; Taeimah, M.; Khattab, R.; Salem, R. The COVID-19 Cytokine Storm; What We Know So Far. *Front. Immunol.* **2020,** *11*, 1446.

Rahman, M. R.; Islam, T.; Gov, E.; Turanli, B.; Gulfidan, G.; Shahjaman, M.; Akhter Banu, N.; Mollah, M.; Haque, N.; Arga, K. Y.; Moni, M. A. Identification of Prognostic Biomarker Signatures and Candidate Drugs in Colorectal Cancer: Insights from Systems Biology Analysis. *Medicina* **2019a,** *55* (1), 20.

Rahman, M. R.; Islam, T.; Turanli, B.; Zaman, T.; Faruquee, H. M.; Rahman, M. M.; Mollah, M. N. H.; Nanda, R. K.; Arga, K. Y.; Gov, E.; Moni, M. A. Network-Based Approach to Identify Molecular Signatures and Therapeutic Agents in Alzheimer's Disease. *Comput. Biol. Chem.* **2019b,** *78*, 431–439.

Rapaport, F.; Zinovyev, A.; Dutreix, M.; Barillot, E.; Vert, J. P. Classification of Microarray Data Using Gene Networks. *BMC Bioinform.* **2007,** *8* (1), 35.

Sakkas, L. I.; Mavropoulos, A.; Perricone, C.; Bogdanos, D. P. IL-35: A New Immunomodulator in Autoimmune Rheumatic Diseases. *Immunol. Res.* **2018,** *66* (3), 305–312.

Sam, Q. H.; Yew, W. S.; Seneviratne, C. J.; Chang, M. W.; Chai, L. Y. A. Immunomodulation as Therapy for Fungal Infection: Are We Closer? *Front. Microbiol.* **2018,** *9*, 1612.

Sarkar, A.; Maulik, U. *Vaccines and Treatment Strategies for SARS-COV-2*. 2020, May 6. https://doi.org/10.31219/osf.io/3qzm2

Schmidt, J.; Stoffels, B.; Moore, B. A.; Chanthaphavong, R. S.; Mazie, A. R.; Buchholz, B. M.; Bauer, A. J. Proinflammatory Role of Leukocyte-Derived EGR-1 in the Development of Murine Postoperative Ileus. *Gastroenterology* **2008,** *135* (3), 926–936.

Shi, Y.; Wang, Y.; Shao, C.; Huang, J.; Gan, J.; Huang, X.; Bucci, E.; Piacentini, M.; Ippolito, G.; Melino, G. COVID-19 Infection: The Perspectives on Immune Responses. *Cell Death Different.* **2020,** *27* (5), 1451.

Sithisarn, P.; Michaelis, M.; Schubert-Zsilavecz, M.; Cinatl, J. Differential Antiviral and Anti-inflammatory Mechanisms of the Flavonoids Biochanin A and Baicalein in H5N1 Influenza A Virus-Infected Cells. Antiviral research **2012,** *97*. doi:10.1016/j.antiviral.2012.10.004.

Suwannarach, N.; Kumla, J.; Sujarit, K.; Pattananandecha, T.; Saenjum, C.; Lumyong, S. Natural Bioactive Compounds from Fungi as Potential Candidates for Protease Inhibitors and Immunomodulators to Apply for Coronaviruses. *Molecules* **2020,** *25* (8), 1800.

Szklarczyk, D.; Franceschini, A.; Wyder, S.; Forslund, K.; Heller, D.; Huerta-Cepas, J.; Simonovic, M.; Roth, A.; Santos, A.; Tsafou, K. P.; Kuhn, M. STRING v10: Protein–Protein Interaction Networks, Integrated over the Tree of Life. *Nucl. Acids Res.* **2015,** *43* (D1), D447–D452.

Wishart, D. S.; Feunang, Y. D.; Guo, A. C.; Lo, E. J.; Marcu, A.; Grant, J. R.; Sajed, T.; Johnson, D.; Li, C.; Sayeeda, Z.; Assempour, N. DrugBank 5.0: A Major Update to the DrugBank Database for 2018. *Nucl. Acids Res.* **2018,** *46* (D1), D1074–D1082.

Xia, J.; Fjell, C. D.; Mayer, M. L.; Pena, O. M.; Wishart, D. S.; Hancock, R. E. INMEX—A Web-Based Tool for Integrative Meta-analysis of Expression Data. *Nucl. Acids Res.* **2013,** *41* (W1), W63–W70.

Xia, J.; Benner, M. J.; Hancock, R. E. NetworkAnalyst-Integrative Approaches for Protein–Protein Interaction Network Analysis and Visual Exploration. *Nucl. Acids Res.* **2014,** *42* (W1), W167–W174.

Xia, J.; Gill, E. E.; Hancock, R. E. NetworkAnalyst for Statistical, Visual and Network-Based Meta-analysis of Gene Expression Data. *Nat. Protocols* **2015,** *10* (6), 823–844.

Zapater, P.; González-Navajas, J. M.; Such, J.; Francés, R. Immunomodulating Effects of Antibiotics Used in the Prophylaxis of Bacterial Infections in Advanced Cirrhosis. *World J. Gastroenterol.* **2015,** *21* (41), 11493.

Zhou, G.; Soufan, O.; Ewald, J.; Hancock, R. E.; Basu, N.; Xia, J. NetworkAnalyst 3.0: A Visual Analytics Platform for Comprehensive Gene Expression Profiling and Meta-analysis. *Nucl. Acids Res.* **2019,** *47* (W1), W234–W241.

CHAPTER 2

COVID-19: Role of Polyphenols as Immunomodulators

KHUSHWINDER KAUR

Department of Chemistry and Centre of Advanced Studies in Chemistry, Panjab University, Chandigarh, Punjab, India

ABSTRACT

Immunomodulators are natural or synthetic substances that maintain the regulatory act of the body by sustaining cell homeostasis. They hold an enormous commitment to prevent lifestyle diseases like cancer, diabetes, neurodegenerative disorders, and so on. They turn on the cytokines, the natural defense mechanism of the body enabling it to reinvigorate itself. It is well established that natural compounds such as polyphenols and flavanoids contribute largely toward immunomodulators. The mechanism of action involve either suppression or stimulation of the immune response of the body to fight against various diseases including cancer, autoimmune diseases, viral infections, and other stages of immune deficiency. Natural immunomodulators offer an inherent advantage over prescribed/artificial drugs of being safe and have no side effects. However, they are usually used in combination with other medicines, thus tweaking the way it works.

2.1 INTRODUCTION

The outbreak of COVID-19 has traumatized the entire world stressing the need for improvement of not only health infrastructure but also the development of strong immune system or immunomodulation. The recent

COVID-19 and Immunomodulation with Special Emphasis on Nutraceutical and Herbal Formulation.
Rajesh K. Kesharwani & Raj K. Keservani (Eds)

data show that more than 3.2 million people have been infected and over 250,000 have died (Nicholas et al., 2020). It has been reported that while most of the people develop mild illness, 15–20% require hospitalization and nearly 5% are critically ill requiring ICU care (Alijotas-Reig et al., 2020). People with comorbidities such as diabetes, respiratory, and digestive infection are at higher risk. The initial response to fight the outbreak of this pandemic was to go in for lockdown so that physical boundaries could be imposed among people and the spread of disease could be slowed. However, gradually the governments have realized that lockdowns to enforce social distancing are not the only solution as these prolonged shutdown have an adverse impact on the worldwide financial system and employment of people. No doubt the most arduous preclusion approach would be a vaccine but it is unlikely to be available on time to the entire human race. While the race for finding the vaccine is on; however, till the time one is able to lay his hand on the safe and secure vaccine to this virus, the need of the hour is to work on developing strong immunity which can withstand the load of virus.

A report recently (Kim et al., 2020) indicated that hospitalized COVID-19 patients have elevated levels of various cytokines. This includes IL-2, IL-7, IL-10, G-CSF IP-10, MCP-1, TNF-α, and so on. The development of various forms of cytokines leads to high mortality. It is further anticipated that damage to the lungs and other organs is actually due to enhanced levels of cytokinases. Such high levels might be associated with the severity of the disease. Similar case studies have been found in case of *severe acute respiratory syndrome (*SARS) and Middle-East Respiratory Syndrome (MERS). Also, a recent finding suggests that the virus reaches the respiratory tract after affecting the nasal and larynx epithelium. This then may go into the blood attacking various organs such as heart, kidney, liver, and so on making it fatal for the patient. This increased level of cytokinases is a cause of worry for the clinicians (Nicholas et al., 2020; Alijotas-Reig et al., 2020; Kim et al., 2020).

Presently, no fixed therapeutic option is available for the treatment of the disease. Therefore, different combinations are being tried to treat patients with COVID-19. This includes antimalarial drugs such as chloroquine and its derivative hydroxychloroquine, remdesivir, infusing patient with the serum of COVID-19 survivor, drug cocktail of antiviral drugs, using drugs that are used for arthritis and other autoimmune diseases. Apart from these, many other combinations are being tried on COVID patients till a fixed therapy is developed based on the condition of the patient and experience of the health-care team (Ming, 2020). The combination is tried with an approach that they lower the levels of cytokines in human body. However, the mechanism of action of most of these drugs on COVID-19 is not known. It has been reported that the most frequently used drugs like chloroquine and hydroxychloroquine have both anti-inflammatory and strong in-vitro antiviral properties. Structural explanation reports indicate that both chloroquine and hydroxychloroquine are weak bases. Therefore, they have the affinity to hoard in acidic organelles such as lysosomes. Here, they can increase endosomal/lysosomal pH therefore inhibiting viral replication. Further, the Toll-like receptor signaling and cyclic guanosine-adenosine synthase stimulation of interferon genes play a major role to suppress the expression of major histocompatibility complex class II, antigen presentation, and immune activation (reducing CD154 expression by T cells) (Schrezenmeier and Dörner, 2020). Thus, chloroquine and hydroxychloroquine can cut down the making of a range of pro-inflammatory cytokines, such as IL-1, IL-6, IF-α, and tumor necrosis factor, which are engaged in the production of cytokine storm (Schrezenmeier and Dörner, 2020). These immunomodulatory effects may show symbiosis with their antiviral effects in the management of COVID-19.

Immunomodulation is the modulation of the immune system by various enzymes, drugs, probiotics, and plant bioactives. It may also be referred to as part of the immune system wherein immune response is modified, augmented, induced, or attenuated. It may be specific or nonspecific. For specific purposes, it comes through behavioral interventions which might occur through focus on education, hygiene, breastfeeding, and vaccination for certain targeted pathogens. Nonspecific immunomodulation implies with developing the ability of the immune system to fight various infections by utilizing plant-based extracts, bacterial lysates, bacterial ribosomal preparations, and so on (Almeida et al., 2020).

The immunomodulatory effect and development of therapeutics from plants have recently gained great importance. This is because plant-based immunomodulators are known to inhibit or stimulate the immune response against various diseases. Particularly, for the treatment of immunological disorders, medicinal plants exhibiting cellular and humoral responses could have enormous inference (Mirshafiey et al., 2004). Currently, due COVID-19 epidemic there is a growing interest for using immune stimulants as supplements in combination with the therapeutic modalities in the treatment of COVID-19. This is because the immune system is involved in the chief role of protecting the body against pathogens and harmful antigens. The chapter focuses on immunomodulation by plant-based extracts with particular emphasis on polyphenols.

2.2 POLYPHENOLS AND THEIR CLASSIFICATION

Polyphenols also known as secondary metabolites of plants have an intrinsic capacity to control the immune system by restraining the cytokine release. This may also affect the other aspects that influence the immune response of the body. Their biological effects are primarily ascribed to the aptness to impound or reduce reactive oxygen and nitrogen species, transport electrons to free radicals, along with activating antioxidant enzymes for improving oxidative stress and inflammation, thus representing potential effects in the deterrence of a variety of diseases such as obesity, diabetes, cardiovascular diseases, cancer, osteoporosis, neurodegenerative diseases, and so on (de Araújo et al., 2021). They, therefore, show anti-inflammatory, antimicrobial, antitumor, and immunomodulatory properties, which in turn can bring vital benefits to human well-being. But their biological properties depend on many other factors such as their concentration in the food, bioavailabilty, bioaccessibility, bioefficacy, and so on. These effects and their mechanistic details have been well documented in literature (Ibrahim et al., 2017; Gasmi et al., 2020).

Besides this, they have the tendency to fight against various viruses such as influenza virus, retrovirus, Epstein–Barr virus, papillomavirus, enterovirus, herpes simplex virus, and other viruses causing respiratory tract-linked epidemics (Gasmi et al., 2020). However, there are limited studies that talk about the effect of polyphenols on viruses particularly COVID-19. But it is anticipated that they can play role in preventing inflammation by mitigating inciting response in adipocytes, immune cells, and macrophages. They have the tendency to alter dendritic cells (DCs) and change them into tolerogenic DCs for altering physical condition and preventing disease (Rahimi et al., 2020). This not only promotes immunity against pathogens but also promotes differentiation of regulatory T cells and suppresses T-cell responses.

Very recently, prebiotic agents have also been identified as polyphenols because of their tendency to interact with gut microbes. It is reported that when the polyphenolic content of blueberry is injected in mice, it normalized lipid metabolism and thus prevented weight gain (Jiao et al., 2019). Further, the function of a laccase–chlorogenic acid recombinant system in the makeup of curds has enhanced the antioxidant levels. Thus, the final product has remarkable nutritional value (Loi et al., 2018). This indicates that the interaction between carbohydrates and polyphenols has been found to improve not only the physiochemical properties of starch, proteins, or the food matrix but also their physiological effects. They can alter the gelatinization, retrogradation, and gelation along with the digestibility of starch. Compounds like tannin can increase crystallinity, bonding temperature, and maximum viscosity of starch. Therefore, they modify the food product by alternating their functional, nutritional, and nutraceutical properties (Du et al., 2019). This indicates that polyphenols play a major role not only in managing disease but also amending the immune reaction of the body to various diseases.

To further understand them in depth polyphenols have been classified on the basis of their carbon structures. Figure 2.1 elucidates the exhaustive arrangement of polyphenols. They are broadly dispersed in fruits and vegetables and nearly 800 structures have already been isolated. They are classified on the basis of their chemical structure, ranging from simple C arrangements such as phenolic acids, to highly polymerized structures, such as tannins. They are usually classified as flavonoids, lignanes, stilbenes, and tannins (Keservani et al., 2016a, 2016b).

2.2.1 STILBENES

Stilbenes are secondary metabolites derived from the phenylpropanoid pathway. They are found in a large number of different plant species and play a key role in the treatment of various diseases. Stilbene synthase is the key enzyme that catalyzes the biosynthesis of stilbenic compounds in plants. Chemically, they have (1,2-diphenylethylene) backbone and exist in two isomeric forms: 1,2-diphenylethylene: (*E*)-stilbene (*trans*-stilbene) and (*Z*)-stilbene (*cis*-stilbene), pterostilbene. The structures have been represented in Figure 2.2. However, (*E*)-stilbene (*trans*-stilbene) is more stable as it is not sterically hindered. The *trans*-isomers possess estrogenic activity and therefore can be used to make nonsteroidal synthetic estrogens. The most common example of *trans*-stilbene is resvaretrol (RSV) and pinosylvin (3,5-dihydroxy-*trans*-stilbene). They are found naturally

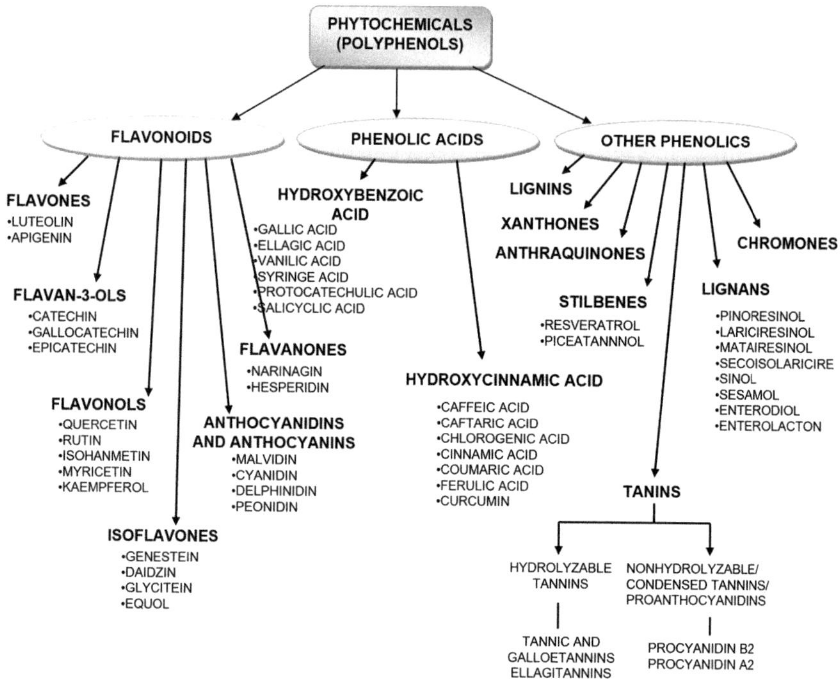

FIGURE 2.1 Classification of polyphenols based on the carbon structures.

in grape wine, sorghum, peanuts, and so on. The natural mechanism of synthesis of stilbenes is still not completely understood (Dai et al., 2012; Fontana et al., 2013).

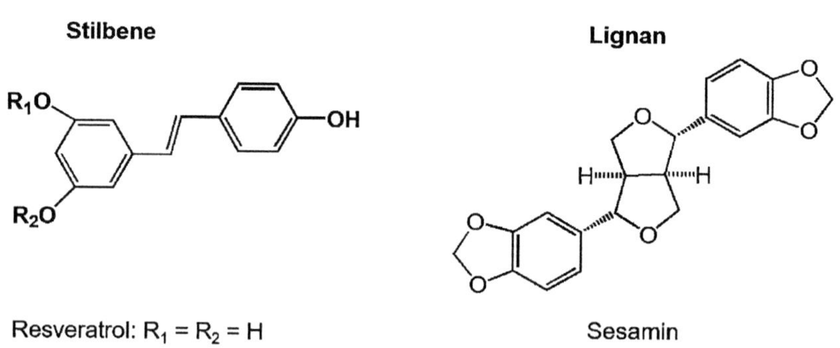

FIGURE 2.2 Structures of stilbene compounds.

2.2.2 FLAVONOIDS

Flavanoids are a class of polyphenols that is present in almost all fruits and vegetables. Besides carotenoids, they are largely accountable for the color of natural foods. They offer antioxidant, anti-inflammatory, anticancer, and cardioprotective effects. Rich sources include onions, green tea, strawberries, apples, almonds, kale, grapes, Brussels sprouts, lettuce, citrus fruit, parsley, and many spices. This class includes flavonoids (flavanol, flavone, flavon-3-ol, anthocyanin, and isoflavone flavanone) and nonflavonoids (gallic acid, hydroxyl cinnamic acid, lignan, stilbene, and curcumin). They constitute the most important group with a common structure of diphenylpropanes (C_6–C_3–C_6), derivatives of flavan and isofalvan.

Based on the carbon structure and level of oxidation on the aromatic ring, they are further classified flavonols, flavones, flavan-3-ols, anthocyanins, flavanones, and isoflavones (Auger et al., 2008; Gardana et al., 2007). They are mainly present in plants in glycosylated forms in the class of quercetin, kaempferol, and myricetin. This includes tea, coffee, fruits, and other grains.

Flavones have a double bond between C2 and C3, like flavonols, with which they differ by the absence of hydroxyl group in the 3 position. This simple discrepancy in the structural plan of flavones and flavonols has very vital consequences in the biogenesis, physiological, and pharmacological function. This also effects the phylogenetic and chemotaxonomic signification of these compounds.

Flavones are broadly dispersed between the higher plants in the form of aglycones or glycosides (Fig. 2.3). Flavanones on the other hand are 2,3-dihydrogenated flavones, whereas flavanonols are 2,3-dihydrogenated flavonols. The basic chemical arrangement of anthocyannins is flavylium cation (2-phenylbenzopyrilium) that links hydroxyl (–OH) and/or methoxyl (–OCH_3) groups, and one or more sugars. They offer various roles in foods particularly in cardioprotection and organoleptic characteristics in food products. Apart from this, other varieties include biflavonoids (dimmers of flavanoids) with linkages at positions 6 and 8 which are considered to be highly reactive, isoflavones and chalcones. The biosynthesis of flavanoids in plants is enhanced due to oxidative stress.

They absorb UVA and UVB that prevents the formation of free radicals. Mechanisms of antioxidant action include (1) inhibition of reactive oxygen species (ROS) formation, (2) scavenging ROS, and (3)

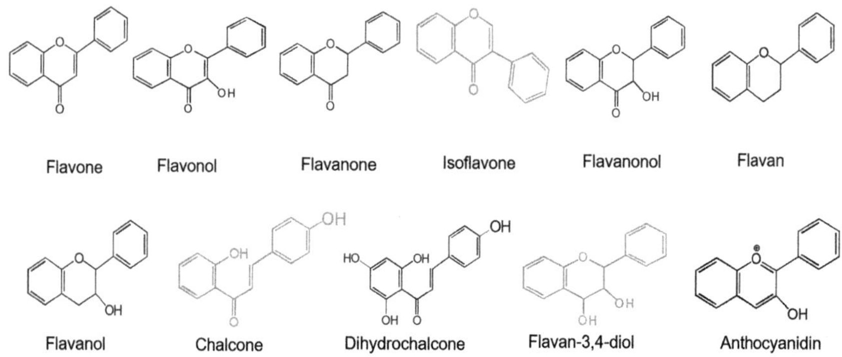

FIGURE 2.3 Representative structures of various flavanoids.

upregulation of defense. They also protect lipids against oxidative stress by various mechanisms.

2.2.3 *PHENOLIC ACIDS*

They are basically nonflavanoid derivatives (Tsao, 2010) of benzoic and cinnamic acid with C1–C6 and C3–C6 backbones (Fig. 2.4). They are usually present as free aglycone or conjugated bound form along with a carbohydrate. The common derivates include benzoic acid, cinnamic acid, caffeic acid, and ferulic acid. They are found in free state in vegetables and fruits, whereas in grains they occur in bound state. They provide more health benefits than using vitamin supplements. Regular intake not only boosts immunity but also provides anti-aging and antioxidant effects. They are found abundantly in cereals, fruits, vegetables, herbs, and others. Not only they act as antioxidants but also participate in changing cell signaling pathways (Keservani et al., 2016b).

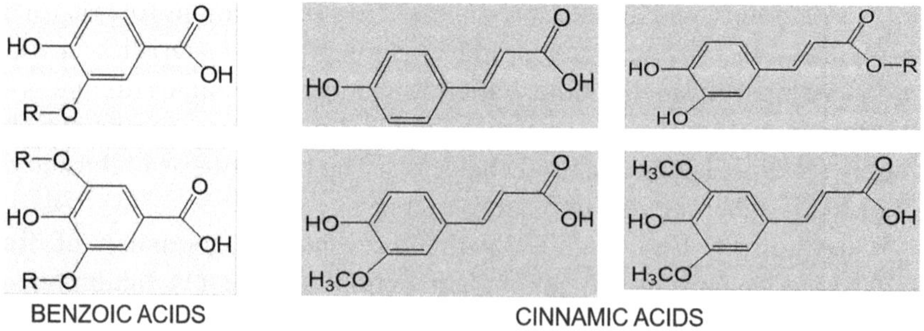

FIGURE 2.4 Representative structures of various phenolic acids.

2.2.4 TERPENOIDS AND OTHER PHYTOCHEMICALS

Terpenoids, also called as isoprenoids, are made from 5-carbon isoprene unit. Molecules with multiples of five carbons mainly with single carbon side chains probably belong to this group. The most important member of terpenoid class includes sterols. They are widely used in the treatment of various diseases. A major steroidal lactone, withaferin A, is present in the medicinal plant; *Withania somnifera*, is consumed around the world as a dietary supplement particularly in Asian countries for treating inflammation and tumors. They are present in the membranes of the cells and affect their fluidity (Yang et al., 2007). Also, lignans result from the condensation of 2–5 molecules of phenylpropane derivatives (C6–C3).

2.3 PROTECTIVE ACTION OF POLYPHENOLS

Polyphenols not only act as antioxidants, anticancer, offer protection against various brain diseases but also have a great immunomodulatory potential, thus contributing to their antiviral and antibacterial properties. They have been found to be effective against various viruses, particularly enveloped viruses such as retrovirus, influenza virus, papillomavirus, herpes virus, and flaviviruses. Sulfated polysaccharides and phenolic compounds found in seaweeds and land plants possess the best antiviral activity. Therefore, investigations into the immunomodulatory potential of these compounds are far more important in the era of COVID-19. The polyphenols like curcumin act on the membranes of enveloped virus effecting membrane fluidity. This then alters the structure of associated glycoproteins, thus making the virus unable to establish a contact with the cells they are to infect. For example, the measles virus (MeV) is an enveloped virus with protected genetic material that has reacquired significance as a pathogen as a consequence of the numerous current outbreaks that have happened in developed countries (Holzmann et al., 2016). Even though the vaccine is available, this illness has not been eradicated; hence, the use of an effective antiviral as a therapy was mandatory to add to hold the outbreak of the disease and finally eliminate it. This involved the strategy of concurrently and aggressively targeting multiple targets. However, this is a much-studied approach in the control of viral diseases (Holzmann et al., 2016). So, this is combined with immunomodulators.

Combining targeted therapies with immunomodulators have demonstrated multiple advantages in this field, such as reduction of drug dose and side effects of antiviral agents, along with the avoidance of the appearance of drug-resistant viruses (Morán-Santibañez et al., 2018).

Not only MeV, the problem is the same with dengue fever. Though many drugs like chloroquine, prednisolone, and lovastatin, and so on have been used in dengue fever to decrease the viral load but not high beneficial effects have been reported till date. The preset treatment line of infection involves fluid revival and compassionate concern in patients with hypovolemic shock. However, many plant extracts laden with poyphenols such as quercetin, curcumin, and so on have been used against the virus. Reports exhibit their potential to restrain infection originating from two viral sterotypes, thus downregulating the outcome of pro-inflammatory cytokines leading to severe dengue pathogenesis (Jasso-Miranda et al., 2019). Polyphenols such as quercetin and fisetin have the tendency to interact with the virus through various mechanisms. They interact with the proteins and inhibit the various pathways of virus replicative cycle. They may also act directly on the cell changing the signaling conduit implicated in inherent reaction. As an example during infection caused by influenza quercetin is known to interact with influenza hemagglutinin protein and then inhibits viral–cell fusion thus activating the transcription of genes implicated in the antiviral reaction. Similar is the case with many other flavanoids such as dihydroquercetin, dihydrofisetin, leucocyanidin, pelargonidin chloride, and catechin. They show activity against various viruses such as HSV, respiratory syncytial virus, poliovirus, and Sindbis virus. The antiviral mechanism involves the inhibition of viral polymerase and binding of viral nucleic acid or viral capsid proteins (Jasso-Miranda et al., 2019).

2.4 IMMUNOMODULATORY EFFECT OF POLYPHENOLS ON VIRAL DISEASES

2.4.1 CURCUMIN

The drug-yielding potential of *Curcuma longa* L. is mainly due to the presence of active constituent curcumin in it. This well-known Indian spice has good immunomodulatory action and offers protection against diseases like cancer, cardiovascular, neurological disorders, autoimmune diseases, and so on. However, various geographical parameters affect the use of curcumin as drug. This involves the accessibility of elevated curcumin-containing genotype and disparity of curcumin content with climatic setting. It interconnects the molecular mechanisms implicated in inflammatory processes such as cytokines and a variety of transcription factors thus downstreaming signaling pathways (Catanzaro et al., 2018; Nelson et al., 2017; Kunnumakkara et al., 2017). It has been known to network with membranes and act as a membrane-disturbing agent. Not only does it changes the membrane structure, it decreases the mitochondrial potential. The hydrophobic properties of membranes favor the intercalation of curcumin into the lipid bilayer, such as in cellular membranes. This suppresses the immunostimulatory function of DC and obstructs the myeloid DC maturation thus disturbing membrane proteins that stimulate the production of T cells and impairs the formation of pro-inflammatory cytokine. All this suggests that it can effect and improve the immune function significantly (Weissenberger et al., 2010; Lin et al., 2011).

It also interrupts viral infection process. It is found to be effective against various influenza viruses such as H1N1, H2N2, H3N2, H5N1, and respiratory syndrome virus. Protection from viruses occurs by multiple mechanisms. This may involve direct targeting of the virus, inhibiting gene expression, blocking the entry of virus, its replication, and propagation, inhibiting pulmonary fibrosis. It may also effect or completely block the attachment of virus with human cell (Liu and Ying, 2020). Pulmonary edema and pulmonary fibrosis are associated with COVID-19 and are referred to as one of the major causes of death as well as long-term damages caused by COVID. It has been established that curcumin could come to rescue to modulate cellular-signaling pathways such as inflammation, apoptosis, RNA replication, inhibitory effects on NF-κB, and several pro-inflammatory cytokines. All this makes curcumin a potential component in the fight against novel coronavirus.

Not only it offers lung protection but also has a role in cardioprotection during COVID-19. Cardiovascular function is impaired during this infection due to the fastening of virus spike protein to angiotensin-converting enzyme 2 (ACE2). The symptoms of lung infection are more prominent in patients having cardiovascular issues too. This is because ACE2 is more expressed in patients with cardiovascular issues. Pang et al. (2015) demonstrated that curcumin significantly decreases mean arterial blood pressure and improves cardiac fibrosis in rats through upregulation of angiotensin II type II receptor, downregulation of angiotensin II type I receptor, an increase of ACE2 in the myocardium. It has the tendency to reduce myocardial ischemia–reperfusion injury through a reduction of c-Jun N-terminal kinase and NF-κB nuclear translocation phosphorylation (Sahebkar and Henrotin 2016). Curcumin has the tendency to offer nephroprotection during COVID-19. This occurs by multiple mechanisms which involve upregulating the ACE2 and ACE2 mRNA, directing improved renal blood flow. It inhibits renal fibrosis at the primary stage by suppressing the inflammation caused by reduced MCP-1, NF-κB, TNF-α, IL-1β, COX-2, and caveolin-1 levels. It also increases the expression of anti-inflammatory factors. Thus, curcumin can offer a protective role as immunomodulator in COVID-19. ARS-CoV papain-like protease (PLpro) significantly induces the generation of ROS and activates TGF-β1-mediated profibrotic response, thus preventing oxidative stress. However, curcumin still struggles with the problems of poor bioavailability, poor solubility, pH stability, and significant differences in in-vitro and in-vivo investigations.

Nutritional blend of curcumin with vitamin C offers a great combination during the era of COVID-19. This has shown results in various hospitalized Indian patients (Manohar et al., 2020). The best formulations of bioavailable curcumin are nanoemulsions. However, a more detailed and planned study is still required in this direction.

2.4.2 RESVERATROL

RSV is another polyphenol that acts as an antiviral agent mainly by inhibiting the replication of viruses (Sato et al., 2013). It is a 14-carbon stilbene skeleton found in plants such as *Vitis vinifera* and *Polygonum cuspidatum*. It has three hydroxyl groups in position 3, 5, and 4′ joined to the two aromatic rings by a double styrene bond. This establishes the presence of *cis-* and *trans*-RSV isomers. In case of MERS-CoV RSV has been found to inactivate the virus in concentration varying from 125 to 250 μM. It inhibited the virus replication at concentrations ranging from 250 to 31.25 μM. It further decreases the viral load at concentrations 250 to 125 μM. Nucleocapsid proteins also exhibited dose-dependent inhibition expression. Therefore, it further inhibited apoptosis. The other evidence for inhibition of apoptosis is inhibition of the caspase-3 expression. In fact, it is anticipated that RSV (i) activates the ERK1/2 and SIR1-signaling pathways, (ii) slows down the MERS-CoV, and (iii) condenses the disease. Among its derivatives, methoxylated, hydroxylated, and halogenated RSV derivatives showed a stronger pharmacological potency and a better pharmacokinetic profile than RSV itself in in-vitro and animal-based models (Cheng et al., 2020). Not only this, the cardioprotective effect of RSV has been established by its ability to identify molecular targets of the intracellular pathways essential to the atherosclerotic process. The cardioprotective processes have therefore been attributed to its high antioxidant potential and free radical scavenging activity. It further increases the NO release during the reperfusion period. There is no clear evidence that increase levels of NO offer cardioprotection but it is anticipated that antioxidant activity of resveratrol prevents the formation more toxic peroxynitrite from interaction of NO with superoxide anion which then contributes to enhanced NO levels (Hung, 2000). It has also been established to have an inhibitory effect in influenza via the blockade of nuclear-cytoplasmic translocation of viral ribonucleoprotein complexes, the decrease in the expression of late viral proteins, and the inhibition of cellular protein kinase C activity and its dependent pathway. Therefore, it has been established that RSV acts on posttranscriptional period of the viral life processes. It has been found to have inhibitory effect on Zika virus also. It inhibits the binding of ZIKV particles to cells and thus prevents its circulation in the blood, thus limiting the severity of the disease (Levy et al., 2020).

RSV processes a strong antioxidant potential depending on the arrangement of functional groups on the carbon structure. This infers that the structure, substitution, number of hydroxyl groups, and others play a major role in antioxidant potential but also metal–ion interaction capabilities of RSV. Not only this, RSV processes excellent antioxidant properties and is a potential candidate for the inhibition of various types of cancer. It has been shown to inhibit carcinogenesis initiation, promotion, and progression (Salehi et al., 2018).

However, RSV suffers from the problem of poor bioavailability and rapid metabolism. As a result, to get the desired therapeutic effects, it has to be administered in high dose. Though it is well tolerated by the body, but concentrations greater than 1 g/kg have been reported to induce significant side effects such as nausea, diarrhea, abdominal pain, effects the normal functioning of thyroid, and so on.

A report on the clinical trial database reveals that a total of 244 human clinical trials (http://clinicaltrials.gov/) have been conducted on potential effects of RSV and its interaction with other molecules. The trials exhibit the potential of RSV on the management of various diseases. It interacts with other medications leading to overexpression of drug transporters and CYP450 enzymes, the major cellular system involved in drug metabolism (Basheer et al., 2017). It can also work in combination to enhance drug absorption. It enhances the oral bioavailability of nicardipine which is associated with polyglycoprotein-mediated efflux as PGP is the major drug transporter (Choi et al., 2009; Shaito et al., 2020).

2.4.3 QUERCETIN

One of the extensively dispersed plant flavonoid present in seeds, grains, vegetables, green tea found in conjugation with residual sugars to form glycosides is known as Quercetin (also known as 3,3′,4′5,7-pentahydroxy-flavone). In plants, it is produced from the phenylpropanoid pathway and is eventually obtained from phenylalanine. It is converted to 4-coumaroyl-CoA, via phenylalanine ammonia-lysate, to cinnamate-4-hydroxylase, and 4-coumaroyl-CoA-ligase. This is then combined with malonyl-CoA in a 1:3 ratio by 7,2′-dihydroxy-4′-methoxyisoflavanol synthase to form tetrahydroxy chalcone which is further converted to naringenin and to eriodyctiol through flavonoid 3′-hydroxylase. Ultimately, eriodyctiol is hydroxylated and converted to quercetin (Fig. 2.5) using flavanol synthase (Winkel-Shirley, 2001). It exhibits anticancer, antibacterial, and antiviral activities along with the offer of cardioprotection, neuroprotection as well as nephroprotection. It has antiviral properties against viruses such as dengue, measles, and so on. It is recently being viewed by many as a potential adjunct in the treatment of COVID-19. In short, it exhibits a great potential of being an immunomoduator. As far as viruses are concerned, it works contrary to curcumin. It does not block the virus entry process but inhibits the replication process by blocking the enzymes such as viral polymerases (Zandi et al., 2011). It reduces the making of pro-inflammatory cytokines/chemokines and the expression levels of MHC class II and costimulatory molecules. It has an inherent affinity to restrain the creation of inflammation-producing enzymes such as cyclooxygenase and lipoxygenase. During COVID infection, it inhibits both transmembrane peptidase serine 2 and host endoproteases furin that are known to cut the SARS-CoV-2 spike protein assisting SARS-CoV-2 infectivity (Kim et al., 1998).

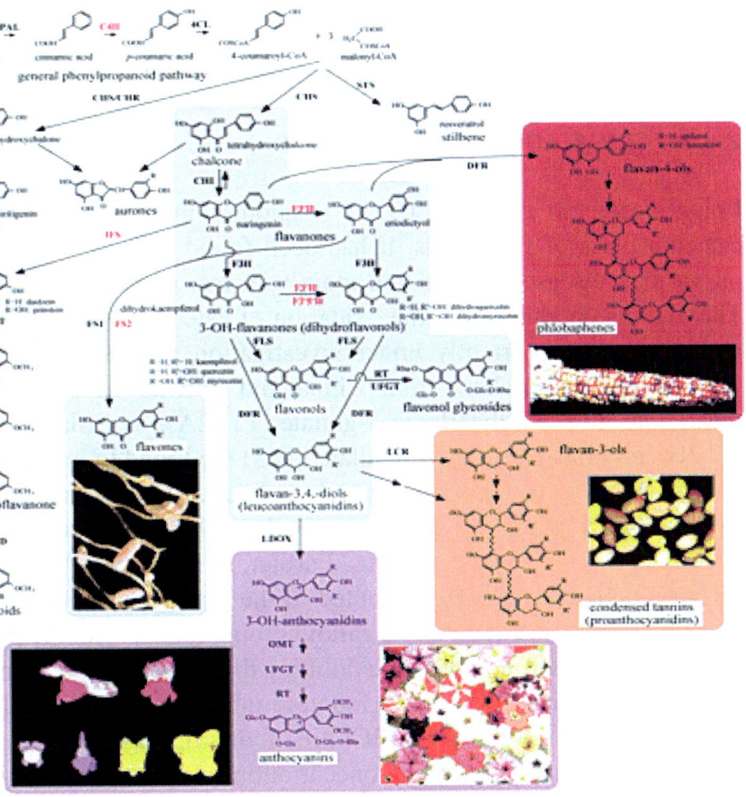

FIGURE 2.5 Biochemical route for the synthesis of flavonoids.

The inhibitory activity of flavonoids against SARS-CoV cysteine proteases was higher as compared to the influence of peptide-derived inhibitors (Park et al., 2017). This inhibitory effect is explained on the basis of strong structural–activity relationships between quercetin and proteases reduce, namely, His41, Gly143, Ser144, Cys145, Glu166, and Gln189. It expresses the formation of H– bonds with O and N atoms of Gln 189 side chain. Also, the N atom of Glu 166 is involved in the formation of the other two H– bonds with flavanoid. This indicates that the four hydroxyl groups of quericitin play great role in inhibitory mechanism and spatial conformation based on sugar moiety and 7-hydroxy site. This allows structural changes through hydrogen-bonding interaction (Chen et al., 2006). However, the pharmaceutical efficacy of quercetin is compromised by low solubility that hampers its absorption, as well as its rapid conjugation with sulfate or glucuronic acid once absorbed, thus leading to poor bioavalibility.

2.4.4 EPIGALLOCATECHIN GALLATE

Epigallocatechin gallate (EGCG) is another important polyphenol of catechin class of flavanoids. It has been found to have valuable effect on various diseases. It is found mainly in tea, especially in green tea. Theaflavins obtained from the oxidation of catechinis found abundantly in black tea are currently under investigation for potential effects on COVID-19. Researchers from China and Taiwan have claimed that theaflavin (TF1), theaflavin-3-gallate (TF2A), theaflavin-3′-gallate (TF2B), and theaflavin-3,3′-digallate (TF3) are found to inhibit COVID-19. These have been recognized as broad spectrum antiviral agents that have no specific site for interaction and exhibit diverse mechanism of action varying from virus to virus. Further, the marked difference in the antiviral activity has been attributed to the number of hydroxyl groups present on the benzene ring and galloyl group, jointly with the pyrogallol group which is accountable for exhibiting diverse action mechanism (Xu et al., 2017). EGCG and TF are found to inhibit one of the vital enzyme 3 chymotrypsin-like protease (3CLpro) found during COVID infection. It inhibits 3 Cl pro at lesser concentration and at the same time also exhibits good binding to the target. This works by forming H– bonds and shows hydrophobic interactions with important sites on the viral S protein. However, EGCG is unstable and shows poor bioavailability when consumed orally (Mhatre et al., 2021). A recent report indicates that theaflavin-3-O-gallate, oolonghomobisflavan-A, and theasinensin-D form stable and stronger bonds with the COVID-19 virus than formed by anti-HIV drugs such as atazanavir, darunavir, and lopinavir (Nature India, 2020).

2.5 CONCLUSIONS

Though the above-written characteristics of polyphenols and their ability to fight corona pandemic sound very interesting, it is tied with limitations. First, only in-vitro studies are available. No in-vivo studies or animal data are available. Therefore, it turns out to be longer journey to change them into effective formulations. Second, the extraction of polyphenols is difficult and needs further studies to find out the composition of active contents. Also, no data are available on the harmful or side effects of polyphenols. Third, polyphenols are large class of compounds and many have been studied, but no evidence is available on which compound to be taken for further studies.

A major question that remains to be answered is to locate the best source of polyphenols; whether they should be available from food/nutraceuticals, synthetic analogs, and extracted phytocomplexes and whether they should be used alone or in blend with already permitted drugs remains to be answered in specific clinical trials. Since it is assumed that these are not as compatible as synthetic drugs, food, and pharmaceutical industries are not very optimistic in performing clinical trials. It is believed that preventive medication is a more reliable approach. Therefore, vigorous pharmacovigilance should be executed by health-care professionals to detect probable unfavorable interactions between recommended and alternative combination medication.

KEYWORDS

- **immunomodulators**
- **polyphenols**
- **quericitin**
- **phenolic acids**
- **curcumin**

REFERENCES

Alijotas-Reig, J.; Esteve-Valverde, E.; Belizna, C.; Selva-O'Callaghan, A.; Pardos-Gea, J.; Quintana, A.; Mekinian, A.; Anunciacion-Llunell, A.; Miró-Mur, F. Immunomodulatory Therapy for the Management of Severe COVID-19. Beyond the Anti-Viral Therapy: A Comprehensive Review. *Autoimmun. Rev.* **2020,** *19*, 102569.

Almeida, C. R.; Bottazzi, B.; De Nardo, D.; Lawlor, K. E. Editorial: Immunomodulation of Innate Immune Cells. *Front. Immunol.* **2020,** *11*, 101.

Annunziata, G.; Zamparelli, M. S.; Santoro, C.; Ciampaglia, R.; Stornaiuolo, M.; Tenore, G. C.; Sanduzzi, A.; Novellino, E. May Polyphenols Have a Role Against Coronavirus Infection? An Overview of In Vitro Evidence. *Front. Med.* **2020,** *7*, 240.

Auger, C.; Mullen, W.; Hara, Y.; Crozier, A. Bioavailability of Polyphenon E Flavan-3-ols in Humans with an Ileostomy. *J. Nutr.* **2008,** *138*, 1535–1542.

Basheer, L.; Schultz, K.; Guttman, Y.; Kerem, Z. In Silico and In Vitro Inhibition of Cytochrome P450 3A by Synthetic Stilbenoids. *Food Chem.* **2017,** *237*, 895–903.

Catanzaro, M.; Corsini, E.; Rosini, M.; Racchi, M.; Lanni, C. Immunomodulators Inspired by Nature: A Review on Curcumin and Echinacea. *Molecules* **2018,** *11*, 2778.

Chen, L.; Li, J.; Luo, C.; Liu, H.; Xu, W.; Chen, G.; Liew, O. W.; Zhu, W.; Puah, C. M.; Shen, X.; Jiang, H. Binding Interaction of Quercetin-3-β-galactoside and Its Synthetic Derivatives with SARS-CoV 3CLpro: Structure–Activity Relationship Studies Reveal Salient Pharmacophore Features. *Bioorg. Med. Chem.* **2006,** *14* (24), 8295–8306.

Cheng, C. K.; Luo, J.-Y.; Lau, C. W.; Chen, Z.-Y.; Tian, X. Y.; Huang, Y. Pharmacological Basis and New Insights of Resveratrol Action in the Cardiovascular System. *Br. J. Pharmacol.* **2020,** *177*, 1258–1277.

Choi, J.-S.; Choi, B.-C.; Kang, K. W. Effect of Resveratrol on the Pharmacokinetics of Oral and Intravenous Nicardipine in Rats: Possible Role of P-Glycoprotein Inhibition by Resveratrol. *Pharmazie* **2009,** *64*, 49–52.

Dai, R.; Ge, H.; Howard, S.; Qiu, W. Transcriptional Expression of Stilbene Synthase Genes Are Regulated Developmentally and Differentially in Response to Powdery Mildew in Norton and Cabernet Sauvignon Grapevine. *Plant Sci.* **2012,** *197*, 70–76.

de Araújo, F. F.; de Paulo Farias, D.; Angélica, I.; Numa, N.; Pastore, G. M. Polyphenols and Their Applications: An Approach in Food Chemistry and Innovation Potential. *Food Chem.* **2021,** *338*, 127535.

Du, J.; Yao, F.; Zhang, M.; Khalifa, I.; Li, K.; Li, C. Effect of Persimmon Tannin on the Physicochemical Properties of Maize Starch with Different Amylose/Amylopectin Ratios. *Int. J. Biol. Macromol.* **2019,** *132*, 1193–1199.

Fontana, A. R.; Antoniolli, A.; Bottini, R. Grape Pomace as a Sustainable Source of Bioactive Compounds: Extraction, Characterization, and Biotechnological Applications of Phenolics. *J. Agric. Food Chem.* **2013,** *61*, 8987–9003.

Gardana, C.; Guarnieri, S.; Riso, P.; Simonetti, P.; Porrini, M. Flavanone Plasma Pharmacokinetics from Blood Orange Juice in Human Subjects. *Br. J. Nutr.* **2007,** *98*, 65–172.

Gasmi, A.; Tippairote, T.; Mujawdiya, P. K.; Peana, M.; Menzel, A.; Dadar, M.; Benahmed, A. G.; Bjørklund, G. Micronutrients as Immunomodulatory Tools for COVID-19 Management. *Clin. Immunol.* **2020,** *220*, 108545.

Holzmann, H.; Hengel, H.; Tenbusch, M.; Doerr, H. W. Eradication of Measles: Remaining Challenges. *Med. Microbiol. Immunol.* **2016,** *205*, 201–208.

Hung, L.-M.; Chen, J.-K.; Huang, S.-S.; Lee, R.-S.; Su, M.-J. Cardioprotective Effect of Resveratrol, a Natural Antioxidant Derived from Grapes. *Cardiovasc. Res.* **2000,** *47*, 549–555.

Ibrahim, S.; Jantan, A. M. I.; Haque, A. Naturally Occurring Immunomodulators with Antitumor Activity: An Insight on Their Mechanisms of Action. *Int. Immunopharmacol.* **2017,** *50*, 291–304.

Jasso-Miranda, C.; Herrera-Camacho, I.; Karem, L.; Mendoza, F.; Dominguez, F.; Vallejo-Ruiz, V.; Guadalupe, G.; Burgos, S.; Pando-Robles, V.; Santos-Lopez, G.; Reyes-Leyva, J. Antiviral and Immunomodulatory Effects of Polyphenols on Macrophages Infected with Dengue Virus Serotypes 2 and 3 Enhanced or Not with Antibodies. *Infect. Drug Resist.* **2019,** *12*, 1833–1852.

Jiao, X.; Wang, Y.; Lin, Y.; Lang, Y. X.; Li, E.; Zhang, X.; Zhang, Q.; Feng, Y.; Meng, X.; Li, B. Blueberry Polyphenols Extract as a Potential Prebiotic with Anti-obesity Effects on C57BL/6 J Mice by Modulating the Gut Microbiota. *J. Nutr. Biochem.* **2019,** *64*, 88–100.

Keservani, R. K.; Sharma, A. K.; & Kesharwani, R. K. Nutraceutical and Functional Foods for Cardiovascular Health. In *Food Process Engineering*; Apple Academic Press: Palm Bay, FL, 2016a, pp 257–278, 291–312. ISBN: 9781771884020.

Keservani, R. K.; Sharma, A. K.; Kesharwani, R. K. Medicinal Effect of Nutraceutical Fruits for the Cognition and Brain Health. *Scientifica* **2016b,** *2016*, Article ID 3109254, 10 p. doi:10.1155/2016/3109254.

Kim, H. P.; Mani, I.; Iversen, L.; Ziboh, V. A. Effects of Naturally-Occurring Flavonoids and Bioflavonoids on Epidermal Cyclooxygenase and Lipoxygenase from Guineapigs. *Prostaglandins Leukot. Essent. Fat Acids* **1998,** *58*, 17–24.

Kim, J. K.; Ota, K.; Sung, N.; Huang, C.; Alsubki, L.; Lee, S.; Han, J. W.; Han, A.; Yang, X.; Saab, W.; Derbala, Y.; Wang, W.-J.; He, Q.; Liao, A.; Takahashi, T.; Cavalcante, M. B.; Barini, R.; Bao, S.; Coulam, C. COVID-19 and Immunomodulation Treatment for Women with Reproductive Failures. *J. Reprod. Immunol.* **2020,** *141*, 103168.

Kunnumakkara, A. B.; Bordoloi, D.; Padmavathi, G.; Monisha, J.; Roy, N. K.; Prasad, S.; Aggarwal, B. B. Curcumin, the Golden Nutraceutical: Multitargeting for Multiple Chronic Diseases. *Br. J. Pharmacol.* **2017,** *174*, 1325–1348.

Levy, E.; Delvin, E.; Marcil, V.; Spahis, S. Can Phytotherapy with Polyphenols Serve as a Powerful Approach for the Prevention and Therapy Tool of Novel Coronavirus Disease 2019 (COVID-19)? *Am. J. Physiol. Endocrinol. Metab.* **2020**. doi:10.1152/ajpendo.00298.2020.

Lin, J.-A.; Chen, J.-H.; Lee, Y.-W.; Lin, C.-S.; Hsieh, M.-H.; Chang, C.-C.; Wong, C.-S.; Chen, J. J.-Y.; Yeh, G.-C.; Lin, Y.-Y. Biphasic Effect of Curcumin on Morphine Tolerance: A Preliminary Evidence from Cytokine/Chemokine Protein Array Analysis. *Evid.-Based Complement. Altern. Med.* **2011**. doi:10.1093/ecam/neq018.

Liu, Z.; Ying, Y. The Inhibitory Effect of Curcumin on Virus-Induced Cytokine Storm and Its Potential Use in the Associated Severe Pneumonia. *Front. Cell Dev. Biol.* **2020,** *8*, 479.

Loi, M.; Quintieri, L.; Fanelli, F.; Caputo, L.; Mulè, G. Application of a Recombinant Laccase-Chlorogenic Acid System in Protein Crosslink and Antioxidant Properties of the Curd. *Food Res. Int.* **2018,** *106*, 763–770.

Manohar, Y.; Haridas, V.; Vasanthakumar, K. C.; Muthu, S.; Thavoorullah, F. F.; Shetty, P. Curcumin: A Wonder Drug as a Preventive Measure for COVID-19 Management. *Indian J. Clin. Biochem.* **2020,** *35* (3), 373–375.

Mhatre, S.; Srivastava, T.; Naik, S.; Patravale, V. Antiviral Activity of Green Tea and Black Tea Polyphenols in Prophylaxis and Treatment of COVID-19: A Review. *Phytomedicine* **2021,** *85*, 153286.

Mirshafiey, A.; Rehm, B. H. A.; Sahmani, A. A.; Naji, A.; Razavi, A. M2000, as a New Antiinflammatory Molecule in Treatment of Experimental Nephrosis. *Immunopharmacol. Immunother.* **2004,** *26*, 611–619.

Morán-Santibañez, K.; Peña-Hernández, M. A.; Cruz-Suárez, L. E.; Ricque-Marie, D.; Skouta, R.; Vasquez, A. H.; Rodríguez-Padilla, C.; Trejo-Avila, L. M. Virucidal and Synergistic Activity of Polyphenol-Rich Extracts of Seaweeds against Measles Virus. *Viruses* **2018,** *10*, 465.

Nature India. Tea Plant Chemicals Block Coronavirus Activity Better Than Anti-HIV Drugs. *Nat. India* **2020**. doi:10.1038/nindia.2020.86. https://www.natureasia.com/en/nindia/article/10.1038/nindia.2020.86

Nelson, K. M.; Dahlin, J. L.; Bisson, J.; Graham, J.; Pauli, G. F.; Walters, M. The Essential Medicinal Chemistry of Curcumin. *J. Med. Chem.* **2017,** *60*, 1620–1637.

Nicholas, E. I.; Sahar, L.-E.; Beth, K. T.; Kristina, T.; Rachel, S. M.; Holtan, S. G.; Dudley, R. A.; Tignanelli, C. J. Immunomodulation in COVID-19. *Lancet Respir. Med.* **2020,** *6*, 544–546.

Pang, X.; Zhang, L.; Bai, F.; Wang, N.; Garner, R. E.; McKallip, R.; Zhao, Z. Attenuation of Myocardial Fibrosis with Curcumin Is Mediated by Modulating Expression of Angiotensin II AT1/AT2 Receptors and ACE2 in Rats. *Drug Des. Dev.*el *Ther.* **2015,** *9*, 6043–6054.

Park, J. Y.; Yuk, H. J.; Ryu, H. W.; Lim, S. H.; Kim, K. S.; Park, K. H.; Ryu, Y. B.; Lee, W. S. Evaluation of Polyphenols from *Broussonetia papyrifera* as Coronavirus Protease Inhibitors. *J. Enzyme Inhib. Med. Chem.* **2017,** *32* (1), 504–515.

Rahimi, K.; Hassanzadeh, K.; Khanbabaei, H.; Haftcheshmeh, S. M.; Ahmadi, A.; Izadpanah, E.; Mohammadi, A.; Sahebkar, A. Curcumin: A Dietary Phytochemical for Targeting the Phenotype and Function of Dendritic Cells. *Curr. Med. Chem.* **2020**. doi:10.2174/0929867327666200515101228.

Sahebkar, A.; Henrotin, Y. Analgesic Efficacy and Safety of Curcuminoids in Clinical Practice: A Systematic Review and Meta-Analysis of Randomized Controlled Trials. *Pain Med.* **2016,** *17*, 1192–1202.

Salehi, B.; Mishra, A. P.; Nigam, M.; Sener, B.; Kilic, M.; Sharifi-Rad, M.; Fokou, P. V. T.; Martins, N.; Sharifi-Rad, J. *Biomedicines* **2018,** *6*, 91.

Sato, F.; Martinez, N. E.; Shahid, M.; Rose, J. W.; Carlson, N. G.; Tsunoda, I. Resveratrol Exacerbates Both Autoimmune and Viral Models of Multiple Sclerosis. *Am. J. Pathol.* **2013,** *183*, 1390–1396.

Schrezenmeier, E.; Dörner, T. Mechanisms of Action of Hydroxychloroquine and Chloroquine: Implications for Rheumatology. *Nat. Rev. Rheumatol.* **2020,** *16*, 155–166.

Shaito, A.; Posadino, A. M.; Younes, N.; Hasan, H.; Halabi, S.; Alhababi, D.; Al-Mohannadi, A.; Abdel-Rahman, W. M.; Eid, A. H.; Nasrallah, G. K.; Pintus, G. Potential Adverse Effects of Resveratrol: A Literature Review. *Int. J. Mol. Sci.* **2020,** *21* (6), 2084.

Tsao, R. Chemistry and Biochemistry of Dietary Polyphenols. *Nutrients* **2010,** *2*, 1231–1246.

Weissenberger, J.; Priester, M.; Bernreuther, C.; Rakel, S.; Glatzel, M.; Seifert, V.; Kögel, D. Dietary Curcumin Attenuates Glioma Growth in a Syngeneic Mouse Model by Inhibition of the JAK1,2/STAT3 Signaling Pathway. *Clin. Cancer Res. Off. J. Am. Assoc. Cancer Res.* **2010,** *16*, 5781–5795.

Winkel-Shirley, B. Flavonoid Biosynthesis. A Colorful Model for Genetics, Biochemistry, Cell Biology and Biotechnology. *Plant Physiol.* **2001,** *126*, 485.

Xu, J.; Xu, Z.; Zheng, W. A Review of the Antiviral Role of Green Tea Catechins. *Molecules* **2017,** *22* (8), 1337.

Yang, H.; Shi, G.; Dou, Q. P. The Tumor Proteasome Is a Primary Target for the Natural Anticancer Compound Withaferin A Isolated from Indian Winter Cherry. *Mol. Pharmacol.* **2007,** *71*, 426–437.

Zandi, K.; Teoh, B. T.; Sam, S. S.; Wong, P. F.; Mustafa, M. R.; Abubakar, S. Novel Antiviral Activity of Baicalein against Dengue Virus. *BMC Complement. Altern. Med.* **2011,** *12*, 214.

Zhao, M. Cytokine storm and immunomodulatory therapy in COVID-19: Role of Chloroquine and Anti-IL-6 Monoclonal Antibodies. *Int. J. Antimicrob. Agents* **2020,** *55*, 105982.

CHAPTER 3

Herbal Formulation and COVID-19

RAJKUMARI LODHI, SATISH SHILPI, RAVI KESHARWANI, UMESH DHAKAD, and KAPIL KHATRI

Department of Pharmacy, Ravishankar College of Pharmacy, Bhopal, India

ABSTRACT

Viral infection is a major threat to humanity around the world. The increasing dominance of viral infection becomes a major issue, necessitating the development of effective treatment options such as vaccines and novel drugs. This chapter discusses the use and role of herbal medicines, as well as their formulation, in the treatment and management of COVID-19 infection. There is no vaccine or specific antiviral drug to prevent or treat COVID-19. However, no vaccination for COVID-19 is available as of yet, and it would be appropriate to consider Ayurveda for boosting natural immunity in the body alongside COVID-19. The ancient science of Ayurveda provides a variety of formulations, treatments, and practices to aid in the strengthening of immunity. A large number of medicinal plants are mentioned in the Indian long-established scheme recognized, because Rasayana (devoted to the improvement of the body's fight) has involved the awareness of scientists from humanity. There are numerous medicinal plants that use immunomodulatory action in an untested model at a precise dose. Ethnopharmacology is a method of investigating the immunomodulatory properties of active

COVID-19 and Immunomodulation with Special Emphasis on Nutraceutical and Herbal Formulation. Rajesh K. Kesharwani & Raj K. Keservani (Eds)

constituents found in medicinal plants, which are considered natural medicines. Because their active ingredient has immunomodulatory properties, herbal combination preparations of Indian traditional medicine may encourage immunomodulation. This hypothesis may be significant to recognize their use besides their toxicity in ancient times as well as today. The lack of treatment strategies forces us to develop novel approaches against COVID-19 infection. Probable vaccines and various specific drug treatments are under study and will take a long time. In this urgent situation (pandemic), the identification of some alternate approaches that can manage the infection effectively is essential. The conventional remedies of herbal plants, for example, tulsi, garlic (lassan), ginger (adrak), turmeric (haldi), cumin seeds (zeera), Cannabis sativa (common hemp). The use of herbal ingredients as immunomodulators is independent of the different approaches to preventing COVID-19 disease.

3.1 INTRODUCTION

Traditional herbal medicines work with the natural mechanism. In the last few decades, herbal medicines are getting attention and play an important role in global health and fitness. It was reported previously that some usual herbal medicines were used that effectively work in the treatment of severe acute respiratory disorder (SARS) in China (Geneva: WHO; 2003). It is also reported that the majority of African people use a variety of conventional herbal medicines for the treatment of different types of viral infections and other diseases (WHO, 2002). Currently, countries, such as China, India, Nigeria, United States of America (USA) have made extensive study investments in conventional herbal medicines (Willcox and Bodeker, 2004). At present, pharmaceutical industries are empowering money to develop effective herbal formulations for the treatment of different types of diseases (Zamiska, 2006). Novartis was eyeing conventional Chinese medicine in 2007. But the lack of literature is a limiting factor in growth of traditional herbal medicinal research works (Zaslawski and Davis, 2005; Nyika, 2006; Emanuel et al., 2004). From ancient times, natural plants have been used for various purposes. Having co-evolved with living things, many of the plant medicines with therapeutic benefits are billions of years older. Medicines derived from young plants have played a fundamental role in the physical condition care of many cultures, both earliest and contemporary (Newman and Cragg, 2007).

3.2 CORONAVIRUS

CoV is an enveloped, positive-sense single-stranded RNA (ssRNA) virus belonging to the Coronaviridae ancestors. The CoV family consists of numerous variants and can cause greater respiratory tract infection, and is also responsible for gastrointestinal tract infection in mammals and animals. In humans, it mainly causes the common cold but can develop complications which include pneumonia and SARS (van der Hoek, 2007). The human coronavirus species, such as HCoV-229E, OC43, NL63, and HKU1 are responsible for severe acute respiratory infection. Coronavirus (SARS-CoV) becomes an international threat that spread the infection to a large number of people in 2003 (Geller et al., 2012).

WHO selected a sixth type of HCoV species and their infection known as (MERS-CoV) Middle East Respiratory Syndrome, which was responsible for high casualty (WHO, 2013). The replication cycle of coronavirus is depicted in Figure 3.1.

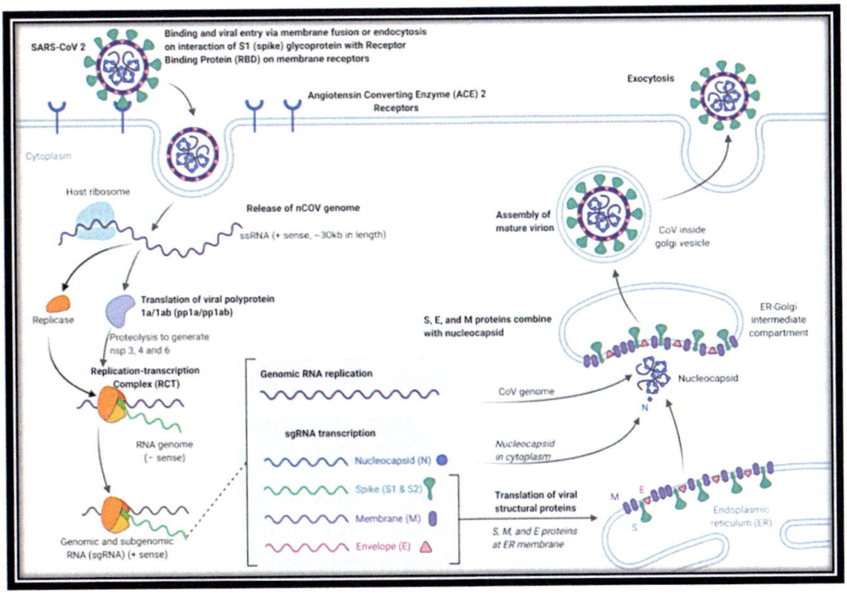

FIGURE 3.1 Replication cycle of coronavirus.

Source: Figure by Rohan Bir Singh, MD. Reprinted from Cascella et al., 2020. https://creativecommons.org/licenses/by-nc-nd/4.0/

3.3 ETIOLOGY

CoVs are a type of RNA viruses having crown-like exterior. The crown-like structure is due to the occurrence of spike glycoproteins on the covering. The orthocoronavirinae is a strain of the Coronaviridae (order Nidovirales), and it is further classified into four genera of CoVs, that is, alpha, Beta, Delta, and Gamma-CoV. In addition, the beta-CoV species are divided into five sub-genera or lineages (Chan et al., 2013). All the genomics of bats and rodents are the genetic material sources of alpha-CoVs and beta-CoVs. On the contrary, avian species appear to represent the genetic material sources of delta-CoVs and gamma-CoVs.

The members of these large ancestors of viruses are responsible for respiratory, hepatic, and neurological diseases in humans and animals, such as camels, cattle, cats, and bats. About 7 CoVs (HCoVs) strains have been found to be capable of infecting humans (Chen et al., 2020).

3.4 TRANSMISSION

The first case of COVID-19 infection was known from Huanan Seafood wholesale Market of Wuhan, the animal to human transmission was presumed as the main system. Therefore, it was accomplished that the virus is transmitted from human to human, and indicative people are the most recurrent resource and reason for spreading COVID-19 infection. A few days after infection, the persons who remain asymptomatic can transmit the virus, and infect another person. The self- quarantine of others is good to prevent the spreading of the infection. Pre- and asymptomatic individuals may transmit and infect 80% of the people with the COVID-19 virus. Primarily restricted family members, healthcare professionals, and other close contacts should maintain at least 6 feet, 1.8 meters of distance from each other. According to research, which involved the study of the viability of the infecting COVID-19 virus on objects and surfaces, it was revealed that SARS-CoV-2 can be found on plastic for up to 2–3 days, on cardboard for up to 1 day, and on copper for up to 4 h (Guo et al., 2020). The transmission cycle of coronavirus is depicted in Figure 3.2.

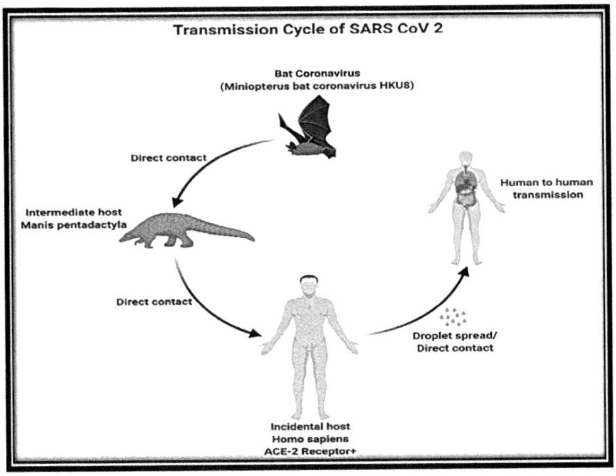

FIGURE 3.2 Transmission cycle of coronavirus.

Source: Figure by Rohan Bir Singh, MD. Reprinted from Cascella et al., 2020. https://creativecommons.org/licenses/by-nc-nd/4.0/

3.5 EPIDEMIOLOGY

The data provided by The World Health Organization Health Emergency Control panel report 8,525,042 determinate cases of coronavirus, which includes 456,973 deaths (as of 1:38 pm CEST, June 20, 2020). To date, COVID-19 cases are found in more than 215 Countries. In Europe, there are 2,509,750 reported cases; Americas 4,163,813; South East Asia 206,200; Africa 208,000; Eastern Mediterranean 878,428. The maximum number of fatal cases had been shown in the US (121,130) and Brazil (49,156). UK (42,589). The most updated information on the epidemiology of this rising deadly infectious disease can be found at the following sources, including The WHO Novel Coronavirus (COVID-19) Situation Board,, The Johns Hopkins Center for Systems Science and Engineering site for Global Cases COVID-19, which uses openly public sources to track the multiplication rate of the COVID-19 virus.

3.6 EVALUATION

Most countries make use of several types of medical and epidemiologic data in order to understand who should have trial carried out. In the US, criteria have been urbanized for persons under analysis (PUI) for COVID-19.

According to the U.S. CDC, most patients who have been known to be confirmed cases of COVID-19 have developed fever and other symptoms of sensitive respiratory illness (e.g., difficulty in breathing, cough, cold). If a patient is a PUI, it is compulsory that a physician is instantly put in place for infection control and preventive measures. At first, they need to test for various sources of respiratory illness.

3.7 DIAGNOSIS

3.7.1 MOLECULAR TEST

It is necessary to collect the sample of expectorated sputum, end tracheal aspirate, or bronchoalveolar lavage from the upper and lower respiratory tract of the patient for conducting molecular tests and the samples are to be stored at 4°C temperature until the test is completed. The compilation of BAL sample should be performed in systematically ventilated persons as lower respiratory tract samples appear to remain positive for a more extended period. In the laboratory, however, the amplification of the heritable material taken out from the mucus or saliva sample is through a reverse polymerase chain reaction (RT-PCR), which involves the synthesis of a double-stranded DNA molecule from an RNA mold. Once the heritable material is enough, then the search is done for those part of the heritable code of the CoV that are conserved.

3.7.2 SEROLOGY

Despite the various antibody test intended, serologic analysis is low in specificity and sensitivity and may obtain dissimilar results from different tests. It was found that there is no cross-reactivity between the autoantibody collected from serum samples from a person with autoimmune disease and COVID-19 antibodies on the other hand; additional research is needed for elucidating many aspects related to disease if immunity will be developed by IgG from future SARS-CoV-2 viral infection.

3.7.3 LABORATORY EXAMINATIONS

In the early stage of the infection, a normal or decreased WBC and decreased lymphocyte count could be demonstrated. Interestingly, lymphopenia appears to be a negative analytical factor. The elevated level of muscle enzymes, lactate dehydrogenase (LDH), liver enzymes, as well as C-reactive protein, can be detected to diagnose the COVID-19 infection. If a bacterial infection is overlapped with COVID-19 then it is necessary to detect the procalcitonin level in the body.

The important neutrophil-to-lymphocyte relative count (NLR), consequent NLR percentage, and ratio of platelet-to-lymphocyte abnormal level in plasma are the indication of major inflammation in the body (Yang et al., 2020). D-dimer value is another important factor which can indicate the level of infection in the body. In serious patients, D-dimer value is increased, decreased blood lymphocytes, and elevated level of amylase, and coagulation disorders are the sign of multi-organ imbalance.

3.8 MEDICATION AND MANAGEMENT OF COVID-19

The exact treatment is not available for COVID-19 viral infection; the currently available vaccines act on the particular variant of the COVID-19 virus. All the current treatments are symptomatic. Oxygen therapy is the only option to maintain the oxygen level in the body in the case of respiratory failure. Noninvasive ventilation is required for severe patients for oxygen treatment. Again, demanding care is required to deal with the complicated form of infection. Regarding ARDS treatment, accumulating information on the pathophysiology of lung damage, help clinicians to develop a new approach to managing respiratory failure. This part of the disease is of fundamental value and has all probability of a critically pretentious curing approach in the untimely stages of the pandemic.

3.8.1 O_2 FAST CHALLENGE

In an affected person with a SpO2 $< 93 >$ 28–30/min, or dyspnea, the supply of O_2 by means of a 40% Venturi mask ought to be accomplished. After a 5–10 min evaluation, if the medical and instrumental image has progressed, the patient maintains the medication and undergoes evaluation within 6 h. If it fails, then a noninvasive remedy is preferred to supply oxygen.

3.8.2 NONINVASIVE VENTILATION

With regards to NIV, the experts' panel, factors out that those strategies accomplished by means of structures with properly affiliated becoming do not create appreciable dispersion of exhaled air, and their use may be taken into consideration at the minimal chance of airborne transmission of the virus (Hui, et al. 2019).

3.8.3 PROTECTIVE MECHANICAL VENTILATION

Special provisions are vital at some stage in intubation. The system must be done by means of a health professional operator who makes use of PPE, including disposable FFP3 or N95 masks, defensive goggles, dressing gown or long coat, hats, socks, and gloves. If possible, speedy collection intubation (RSI) must be accomplished. Preoxygenation (100% O_2 for 5 min) must be accomplished through the continuous positive airway pressure (CPAP) method.

3.8.4 OTHER THERAPIES

3.8.4.1 CORTICOSTEROIDS

Among distinctive recovery strategies, Despite the reality that systemic corticosteroids for the treatment of viral pneumonia or acute respiration distress syndrome (ARDS) are now not recommended, in severe cases of CARDS, the corticosteroid drugs are commonly used (e.g., methylprednisolone 1 mg/kg/day). A state-of-the-art large-size RCT (the RECOVERY trial) validated that dexamethasone reduces deaths by one-third among significantly ill COVID-19 patients (Ledford, 2020).

3.8.4.2 ANTIVIRAL AGENTS

Although no antiviral medications were passed, numerous strategies were proposed, including lopinavir/ritonavir (400/100 mg by an oral route in each 12 h) (Bimonte et al., 2020). Preclinical research approved that remdesivir antiviral drug (GS5734) an inhibitor of ribosome nucleic acid polymerase with in vitro recreation in opposition to a couple of RNA viruses such as Ebola might be powerful for each prophylaxis and medication of COVID-19 infections (Gordon et al., 2020).

3.8.4.3 ANTIVIRAL/IMMUNOMODULATORY DRUGS

Hydroxychloroquine (200 mg each 12 h) and Chloroquine (500 mg each 12 h) have been proposed as immunomodulatory medicine. Gautret et al. studied the effect of hydroxychloroquine which minimizes the viral load till viral disappearance. In vivo and in vitro research, indeed, have proved that macrolides might also additionally mitigate infection and modulatory effects on the immune system (Zarogoulidis et al., 2012).

3.8.4.4 SEROTHERAPY

Antibodies collected from the infectious blood of healed people who are suffering from COVID-19 constitute a healing choice which is presently under study. It is calculated that the calculative dose of antibodies important for the remedy of a single patient with SARS-CoV-2, calls for the removal of antibodies accomplished from a minimum of three persons recovered from the COVID-19 infection. A trial has been launched (June 11, 2020) for proving an antibody cocktail for the avoidance and medication of COVID-19.

3.8.4.5 ANTICOAGULANT

Because COVID-19 sufferers have a higher incidence of venous thromboembolism and anticoagulant treatment is associated with reduced ICU mortality, it is far advised that patients ought to obtain thromboprophylaxis. Moreover, in the case of recognized thrombophilia or thrombosis, complete healing-depth anticoagulation is indicated (Kollias et al., 2020).

3.8.4.6 INFLAMMATION INHIBITORS

The utilization of tocilizumab is suggested in addition to conventional treatments. It is a humanized IgG1 monoclonal antibody, directed in the direction of the IL-6 receptor and normally used in the treatment of rheumatoid arthritis, juvenile arthritis, big molecular arthritis, Castleman's syndrome, and for handling toxicity due to immune checkpoint inhibitors. Moreover, in the US, a Phase 2/3, randomized, double-blind, placebo-managed study has taken a look on sarilumab, which is an another anti-IL-6 receptor antibody; the study is ongoing (Buonaguro et al., 2020).

3.8.4.7 OTHER THERAPIES

When the ailment outcomes in complicated scientific photographs of MOD, organ function support similar to breathing help, is highly necessary. Extracorporeal membrane oxygenation (ECMO) for persons with refractory hypoxemia in spite of lung-protective ventilation ought to benefit attention after a case-by-case analysis. It may be advised for people with negative outcomes to inclined position ventilation.

3.9 PREVENTION

Preventive measures are the modern-day method to restrict the spread of cases. Because a deadly disease will boom so large as R0 is greater than 1 (COVID-19 is 2.2), preventive measures need to be focussed on decreasing the rate to heavy less than 1. Curative techniques are centered on the separation of persons and cautious contamination control, consisting of suitable measures to be followed in the course of the analysis and the supply of clinical care to an inflamed patient. For instance, droplet, touch, and airborne precautions ought to be followed in the course of the specimen collection; and sputum induction ought to be avoided. Wash your fingers often, especially after touching inflamed patients or contact with their environment. Avoid unprotected contact with farm or wild animals. People with symptoms and signs of acute airway infection must maintain their distance, cover coughs or sneezes with disposable tissues or clothes, and wash their hands. Individuals who might be immune-compromised have to avoid public gatherings. The most critical technique is to regularly wash hands and use portable hand sanitizer and avoid contact with their face and mouth after interacting with a likely inflamed environment (Kucharski et al., 2020). Healthcare professionals who care for infected patients ought to utilize contact and airborne precautions to use PPE kits.

3.10 THE VACCINE

Meanwhile, medical study is progressing to develop a Sars-CoV-2 vaccine. There are more than 100 candidate vaccines in improvement worldwide; of these, 8–10 vaccines are under clinical research. In this "vaccine gaming," Chinese investigators seem to be ahead, having finished a phase I investigation. Nevertheless, numerous investigations are ongoing, especially in the US, and the UK.

3.10.1 *THIS FIRST-IN-HUMAN TRIAL*

The outcomes of phase I medical trial carried out in a single center in Wuhan (China), designed to evaluate the protection, reactogenicity, and immunogenicity of a recombinant adenovirus type-5 (Ad5) vectored COVID-19 vaccine expressing the spike glycoprotein have been published. Between March 16–27, 2020, 108 healthy adults aged 18–60 years have been consecutively enrolled and assigned to one of the three study groups in step with the dose of vaccine administered (intramuscular injection). The primary very last effects were modified into the evaluation of damaging events in the 7 days following vaccination. Safety was modified into assessed over 28 days after vaccination (Zhu et al., 2020).

3.10.2 *OTHER ONGOING INVESTIGATIONS*

A Chinese phase II, randomized, double-blinded, placebo-controlled clinical trial was designed to assess the immunogenicity and protection of Ad5-CoV which encodes for a full-duration spike protein of SARS-CoV-2. the predicted completion date of the study date is January 31, 2021 (NCT04341389). Even though the RBD is an alternative, the candidate vaccines cover spike collection. This Phase half, randomized, placebo-controlled, observer-blind, dose-finding, examination will result in March 2023. Another Phase I examination was designed to evaluate the protection, tolerability, and immunological profile of a vaccine administered via intradermal injection observed via electroporation which is a method used to facilitate the passage of medication into the molecular membrane, by using a particular system (NCT04336410).

3.11 POLYHERBAL FORMULA: CONCEPT OF AYURVEDA

Ayurveda is one of the conventional medicinal structures with longtime records of many centuries. Ayurveda is one of the ancient sciences prevailing for many centuries. Originated in India, lots of years in the past,

Ayurveda is called the mother of All Healing (A quick creation and manual 2003). Etymologically speaking, itis the mixture of the Sanskrit phrases ayur (lifestyles) and veda (technological know-how or understanding), this means the technological know-how of lifestyles, specializing in bringing concord and stability in all regions (U.S. Department of Health and Human Services, 2005).

3.11.1 SINGLE NATURAL AS AGAINST TO POLYHERBAL FORMULA

Drug formula in Ayurveda is primarily based totally on principles: Use as an unmarried drug and use of multiple drugs, wherein the latter is called PHF. This key conventional healing natural method exploits the combining of numerous medicinal herbs to reap more healing effectiveness, generally called polypharmacy or polyherbalism. The Sarangdhar Samhita has highlighted the polyherbalism (Srivastava et al., 2013). In the conventional system of Indian medicinal drugs, plant formulations and mixed extracts of flowers are selected in place of personal ones. It is understood that Ayurvedic herbals are organized in some of the dosage forms, wherein frequently, they are PHF (Jayakumar, 2010; Parasuraman et al., 2010). There are some Ayurvedic herbal mixtures to be referred to here: Combination of ginger with black pepper and long pepper complements their heating and mucous-decreasing effects; sour and unthreatening herbs are mixed with hotter herbs (mixture of neem and ginger) to definitely offset any severe effects. Cumin, black pepper, and asafoetida are used collectively historically to lessen bloating because of vulnerable digestion; while guduchi and turmeric mixture serves as a booster of one's immunity (Pole, 2013; Thyagarajan et al., 2002).

3.12 MEDICINAL HERBAL PLANTS

3.12.1 OCIMUM SANCTUM LINN (TULSI)

3.12.1.1 A POTENT ADAPTOGEN

Tulsi (Fig. 3.3) acknowledged in English as Holy Basil and botanically known as *Ocimum sanctum* is defined as a medicinal ayurvedic plant in Ancient literature reviews. Tulsi is also known as "Elixir of Life" because it promotes durability. It is an essential representation of the Hindu spiritual way of life and is found in most of the Indian houses and is worshipped (Kumar et al., 2012; Sanctum, 2010; Pandey and Madhuri, 2010). The name tulsi in Sanskrit way "The incomparable One," has given varieties, Krishna Tulsi (black) and Rama Tulsi (green) (Mondal et al., 2009; Goyal and Kaushik 2011) Their chemical materials are comparable, however, Krishna Tulsi possesses excellent medicinal price as cited in Charaka Samhita (historic Indian literature). It is a herb that is bestowed with great antimicrobial constituents and is used to deal with loads of ailments starting from diabetes, arthritis, bronchitis, pores, and skin sicknesses. The use of remedial plants in conventional remedies has been defined in the literature and the relationship dates back a thousand years (Chang et al., 2016). Books on Ayurvedic remedies, written in the Vedic period (3500–1600 B.C.) describe practices, which include the usage of medicinal plants, that shaped the premise of all different clinical sciences advanced in India (Pattanayak et al., 2010). Tulsi is possibly one of the quality examples of Ayurveda's holistic way of life technique to fitness. Tulsi tastes warm and sour and is stated to go in the deep tissues by penetration, tissues which are dry secretions and normalize kapha and vata. Routine intake of tulsi is stated to save you from disease, gives well-known fitness, health, and durability, and helps in managing the stresses of each day life. Tulsi is likewise credited with giving sweetness to the voice and intelligence, stamina, and a relaxed emotional disposition and fostering beauty (Singh et al., 2010; Mahajan et al., 2013; Mohan et al., 2011; Pattanayak et al., 2010). In addition to those fitness-selling residences, tulsi is usually recommended as a remedy for quite a number of situations which includes anxiety, indigestion, diarrhea, cough, fever, asthma arthritis, sicknesses, eye sicknesses otalgia, hiccups, emesis, gastric, genitourinary and cardiac problems, lower back pain, pores and skin sicknesses, insect, warms, scorpion snake bites, and malaria (Singh et al., 2010; Mohan et al., 2011; Pattanayak et al., 2010; Mondal et al., 2009). It is also acknowledged to sell immune machine function (Mondal et al., 2011). A decoction prepared from this medicinal plant is immunomodulatory, and possesses analgesic, hepatoprotective, antipyretic properties; it is used in malarial fever (Gupta and Prakash, 2002). Tulsi has been additionally used as a pot herb in folklore studies for some illnesses and sicknesses (Khosla, 1995). In every other look, the immunomodulatory impact of *O. sanctum* L. seed oil (OSSO) was evaluated in each non-stressed and stressed animal (Mediratta et al., 2002). *Ocimum sanctum* L. seed oil (3 ml/kg, Ip) produced a huge increase in anti-sheep red blood cells (SRBC) antibody titer and a lower in percent histamine launch from peritoneal mast cells of sensitized rats (humoral immune responses) and reduction in footpad thickness and percent leucocyte migration inhibition (cell-mediated immune responses).

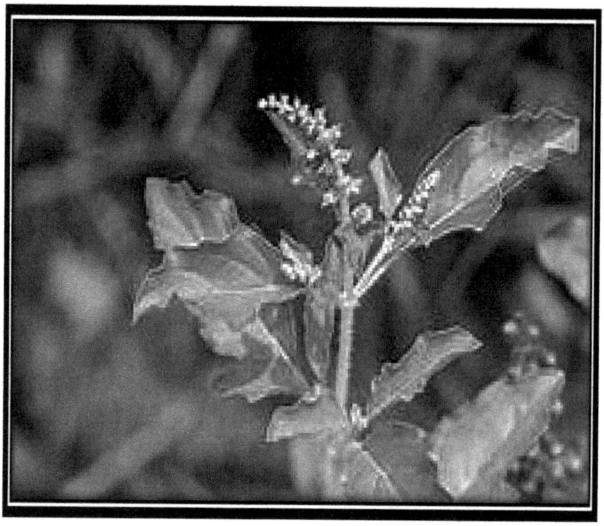

FIGURE 3.3 Tulsi.

3.12.1.2 INFECTION PROTECTION

Modern studies have revealed that tulsi has many types of antifungal, antibacterial, and also antiviral properties (Vasudevan et al., 1999) that act against many pathogens chargeable for human infections. Tulsi has additionally been proven to reinforce defenses toward infective threats by improving immune responses in nonstressed and stressed animals (Mediratta et al., 2002; Hemalatha et al., 2011; Tripathi et al., 2008; Goel et al., 2010; Pavaraj et al., 2011; Chitra and Krishnaveni, 2011) and wholesome humans (Mondal et al., 2011) While no human trials were available, there is an experimental proof that tulsi may also assist in the remedy of numerous human bacterial infections which include urinary tract infections (Ali and Dixit, 2012), numerous cases of pneumonia (Saini et al., 2009), and fungal infections (Deo et al., 2011; Balakumar et al., 2011; Das et al., 2010; Chandra et al., 2011) in addition to mosquito-borne sicknesses which include dengue, malaria and filariasis (Rajamma et al., 2011; Gbolade and

Lockwood, 2008; Inbaneson et al., 2012). In numerous reviews (Prakash and Gupta, 2005; Pattanayak et al., 2010), the healing price of tulsi leaves is attributed specifically to eugenol. Eugenol was identified as a main component (67%) of the important oil of *Ocimum gratissimum*, and can be chargeable for the antibacterial properties of that oil.

3.12.2 NEEM (AZADIRACHTA INDICA)

3.12.2.1 A POTENT ADAPTOGEN

Neem (Fig. 3.4) is an all-powerful tree and a sacred present of nature. Neem tree is cultivated inwards the Indian supercontinent. Today it is far acknowledged through the botanical call *Azadirachta indica* (*A. indica*) A. Juss. Neem has been used exceptionally by the public to deal with numerous illnesses earlier than the supply of written information which recorded the start of history. Since antiquated times, neem has been utilized by humankind. Hence, it is actually the unfastened tree of India (Neem Foundation, 2012). The neem tree is an unbelievable plant that has been announced as the Tree of the 21st century by the United Nations (United Nations Environment Program, 2012). The US National Academy

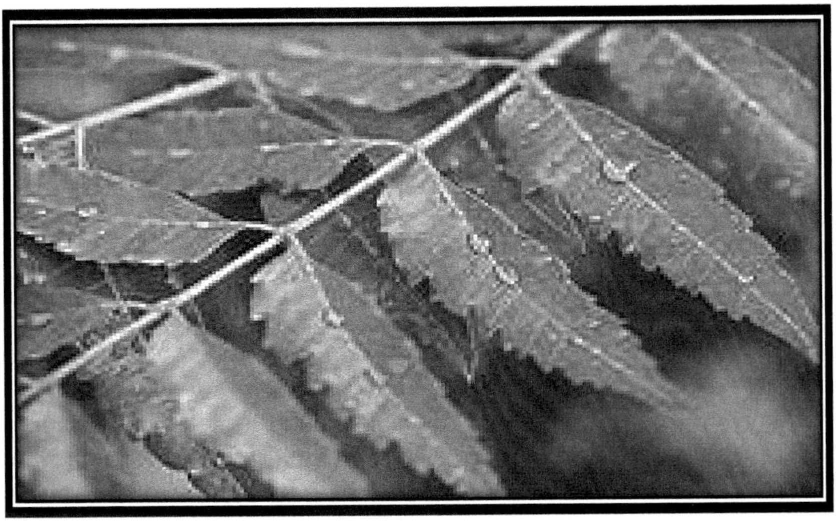

FIGURE 3.4 Neem.

of Science posted a document in the year of 1992, that authorized the neem as Neem: A tree for fixing worldwide problems (NAS, 1992). We all know that the neem plant is an evergreen tree cultivated in the Indian supercontinent and is ordinarily called Indian neem or Indian lilac (Chopra et al., 1956; Drabu et al., 2012). The natural agent, *Azadirachta indica* (Neem) has an extract which expresses an antibacterial property (Siswomihardjo et al., 2007; Mahfuzul et al., 2007). *Azadirachta indica* (Neem) belongs to the family Meliaceae. Extracts from neem are claimed to have tremendous health effects (Subapriya and Nagini, 2005; Lakshmi et al., 2015; Ahmad and Beg, 2001; Atawodi and Atawodi, 2009).

3.12.2.2 DRUGS FROM NATURE

The World Health Organization (WHO) assesses that 80% of the populace residing in the growing global locations is predicated to be completely on the conventional remedy for his or her number one healthcare. Researchers generally agree that herbal products derived from plants and other organisms are the most consistently successful source of ideas for new drugs. Drug discovery scientists regularly talk over with those thoughts as leads, and chemical substances which have applicable residence in laboratory examinations are known as lead compounds (Sashidhara et al., 2012). Plants have become the basis of conventional remedy tools at some stage in the field for heaps of years and retain to offer humankind new medicinal remedies. The tree particularly withinside the Indian subcontinent and has appreciably contributed to the improvement of various conventional compositions of medicines (Davis, 2012).

3.12.2.3 ULTRAMODERN MEDICINAL USES OF NEEM IN MANKIND

As we all know that the Neem (*A. indica*) is a divine (medicinal) tree specifically cultivated in Indian subcontinent and it is far normally called neem (Puri, 1999; Upma et al., 2011). All the elements of *A. indica* tree are normally utilized in conventional Indian remedies for family treatments of numerous human sicknesses (Botelho et al., 2008). In India, people have been respecting the neem tree (*A. indica*) for a long time. For centuries, hundreds of thousands of people have brushed their tooth enamel with neem twigs to clean their teeth, used neem face packs for pores and skin problems, leaf juice was utilized, consumed neem tea as a tonic, and positioned neem leaves in their books, grain bins, cupboards, beds, and closets to preserve the items from difficult bugs. The tree has relieved such a lot of one-of-a-kind pains, fevers, infections, and different lawsuits that it has been known as the rural pharmacy. In India non-urbanized population regularly used water. The concoction of neem leaves has been used for the prevention and medicinal remedy of numerous illnesses. Research undertaken at the University of Nigeria confirmed the medicinal properties of fractionated acetone/water neem leaf extract (Anyaehie, 2009). Tests performed by the King Institute of Preventive Medicine, Chennai in December 2012 discovered that the Siddha neem preparation reduced the symptoms and speeded up the restoration of patients suffering from dengue (Narayan, 2012). In India, numerous components of neem (leaf, bark, and seeds) are used as a conventional remedy. Different elements of neem were proven to showcase huge pharmacological activities which include antibacterial (Elavarasu et al., 2012) and antiviral (Xu et al., 2012) properties.

3.12.2.4 ANTIBACTERIAL ACTIVITY

Recent research has shown the isolation and identification of the antibacterial capability compound from petroleum ether extract of neem oil (Zhang et al., 2010). Zhong et al. (2010) showed an antibacterial capacity of 9-octadecanoic acid-hexadecanoic acid-tetrahydrofuran-3,4-diyl ester from neem oil (Elavarasu et al., 2012) and studied in vitro antiplaque microbial compounds of neem oil.

3.12.2.5 ANTIVIRAL

Galhardi et al. studied the in vitro antiviral assets of *Azadirachta indica* polysaccharides against poliovirus. Saha et al. examined the water-extracted polysaccharides from *A. indica* leaves and revealed that they possess anti-bovine herpes virus type 1 (BoHV-1) property. The research of Xu et al. confirmed the in vitro antiviral interest of neem seed kernel extracts toward duck plague virus. Tiwari et al. confirmed the in vitro antiviral interest of neem (*A. indica* L.) bark extract toward herpes simplex virus type infection.

3.12.2.6 NEEM AND THE IMMUNE SYSTEM

Various constituents of the neem plant (*Azadirachta indica*) have such immunomodulatory residences (Biswas et al., 2002) and had been proven to stimulate T cells (Upadhyay et al., 1992), B cells (Sadekar et al., 1998), and macrophages (Ray et al., 1996). We have mentioned in advance the immunoprophylactic characteristic of a secure preparation (Haque et al., 2006) from neem leaf (NLP) to save humans from murine Ehrlich's carcinoma and B16 melanoma (Baral, 2004).

3.12.3 CANNABIS SATIVA: MARIJUANA

3.12.3.1 MARIJUANA

Cannabis sativa (Fig. 3.5) is a medicinal flowering plant indigenous to Eastern Asia, and it now has sophisticated dispensation because of massive cultivation (Mary-Lou et al., 1991). It has been cultivated during autochthonous, recorded history, used as a source of commercial fiber, seed oil, food, recreation, non-secular, and religious moods and medicine. Each part of the plant is harvested differently, relying on the purpose of its use. The species come to be first categorized by Carl Linnaeus in 1753 (Greg Green et al., 2005). The word "sativa" means things which might be cultivated. Medical marijuana refers to the factors of the hashish plant used as a physician-endorsed form of herbal treatment or as a remedy. In America, presently, the use of remedial marijuana has surged in the 16

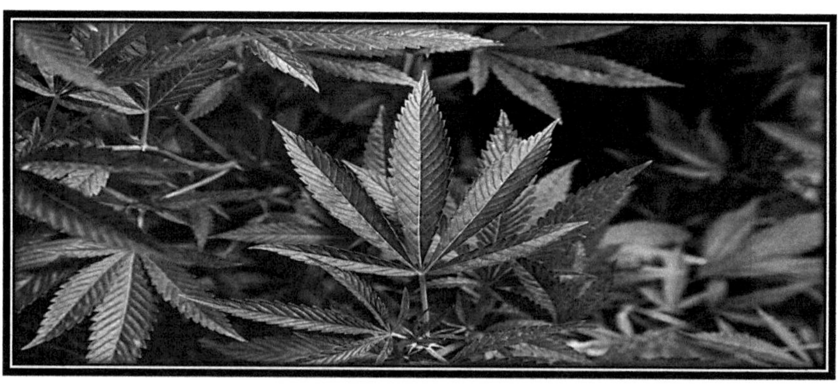

FIGURE 3.5 Cannabinoid.

states and District of Columbia that have a permit for its use. The hashish plant has extended information of use as a medicine dating back to 2737 b.c. (Ben Amar, 2006). *Cannabis sativa* includes over 80 unique chemical additives (Molina, Console-Bram et al., 2012). The well-characterized CBs have their very own unique physiological compounds. The psychoactive outcomes of cannabinoids are associated with CB1; CB2 specially mediates immunomodulatory and anti-inflammatory actions (Miller and Stella, 2008).

3.12.3.2 *CANNABINOID* BROUGHT ABOUT *IMMUNOMODULATION*

The mechanism of cannabinoid-precipitated immunoregulatory roles for cannabinoids has been noted in infectious ailments (Hernández-Cervantes et al., 2017), and *C. sativa* has been identified as a herbal product with a capability of controlling bacterial infections, which includes a study antibacterial interest toward antibiotic-resistant strains (Appendino et al., 2008), a link among CBD, and bacterial MV release, now hitherto has not been investigated. The mechanism of cannabinoid-prompted immunomodulation has been studied in every in vitro and in vivo system; but, many more questions remain unanswered. It is thought that cannabinoids bind to CB1 and CB2 inhibiting adenylate cyclase interest and curing forskolin-stimulated cyclic AMP activation. In that manner, it results in the decreased interest of protein kinase A and ultimately lesser binding of transcription factors to CRE consensus sequences (Condie et al., 1996; Rieder et al., 2010). Cannabinoids certainly modulate immune responses in the course of inflammatory strategies and their immunomodulatory outcomes have been studied in masses of illness models collectively with diabetes, rheumatoid arthritis, and others. Results of animal studies show that cannabinoids exert their immunomodulatory residences in four ways: (1) apoptosis induction, (2) molecular proliferation suppression, (3) pro-inflammatory inhibition cytokines/chemokine biosynthesis and increase in anti-inflammatory cytokines, and (4) regulatory T cells induction (Rieder et al., 2010). Identifying drugs effective withinside the brand new coronavirus illness 2019 (COVID-19) is critical, pending a vaccine for SARS-CoV2. Cannabidiol (CBD) is a non-psychotropic phytocannabinoid, it has the capability to limit the severity and improvement of the ailment for several reasons: (1) *Cannabis sativa* extracts can downregulate the expression of the two key receptors for SARS-CoV2 in severe models of human epithelia, (2) cannabidiol exerts a widespread style of immunomodulatory and anti-inflammatory outcomes, and it can mitigate the out of control cytokine production liable for acute lung injury, (3) being a PPAR agonist, it can show a proper antiviral activity (Giuseppe Esposito et al. 2020).

3.13 MEDICINAL HERBAL SPICES

3.13.1 ALLIUM SATIVUM

Garlic (Fig. 3.6) in English and *Allium sativum* is the botanical name. It belongs to the family Alliaceae (Garagusi and Delahaan, 1985). It has specific minerals together with K, Cu, Ca, Fe, and Mg, and consists of various nutrients. This plant consists of water-soluble compounds like organosulfur, for example, S-allyl cysteine (SAC), S-ethyl cysteine (SEC), and S-propyl cysteine (SPC) (Suleria et al., 2015). The human immune system has a primary function in protecting against several viral sickness and probably against malignant cells. The immune system regulates itself via helper and suppressor cells and soluble products. Nutrients and specific components of spices have the functionality to have an impact on nearly all constituents of the immune gadget (Kandil et al, 1987), the connection between the immune gadget and nutrients positioned in spices has been reviewed comprehensively, which indicates that spices play a contributory function in improving immune characteristic (Kandil et al, 1987). Garlic's immoderate vitamin-C content material and antimicrobial residences make it a usable and sturdy immune system booster and it is very effective against bacterial, viral, fungal, and parasitic infections (Kyo et al., 2001). There is a growing body of evidence that garlic possesses vital immune improvement and anticancer activity (Fleischauer et al., 2000). While the maximum of the observed layout has been completed on animals or in vitro, the clinical studies that have been accomplished are showing significant results. According to Stall and Seebeck (1951), preliminary studies in humans, using standardized garlic powder preparation, have shown extensive outcomes on immunoreactions and phagocytosis.

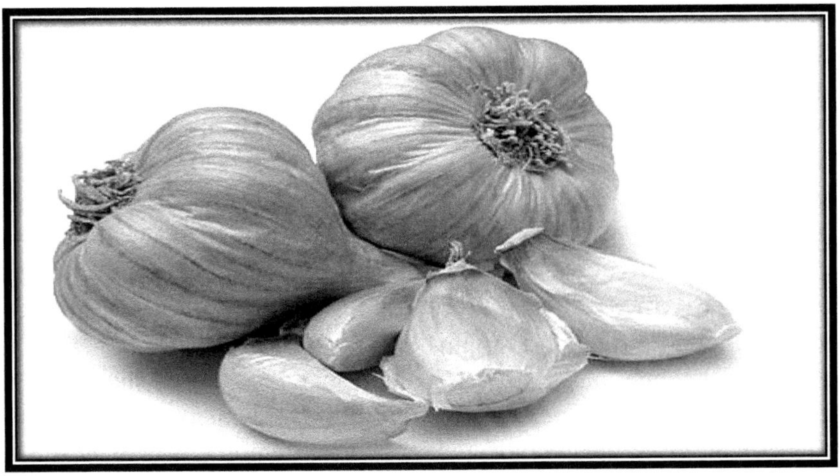

FIGURE 3.6 *Allium sativum.*

3.13.2 MEDICAL SIGNIFICANCE

Many research has proven proof of a widespread reduction of the hazard of growing continual sicknesses (e.g., cardiovascular, cancer, obesity, diabetes, excessive blood pressure, platelet aggregation, LDL cholesterol lowering) related to garlic consumption (Lanzotti et al., 2005; Amagase et al., 2001; Gardner et al., 2001; Lawson et al., 1992; Hussain et al., 1990). Together with healing functions, garlic possesses extra organic activities along with antibacterial, antifungal, and antioxidant properties (Tagoe et al., 2011; Korukluoglu, 2007; Shrestha et al., 2016), ensuing garlic being one of the maximum essential veggies worldwide (FAO, 2016). The clinical significance of extracts of *A. sativum* and *A. cepa* had been properly detailed (Kandil et al., 1987; Kyo et al., 2001). Our look at similarly bolstered it via displaying that there appeared to be a robust connection between the extracts of those plants and the immune system. A study found that widespread enhancement of CD4 and different immunological cells studied of *A. sativum*, *A. cepa* dealt with rats. The post-healing matter of those parameters changed additionally substantially reduced in comparison to without manipulating organization values. The significant increase within the matter of the immunological cells studied can be attributed to the extracts' inherent immunostimulatory properties. Natural products are a primary supply of the latest herbal capsules available and their use as an opportunity medication for the remedy of numerous sicknesses has been multiplied withinside the previous few decades (Vuorelaa et al., 2004; Ansari et al., 2006). In the assessment of the formulated capsules, the herbs and spices have fewer side effects. They also are inexpensive, display higher affected person tolerance and are without difficulty to be had for low socioeconomic populations (Adeshina et al., 2011). In recent years, because of their beneficial effects, the use of spices or herbs has been steadily increasing, not only in developing countries, but also in developed countries (Duman-Aydyn, 2008). The role of medicinal plants in the immune system is gaining a whole lot of interest. The generation of natural medication as a multiple-element agent is anticipated to modulate the complicated immune system in this manner so that it will save you from contamination as opposed to remedy and remedy the disorder. With these types of elements retained in mind, the existing evaluation specializes in an outline of some of the medicinal plants and their immunomodulatory properties. The period of immunity defines the body's herbal protection system against a wide array of sicknesses and disorders. Remarkably, state-of-the-art and superior among vertebrates, the complicated immune system is successful to generate an endless style of cells and molecules to arrest a massive spectrum of infections and unwanted materials. Immunomodulators seek support from materials which can induce, amplify, and inhibit any element or segment of the immune system. Immunostimulators and immunosuppressants are sorts of immunomodulators that are recognized for use. Immunopharmacology is a more modern department of pharma.

3.13.3 GINGER (ADRAK)

Zingiber officinale (Ginger) (Fig. 3.7) is a medicinal flowering plant whose rhizome, root, or ginger is broadly used as a spice and a medicine (Ginger, NCCIH Herbs at a Glance, 2016). Ginger, a famous and historically used plant is broadly consumed for its extraordinary functions in medication, cooking, grocery, and clinical research considering that its income and cost had been proven in extraordinary articles, tests, and research works (Benzie et al., 2011; Altman and Marcussen, 2001).

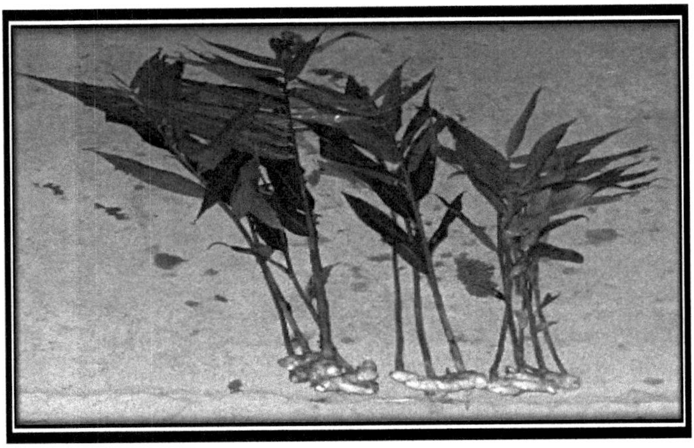

FIGURE 3.7 Garlic.

Antibacterial properties of ginger extracts have been assessed against *Escherichia coli, Pseudomonas aeruginosa*, and *Salmonella typhimurium*) and Gram-positive (*Bacillus subtilis, Staphylococcus aureus, Listeria monocytogenes*) microorganisms strain using the diffusion method (Sacchetti et al., 2005). Since historic times, it has been broadly used as a medicinal herb and spice (The American Family Physician, 2007). Because of the presence of phytochemical components and its use as a useful healing agent, it has been contributing pivotal roles towards an extensive variety of diseases, such as asthma, diabetes, stroke, constipation, and others (Mascolo et al., 1989; Kumar et al., 2013). A systematic exploration of this herb is generating useful outcomes. Among natural extracts, the inhibitory impact of ginger (*Zingiber officinale*) extract on microorganisms has been properly documented. Previous research found the antimicrobial consequences of ginger extract against *Pseudomonas aeruginosa, Staphylococcus aureus*, and *Escherichia coli* (Ogodo and Ekeleme, 2013; Azu and Onyeagba, 2007). *Zingiber officinale*, Ginger, is a spice of meals that has been diagnosed as a nutraceutical by the American Diabetic Association (Motawi et al., 2011; Bloch and Thomson, 1995). Nutraceuticals are purposeful meals that offer essential fitness advantages that consist of prevention and remedy for disorder conditions (Motawi et al., 2011; Bloch and Thomson, 1995; Langner et al., 1998). Ginger extract has greater efficiency due to its less utilization in food in comparison to ginger root powder. This trial has been designed to analyze the side effects of ginger extract on manufacturing performance, antioxidant capability, immunity, and additionally infection of laying hens, attempting to find a herbal and powerful feed additive in broiler diets.

3.13.4 TURMERIC (HALDI, CURCUMA LONGA)

Curcuma longa (*C. longa*) (Fig. 3.8) Linn, normally called turmeric, is a perennial plant belonging to the family Zingiberaceae. It is a not unusual place component in lots of health dietary supplements in Asia, being utilized in diverse healing programs inclusive of blood purifying, wound healing, and inflammatory problems, and holds a distinguished role in conventional Indian medicinal system (Khanna, 1999) The scalded and dried rhizome presents the crude drug Curcumae longae rhizoma, in any other case called turmeric root (Knoss and Chinou, 2012; Knoss, 2008). As a natural medicinal drug, it has been used to deal with inflammatory processes, liver problems, dyspepsia, peptic ulcer, infections, mycoses, wounds, pores, and skin problems.

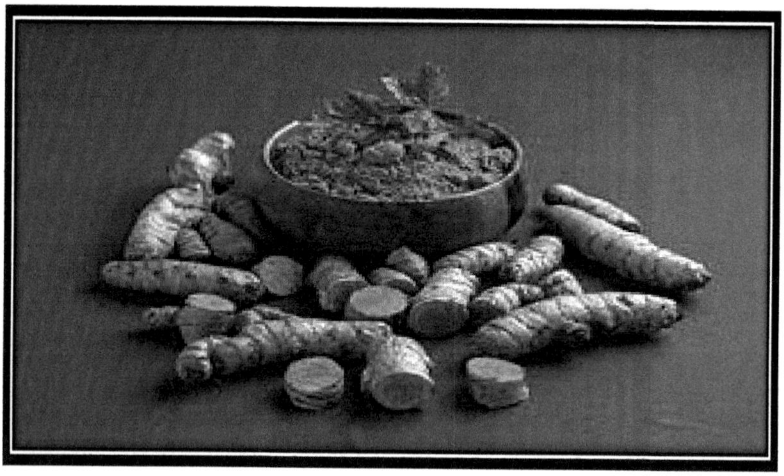

FIGURE 3.8 Turmeric.

3.13.4.1 ANTIVIRAL ACTIVITY

Lack of potential therapeutics for the maximum of viral diseases, the emergence of antiviral drug resistance, and the excessive cost of a few antiviral remedies necessitate locating new powerful antiviral compounds

(Tomei et al., 2005; Lemoine et al., 2013). Additionally, the present antiviral remedies are not constantly properly tolerated or pretty powerful and satisfactory (De Clercq, 2002). Hence, the growing requirement for antiviral materials can be extra-highlighted. Plants as a wealthy source of phytochemicals with distinctive biological activities inclusive of antiviral activities are in the interest of scientists (Jassim and Naji, 2003; Zorofchian et al., 2013). It has been validated that curcumin as a plant spinoff has an extensive variety of antiviral activity in opposition to distinctive viruses. Additionally, polysaccharide-containing *C. longa* extracts had been proven to have antidiabetic, antitumor, antidepressant, antioxidant, antimicrobial, antifertility, immune-modulatory, and hepatoprotective activity (Yue et al., 2010, Mohankumar and McFarlane, 2011; Deshpande et al., 1998; Yu et al., 2002; Selvam et al., 1995; Anbu Jeba Sunilson et al., 2009; Mishra and Singh, 2009; Subramanian and Selvam, 1999). While anti-inflammatory and immune-modulatory activities of curcuminoids had been studied extensively, very constrained reviews on polar extracts (containing polysaccharides) of *C. longa* are available. In this context, we evolved an aqueous primarily based extract of *C. longa*, without curcuminoids, standardized to polysaccharides (NR-INF-02), and evaluated for irritation-associated health conditions.

3.13.5 NIGELLA SATIVA L. (BLACK CUMIN) JEERA

Plants of Jeera (Fig. 3.9) have long been used as a basis of conventional medication inside the records of mankind and additionally act as assets of current drug treatments. According to the World Health Organization (WHO), more than 3-fourths of the groups in resource-constrained international locations depend on remedial plants for their PHC needs because more than 60–60.13% of societies are not able to have access to allopathic drug treatments (WHO, 2017; Jamshidi-Kia et al., 2018)

3.13.5.1 PHARMACOLOGICAL ACTIVITIES OF NIGELLA SATIVA

Medicinal plants had been used for curing illnesses in many nations in distinctive indigenous structures of drugs in addition to people's medicinal drugs. Essential oils are having terpenic combinations obtained from diverse elements of plants through steam distillation or different methods (Daferera et al., 2000). Since those oils are "eco-friendly" and harmless

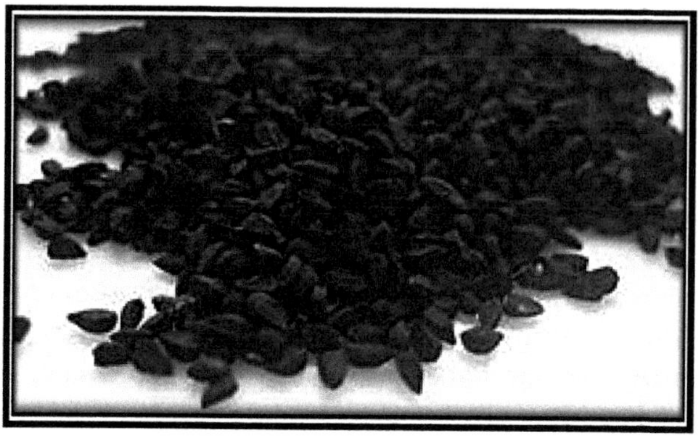

FIGURE 3.9 Black cumin.

to humans, at present, there is growing attention, each in industry and educational research, toward remedial plants and their inhibitory properties against pathogenic and fungi food spoilage (Fan and Chen, 1999)

3.13.5.2 ANTIMICROBIAL ACTIVITY

Antimicrobials had been the bases of scientific medicinal drugs in view that the second half of the 20th century and feature stored distinguished a variety of humans from critical microbial infections. Nevertheless, withinside the past 20th century and the earliest 21st century, it has perceived the appearance and substance of antimicrobial resistance in harmful microorganisms at some point of the globe (Condie et al., 1996; Ventola, 2015). The ever-growing terrorization of infections spread by microorganisms and antimicrobial-resistant microorganisms needs an international conflict to find out for novel solutions that are probably grounded in herbal products inclusive of plants, which can be decided on the premise of famed ethnomedicinal use (Andrade et al., 2015; Theuretzbacher, 2012). Among the inspiring herbal plants, black cumin and green cumin are the ones that displayed robust antiparasitic, antibacterial, antifungal, and antiviral actions.

3.13.5.3 ANTIBACTERIAL ACTIVITY

Many biological activities of *N. sativa* seeds had been suggested, inclusive of antibacterial, antifungal, antitumor, and hypotensive (Ferdous et al., 2006; Hanafy and Hatem, 1991; Worthen et al., 1998; Zaoui et al., 2000).

Thymoquinone turned into the bioactive constituent of the unstable oil of *N. sativa* (El-Dakhakhany, 1963). Moreover, it has been suggested that TQ has antibacterial efficiency, and its activity can enhance antibiotic actions, particularly against *S. aureus* (Halawani, 2009).

3.13.5.4 ANTIFUNGAL ACTIVITY

As noted above, diverse research had been performed to assess the antifungal activity of *N. sativa*; however, its genuine mechanism of action was not properly established. Furthermore, only a little information had been documented on the morphological modifications of harmful germs and/or toxic fungi grown withinside the presence of *N. sativa* oils. In a research carried out by Khosravi et al. (2011), the required essential oil of *N. sativa* of various origins has been suggested to possess slightly inhibitory action against pathogenic harmful strains of yeasts, dermatophytes filamentous fungi together with aflatoxin-generating fungi. The *N. sativa* remedy focused on the molecular wall, membranous organelles, and plasma membrane, particularly withinside the nuclei and mitochondria as had been obtrusive in the morphology of those toxigenic fungi (Shokri, 2016).

3.13.5.5 ANTIVIRAL ACTIVITY

N. sativa seed oil was shown to suppress viral load in murine model: Cytomegalovirus inflamed mice to undetectable level withinside the liver and spleen in 10 days by intraperitoneal administration. This was because of the increase in the numebr and functions of CD4+ve T cells and increased production of interferon- (INF-) gamma (Forouzanfar et al., 2014).

3.14 HEALTH BENEFITS OF NATURAL FORMULATION

The destiny of drugs is rooted withinside the past, earlier than chemists undertook to synthesize artificial silver bullets for all that illnesses, and earlier than pharmaceutical companies hitched our collective health to what has come to be for them a multibillion-dollar wagon. In the past, nearly all of the drug treatments had been from plants; the plant being man's best chemist for ages. Herbs are staging a comeback, the natural renaissance' is occurring all around the globe and increasingly humans are paying attention to natural remedies to deal with diverse kinds of illnesses in the region of mainstream medicinal drugs.

There are three foremost motives for the recognition of natural drug treatments:

1. There is a developing challenge over the reliance on and safety of medicine and surgical treatment.
2. Modern medicinal drug is failing to efficaciously deal with the various maximum not unusual place health conditions.
3. Many herbal measures are being proven to supply better outcomes than drugs or surgical treatment without the aspect effects (Herbal drug treatments nowadays and the roots of current pharmacology, 2009).

Also, there is growing proof that many current drug remedies actually suppress signs and symptoms and forget about the underlying ailment processes. In contrast, many herbal products seem to address the reason for many illnesses and yield advanced scientific outcomes. Unfortunately, many physicians and sufferers are not conscious that those herbal options exist. But studies on this area is a by no means an ending process (Smith et al., 2009). From the affected person's perspective, it is far taken into consideration very applicable to consist of natural or botanical extracts as a part of the clinical intervention primarily based totally on the popularity that the natural intervention is taken into consideration to be herbal and that the exercise can also additionally had been a part of the subculture for lots generations. In this regard, the use of plants and plant extracts to deal with a selected ailment and/or ailment signs and symptoms seems to have been a part of hospital treatment as determined for hundreds of years. Although the use of plant extracts is not a main thing of hospital treatment as practiced in Western populations, it is far nevertheless extraordinarily famous in massive numbers of the world's population, mainly in Asia and Europe (Griggs, 1981).

3.15 QUALITY SAFETY AND SCIENTIFIC EVIDENCE

Herbal/traditional drug products are derived from any plant part (leaves, roots, flowers), and in any form like crude drug, in synthetic form, as extract, or any other form taken as a curative treatment (Merriam-Webster.com, 2018). Although traditional drug products have been used for centuries in many countries, such as Latin America, Asia, and Africa, traditional drugs have been commonly used in antiquated years for treatment and prevention, cure of illness, and health promotion as well as for the enhancement of life cycle and the quality of life. It is only over the past decades that the use of traditional drugs has attracted the attention in the Western world (Koren et al., 1990). Despite the lack of robust efficacy and safety data, the use of herbal medicinal products is widespread and increasing throughout North America and Europe (Falci et al., 2016; Rashrash et al., 2017; Eisenberg et al., 1998; Pokladnikova and Selke-Krulichova, 2016; Wu et al., 2014).

However, there is a lack of a scientific method to evaluate their potency and effectiveness. The holistic method of healthcare makes traditional medicine very effective and makes them useful to many people, but it also makes clinical assessment and it is very challenging due to the fact that a lot of elements need to be taken into account. Herbal tablets are in large use, and despite the fact that many consider that herbal drugs are secure to the human being, they may be regularly applied in combination and are drawn from plant reassets with their very own variability in species, growing conditions, and biologically active constituents. Traditional drug extracts can be contaminated, adulterated, and might consist of toxic or poisonous compounds. The first-rate manipulate of herbal drugs has an immediate effect on their protection and potency (Ernst et al., 2005; Ribnicky et al., 2008). But, there is a report about the composition and the first-rate of most natural tablets now is no longer handiest because of a lack of approved guidelines or government requirements; however, additionally because of a lack of approved or widespread studies, techniques for assessing herbal tablets (WHO, 2001; Kantor, 2009). In addition, there is little or no studies on whole natural combos due to the fact that the drug approval method does now no longer accommodate undifferentiated combos of herbal chemicals. Isolation of every active component from every herb can be immensely time-consuming at a better cost, making it now no longer cost-effective for manufacturers (Richter, 2003).

3.16 RESEARCH NEEDS

The report of the World Health Organization (WHO, 2000) showed the use of herbal medicines or phytomedicines globally. This expanded use has not been restricted to low-income countries where the use of herbal or traditional drugs has been part of their culture but has gained priority in developed countries. Phytomedicine is often used interchangeably with herbal medicines or botanicals. Herbal medicines involve the use of the whole plant body like seeds, berries, leaves, bark, roots, or flowers for clinical use (the University of Maryland Medical Center, 2013). Research interests within the discipline of herbal medicine treatment are huge but are balanced by the capability of health benefits and the significant length of the market. Research into the quality, safety, molecular effects, and medical efficacy of several herbs in not unusual place usage is needed. There is evidence for the efficacy of healing effects of decided herbs and is commonly based totally on experiments demonstrating an organic pastime in an applicable in vitro bioassay or experiments using animal models. In a few cases, that has supported epidemiological studies and a number of intervention experiments on humans by both (WHO 2001). There are three more vital regions of research and they can be described as

1) Quality and standardization of herbal medicine.
2) Assessments and action and preclinical pharmacological.
3) Clinical efficacy and safety index of herbal drug.

3.17 CONCLUSION

Vegetal researchers and other herbal researchers have used plants and herbs since the infancy of mankind and are still used worldwide for the treatment of disease and health promotion. Studies on immunomedicinal herbs will hugely contribute to the well-being of humankind's need for herbal treatment for immunomodulation without any use of allopathic or synthetic drugs and minimize the adverse effects of any allopathic or synthetic drugs. In this Covid pandemic situation, no permanent treatment is available, but some herbal remedies are there by which we can boost our immunity. Some plants play an important role as immunomodulator, such as (tulsi) *Ocimum sanctum* Linn, garlic, ginger, turmeric, black cumin, and *Cannabis sativa* (Common hemp). These plants have been previously discovered by many researchers for their many types of activities like immunomodulatory activities and others. These plants have various types of medicinal activities, such as anticancer activity, immunomodulatory activity. Allopathic treatment is very effective and is also good; but sometimes and in some patients, these drugs show some adverse effects like toxicity. That is why we use herbal therapies, herbal drugs; these herbal drugs are free from side effects and toxicity.

KEYWORDS

- **viral infection**
- **COVID-19**
- **herbal plants**
- **herbal formulation**

REFERENCES

A Brief Introduction and Guide. 2003. http://www.ayurveda.com/pdf/intro_ayurveda.pdf (accessed Jun 22, 2013).

Adeshina, G. O.; Jibo, S.; Agu, V. E.; Ehinmidu, J. O. Antibacterial Activity of Fresh Juices of Allium Cepa and Zingiber Officinale Against Multidrug Resistant Bacteria. *Int. J. Pharma Biosci.* **2011,** *2*, 289–295.

Ahmad, I.; Beg, A. Z. Antimicrobial and Phytochemical Studies on 45 Indian Medicinal Plants Against Multi-drug Resistant Human Pathogens. *J. Ethnopharmacol.* **2001,** *74*, 113–123.

Ali, H.; Dixit, S. *In Vitro* Antimicrobial Activity of Flavonoids of *Ocimum Sanctum* with Synergistic Effect of Their Combined Form. *Asian Pac. J. Trop. Dis.* **2012,** *2*, S396–S398.

Altman, R. D.; Marcussen, K. C. Effects of a Ginger Extract on Knee Pain in Patients with Osteoarthritis. *Arthritis Rheum.* **2001,** *44*, 2531–2538.

Amagase, H.; Petesch, B. L.; Matsuura, H.; Kasuga, S.; Itakura, Y. Intake of Garlic and Its Bioactive Components. *J. Nutr.* **2001,** *131*, 955S–962S.

Anbu Jeba Sunilson, J.; Suraj, R.; Rejitha, G.; Anandarajagopal, K.; Anita Gnana Kumari, A. V.; Promwichit, P. *In Vitro* Antimicrobial Evaluation of *Zingiber Officinale, Curcuma Longa* and *Alpinia Galanga* Extracts as Natural Food Preservatives. *Am. J. Food Technol.* **2009,** *4*, 192–200.

Andrade, P. H. M.; Schmidt Rondon, E.; Carollo, C. A., et al. Effect of Powdered Shells of the Snail *Megalobulimuslopesi* on Secondary-Intention Wound Healing in an Animal Model. *Evid. Based Complement. Alternat. Med.* **2015,** *2015*, 9.

Ansari, M. A.; Ahmed, S. P.; Haider, S.; Ansari, N. L. Nigella Sativa: A Non-conventional Herbal Option for the Management of Seasonal Allergic Rhinitis. *Pak. J. Pharm.* **2006,** *23*, 31–35.

Anwar, F.; Anwar, F.; Muhammad, G., et al. Capparis Spinosa L.: A Plant with High Potential for Development of Functional Foods and Nutraceuticals/Pharmaceuticals. *Int. J. Pharmacol.* **2016,** *12*(3), 201–219.

Anyaehie, U. B. Medicinal Properties of Fractionated Acetone/Water Neem (*Azadirachta Indica*) Leaf Extract from Nigeria: A Review. *Niger J. Physiol. Sci.* **2009,** *24*(2), 157–159.

Appendino, G.; Gibbons, S.; Giana, A.; Pagani, A.; Grassi, G.; Stavri, M.; Smith, E., et al. Antibacterial Cannabinoids from *Cannabis Sativa*: A Structure-activity Study. *J. Nat. Prod.* **2008,** *71*, 1427–1430. 10.1021/np8002673.

Atawodi, S. E.; Atawodi, J. C. Azadirachta Indica (Neem): A Plant of Multiple Biological and Pharmacological Activities. *Phytochem. Rev.* **2009,** *8*, 601–620.

Azu, N. C.; Onyeagba, R. A. Antimicrobial Properties of Extracts of Allium Cepa (Onions) and Zingiber Officinale (Ginger) on Escherichia coli: Salmonella Typhi, and Bacillus Subtilis. *Int. J. Trop. Med.* **2007,** *3*(2), 8148.

Balakumar, S.; Rajan, S.; Thirunalasundari, T.; Jeeva, S. Antifungal Activity of *Ocimum Sanctum* Linn. (Lamiaceae) on Clinically Isolated Dermatophytic Fungi. *Asian Pac. J. Trop. Med.* **2011,** *4*, 654–657.

Baral, R. N.; Chattopadhyay Neem (Azadirachta Indica) Leaf Mediated Immune Activation Causes Prophylactic Growth Inhibition of Murine Ehrlich Carcinoma and B16 Melanoma. *Int. Immunopharmacol.* **2004,** *4*, 355–366.

Ben Amar, M. Cannabinoids in Medicine: A Review of Their Therapeutic Potential. *J. Ethnopharmacol.* **2006,** *105*, 1–25.

Benzie, I. F.; Wachtel-Galor, S.; Bode, A. M.; Dong, Z. *The Amazing and Mighty Ginger*, 2nd ed. Ch. 7; CRC Press: New York, 2011.

Bimonte, S.; Crispo, A.; Amore, A.; Celentano, E.; Cuomo, A.; Cascella, M. Potential Antiviral Drugs for SARS-Cov-2 Treatment: Preclinical Findings and Ongoing Clinical Research. *In Vivo (Athens, Greece)* **2020,** *34*(3 Suppl), 1597–1602.

Biswas, K.; Chattopadhyay, I.; Banerjee, R. K.; Bandopadhyay, U. Biological Activities and Medicinal Properties of Neem (Azadirachta Indica). *Curr. Sci.* **2002,** *82*, 1336–1345.

Bloch, A.; Thomson, C. A. Position of the American Diabetic Association: Phytochemicals and Functional Foods. *J. Am. Diet Assoc.* **1995,** *95*, 406–493.

Botelho, M. A.; Santos, R. A.; Martins, J. G.; Carvalho, C. O.; Paz, M. C.; Azenha, C.; et al. Efficacy of a Mouth Rinse Based on Leaves of the Neem Tree (*Azadirachta Indica*) in the Treatment of Patients with Chronic Gingivitis: A Double Blind, Randomized, Controlled Trial. *J. Med. Plant Res.* **2008,** *2*(11), 341–346.

Buonaguro, F. M.; Puzanov, I.; Ascierto, P. A. Anti-IL6R Role in Treatment of COVID-19-related ARDS. *J. Transl. Med.* **2020,** *18*(1), 165.

Cascella, M.; Rajnik, M.; Cuomo, A. et al. Features, Evaluation and Treatment Coronavirus (COVID-19). Stat Pearls [Internet]. Treasure Island (FL): Stat Pearls Publishing, 2020. https://www.ncbi.nlm.nih.gov/books/NBK554776/

Chan, J. F.; To, K. K.; Tse, H.; Jin, D. Y.; Yuen, K. Y. Interspecies Transmission and Emergence of Novel Viruses: Lessons from Bats and Birds. *Trends Microbiol.* **2013,** *10*, 544–555.

Chandra, R.; Dwivedi, V.; Shivam, K.; Jha, A. K. Detection of Antimicrobial Activity of *Ocimum Sanctum* (Tulsi) and Trigonella foenum Graecum (Methi) Against Some Selected Bacterial and Fungal Strains. *Res. J. Pharm. Biol. Chem. Sci.* **2011,** *2*, 809–813.

Chang, J. D.; Mantri, N.; Sun, B.; Jiang, L.; Chen, P.; Jiang, B. et al. Effects of Elevated CO2 and Temperature on *Gynostemma pentaphyllum* Physiology and Bioactive Compounds. *J. Plant Physiol.* **2016,** *19*, 41–52.
Chen, Y.; Liu, Q.; Guo, D. Emerging Coronaviruses: Genome Structure, Replication, and Pathogenesis. *J. Med. Viral* **2020,** *92*(4), 418–423.
Chitra, G.; Krishnaveni, N. Immunostimulatory Effect of *Ocimum Sanctum* Leaf Extract on the Indian Major Carp, *Catlacatla. Plant Archives* **2011,** *11*, 213–214.
Chopra, R. N.; Nayer, S. L.; Chopra, I. C. *Glossary of Indian Medicinal Plants*; CSIR: New Delhi, 1956.
Condie, R.; Herring, A.; Koh, W. S.; Lee, M.; Kaminski, N. E. Cannabinoid Inhibition of Adenylate Cyclase-mediated Signal Transduction and Interleukin 2 (IL-2) Expression in the Murine T-cell Line: EL4.IL-2. *J. Biol. Chem.* **1996,** *271*, 13175–13183.
Daferera, D. J.; Zirgas, B. N.; Polission, M. G. GC-MS Analysis of Essential Oil from Some Greek Aromatic Plants and Their Fungitoxicity on Penicillium Digitatum. *J. Agric. Food Chem.* **2000,** *48*, 2576–2581.
Das, J.; Buragohain, B.; Srivastava, R. B. *In Vitro* Evaluation of Ocimum Sanctum Leaf Extract Against Dermatophytes and Opportunistic Fungi. *Asian J. Microbiol. Biotechnol. Environ. Sci.* **2010,** *12*, 789–792.
Davis, A. Medicines by Design. NIH Publication No. 06-474 (cited 2012-10-03). 2012. http://www.vigyanprasar.gov.in/Radioserials/Natural%20products%20as%20drugs-%20by%20K%20V%20Sashidhara,%20CDRI.pdf (accessed Sep 10, 2012).
De Clercq, E. Strategies in the Design of Antiviral Drugs. *Nat. Rev. Drug Discovery* **2002,** *1*(1), 13–25.
Delaha, E. C.; Garagusi, V. F. Inhibition of Mycobacteria by Garlic Extract (Allium Sativum). *Antimicrob. Agents Chemother.* **1985,** *27*, 485–486.
Deo, S. S.; Inam, F.; Mahashabde, R. P. Antimicrobial Activity and HPLC Fingerprinting of Crude Ocimum Extracts. *E-J. Chem.* **2011,** *8*, 1430–1437.
Deshpande, S. S.; Ingle, A. D.; Maru, G. B. Chemopreventive Efficacy of Curcumin-free Aqueous Turmeric Extract in 7,12-dimethylbenz a Anthracene-induced Rat Mammary Tumorigenesis. *Cancer Lett.* **1998,** *123*, 35–40.
Drabu, S.; Khatri, S.; Babu, S. Neem: Healer of All Ailments. *Res. J. Pharm. Biol. Che. Sci.* **2012,** *3*, 120–126.
Duman-Aydyn, B. Investigation of Antibacterial Effects of Some Medicinal Plants and Spices on Food Pathogens. *Kafkas Univ. Vet. Fak. Derg.* **2008,** *14*, 83–87.
Eisenberg, D. M.; Davis, R. B.; Ettner, S. L.; Appel, S.; Wilkey, S.; Van Rompay, M., et al. Trends in Alternative Medicine Use in the United States, 1990–1997: Results of a Follow-up National Survey. *JAMA* **1998,** *280*, 1569–1575.
Elavarasu, S.; Abinaya, P.; Elanchezhiyan, S.; Thangakumaran, S.; Vennila, K.; Naziya, K. B. Evaluation of Anti-plaque Microbial Activity of *Azadirachta Indica* (Neem Oil) *In Vitro*: A Pilot Study. *J. Pharm. Bioallied Sci.* **2012,** *4*(2), 394–396.
Elavarasu, S.; Abinaya, P.; Elanchezhiyan, S.; Thangakumaran, Vennila, K.; Naziya, K. B. Evaluation of Anti-plaque Microbial Activity of *Azadirachta Indica* (Neem Oil) *In Vitro*: A Pilot Study. *J. Pharm. Bioallied Sci.* **2012,** *4*(Suppl 2), S394–S396.
El-Dakhakhany, M. Studies on the Chemical Constitution of Egyptian *N. Sativa* L. Seeds. *Planta Med.* **1963,** *11*, 465–470.

Emanuel, E. J.; Wendler, D.; Killen, J.; Grady, C. What Makes Clinical Research in Developing Countries Ethical: The benchmarks of Ethical Research. *J. Infect. Dis.* **2004,** *189*, 930–937.

Ernst, E.; Schmidt, K.; Wider, B. CAM Research in Britain: The Last 10 Years. *Complement Ther. Clin. Pract.* **2005,** *11*, 17–20.

Evans, S. Changing the Knowledge Base in Western Herbal Medicine. *Soc. Sci. Med.* **2008,** *67*, 2098–2106.

Falci, L.; Shi, Z.; Greenlee, H. Multiple Chronic Conditions and Use of Complementary and Alternative Medicine Among US Adults: Results from the 2012 National Health Interview Survey. *Prev. Chronic Dis.* **2016,** *13*, E61.

Fan, J. J.; Chen, J. H. Inhibition of Aflatoxin-producing by Welsh Onion Extracts. *J. Food Prot.* **1999,** *62*, 414–417.

FAO. *FAO Statistic Pocket Book.* Food & Agriculture Organization: Rome, Italy, 2016.

Ferdous, A. J.; Islam, S. N.; Ahsan, M.; Hasan, C. M.; Ahmed, Z. U. In Vitro Antibacterial Activity of the Volatile Oil of *Nigella Sativa* Seeds Against Multiple Drug-resistant Isolates of *Shigella Spp*. and Isolates of *Vibrio Cholerae* and *Escherichia Coli*. *Phytother. Res.* **2006,** *6*, 137–140.

Fleischauer, A. T.; Poole, C.; Arab, L. Garlic Consumption and Cancer Prevention: Meta-analyses of Colorectal and Stomach Cancers. *Am. J. Clin. Nutr.* **2000,** *72*(4), 1047–1052.

Forouzanfar, F.; Fazly Bazzaz, B. S.; Hosseinzadeh, H. Black Cumin (Nigella Sativa) and Its Constituent (Thymoquinone): A Review on Antimicrobial Effects. *Iran J. Basic Med. Sci.* **2014,** *17*(12), 929–938.

Galhardi, L. C.; Yamamoto, K. A.; Ray, S.; Ray, B.; Linhares, R. E.; Nozawa, C. The *In Vitro* Antiviral Property of *Azadirachta Indica* Polysaccharides for Poliovirus. *J. Ethnopharmacol.* **2012,** *142*(1), 86–90.

Gardner, C. D.; Chatterjee, L. M.; Carlson, J. J. The Effect of a Garlic Preparation on Plasma Lipid Levels in Moderately Hypercholesterolemic Adults. *Atherosclerosis* **2001,** *154*, 213–220.

Gattinoni, L.; Coppola, S.; Cressoni, M.; Busana, M.; Rossi, S.; Chiumello, D. COVID-19 Does Not Lead to a "Typical" Acute Respiratory Distress Syndrome. *Am. J. Respir. Crit. Care Med.* **2020,** *201*(10), 1299–1300.

Gautret, P.; Lagier, J. C.; Parola, P.; Hoang, V. T.; Meddeb, L.; Mailhe, M.; Doudier, B.; Courjon, J.; Giordanengo, V.; Vieira, V. E.; Tissot Dupont, H.; Honoré, S.; Colson, P.; Chabrière, E.; La Scola, B.; Rolain, J. M.; Brouqui, P.; Raoult, D. Hydroxychloroquine and Azithromycin As A Treatment of COVID-19: Results of an Open-label Non-randomized Clinical Trial. *Int. J. Antimicrob. Agents* **2020,** *56*(1), 105949.

Gbolade, A. A.; Lockwood, G. B. Toxicity of *Ocimum Sanctum* L. Essential Oil to *Aedes Aegypti* Larvae and Its Chemical Composition. *J. Essent. Oil-Bear Plants* **2008,** *11*, 148–153.

Geller, C.; Varbanov, M.; Duval, R. E. Human Coronaviruses: Insights into Environmental Resistance and Its Influence on the Development of New Antiseptic Strategies. *Viruses* **2012,** *4*, 3044–3068.

Ginger, NCCIH Herbs at a Glance. US NCCIH. *1 September 2016*. Retrieved 2 February 2019.

Giordano, J.; Engebretson, J.; Garcia, M. K. Challenges to Complementary and Alternative Medical Research: Focal Issues Influencing Integration Into a Cancer Care Model. *Integr. Cancer Ther.* **2005,** *4*, 210–218.

Goel, A.; Singh, D. K.; Kumar, S.; Bhatia, A. K. Immunomodulating Property of *Ocimum Sanctum* by Regulating the IL-2 Production and Its mRNA Expression Using rat's Splenocytes. *Asian Pac. J. Trop. Med.* **2010,** *3*, 8–12.

Goldman, P. Herbal Medicines Today and The Roots of Modern Pharmacology. *Ann. Intern. Med.* **2001,** *135*, 594–600. Available from: http://annals.highwire.org/cgi/reprint/135/8_Part_1/594.pdf (accessed Oct 15, 2009).

Gordon, C. J.; Tchesnokov, E. P.; Feng, J. Y.; Porter, D. P.; Gotte, M. The Antiviral Compound Remdesivir Potently Inhibits RNA-dependent RNA Polymerase from Middle East Respiratory Syndrome Coronavirus. *J. Biol* **2020,** *95*(15), 4773–4779.

Goyal, P.; Kaushik, P. In Vitro Evaluation of Antibacterial Activity of Various Crude Leaf Extracts of Indian Sacred Plant: Ocimum Sanctum L. *British Microbiol. Res. J.* **2011,** *1*(3), 70–78.

Guo, Z. D.; Wang, Z. Y.; Zhang, S. F.; Li, X.; Li, L.; Li, C.; Cui, Y.; Fu, R. B.; Dong, Y. Z.; Chi, X. Y.; Zhang, M. Y.; Liu, K.; Cao, C.; Liu, B.; Zhang, K.; Gao, Y. W.; Lu, B.; Chen, W. Aerosol and Surface Distribution of Severe Acute Respiratory Syndrome Coronavirus 2 in Hospital Wards, Wuhan, China. *Emerging Infect. Dis.* **2020,** *26*(7), 1583–1591.

Gupta, S. K.; Prakash, J.; Srivastava, S. Validation of Traditional Claim of Tulsi, *Ocimum Sanctum* Linn. As a Indian Medicinal Plant. *J. Exp. Biol.* **2002,** *40*, 765–773.

Halawani, E. Antibacterial Activity of Thymoquinone and Thymohydroquinone of *Nigella sativa* L. and Their Interaction with Some Antibiotics. *Adv. Biol. Res.* **2009,** *3*, 148–152.

Hanafy, M. S.; Hatem, M. E. Studies on the Antimicrobial Activity of *Nigella Sativa* Seed (Black Cumin). *J. Ethnopharmacol.* **1991,** *34*, 275–278.

Haque, E.; Mandal, I.; Pal, S.; Baral, R. N. Prophylactic Dose of Neem (Azadirachta Indica) Leaf Preparation Restricting Murine Tumor Growth is Nontoxic, Hematostimulatory and Immunostimulatory. *Immunopharmacol Immunotoxicol.* **2006,** *28*, 33–50.

Hemalatha, R.; Babu, K. N.; Karthik, M.; Ramesh, R.; Kumar, B. D.; Kumar, P. U. Immunomodulatory Activity and Th1/Th2 Cytokine Response of *Ocimum Sanctum* in Myelo Suppressed Swiss Albino Mice. *Trends Med. Res.* **2011,** *6*, 23–31.

Hernández-Cervantes, R.; Méndez-Díaz, M.; Prospéro-García, Ó.; Morales-Montor, J. Immunoregulatory Role of Cannabinoids During Infectious Disease. *Neuroimmunomodulation* **2017,** *24*, 183–199. 10.1159/000481824.

Hui, D. S.; Chow, B. K.; Lo, T.; Tsang, O. T. Y.; Ko, F. W.; Ng, S. S.; Gin, T.; Chan, M. T. V. Exhaled Air Dispersion During High-flow Nasal Cannula Therapy *versus* CPAP *via* Different Masks. *Eur. Respir. J.* **2019,** *53*(4).

Hussain, S. P.; Jannu, L. N.; Rao, A. R. Chemopreventive Action of Garlic on Methylcholanthrene-induced Carcinogenesis in the Uterine Cervix of Mice. *Cancer Lett.* **1990,** *49*, 175–180.

Inbaneson, S. J.; Sundaram, R.; Suganthi, P. *In Vitro* Antiplasmodial Effect of Ethanolic Extracts of Traditional Medicinal Plant Ocimum Species Against Plasmodium Falciparum. *Asian Pac. J. Trop. Med.* **2012,** *5*, 103–106.

Jamshidi-Kia, F.; Lorigooini, Z.; Amini-Khoei, H. Medicinal Plants: Past History and Future Perspective. *J. Herbmed Pharmacol.* **2018,** *7*(1), 1–7.

Jassim, S. A. A.; Naji, M. A. Novel Antiviral Agents: A Medicinal Plant Perspective. *J. Appl. Microbiol.* **2003,** *95*(3), 412–427.

Jayakumar, R. V. Herbal Medicine for Type-2 Diabetes. *Int. J. Diabetes Dev. Ctries* **2010,** *30*(3), 111–112.

Kandil, O. M.; Abdellah, T. H.; Elkadi, A. Garlic and the Immune System in Humans: Its Effects on Natural Killer Cells. *Fed. Pro.* **1987,** *46*, 441.

Kandil, O. M.; Abdellah, T. H.; Elkadi, A. Garlic and the Immune System in Humans: Its Effects on Natural Killer Cells. *Federal Procedures* **1987,** *46*, 441.

Kantor, M. The Role of Rigorous Scientific Evaluation in the Use and Practice of Complementary and Alternative Medicine. *J. Am. Coll. Radiol.* **2009,** *6*, 254–262.

Khanna, N. M. Turmeric, Nature's Precious Gift. *Curr. Sci.* **1999,** *76*, 1351–1356.

Khosla, M. K. Sacred Tulsi (*Ocimum Sanctum* L.) in Traditional Medicine and Pharmacology. *Anc. Sci. Life* **1995,** *15*, 53–61.

Knoss, W.; Chinou, I. Regulation of Medicinal Plants for Public Health—European Community Monographs on Herbal Substances. *Planta Med.* **2012,** *78*, 1311–1316.

Knoss, W.; Stolte, F.; Reh, K. The Regulatory Framework for Complementary and Alternative Medicines in Europe. *Bundesgesundheitsblatt Gesundheits for Seining Gesund-heitsschutz* **2008,** *51*, 771–778.

Kollias, A.; Kyriakoulis, K. G.; Dimakakos, E.; Poulakou, G.; Stergiou, G. S.; Syrigos, K. Thromboembolic Risk and Anticoagulant Therapy in COVID-19 Patients: Emerging Evidence and Call for Action. *Br. J. Haematol.* **2020,** *189*(5), 846–847.

Koren, G.; Randor, S.; Martin, S.; Danneman, D. Maternal Ginseng Use Associated with Neonatal Androgenization. *JAMA* **1990,** *264*, 2866.

Korukluoglu, R. I. A. M. Control of Aspergillus Niger with Garlic, Onion and Leek Extracts. *Afr. J. Biotechnol.* **2007,** *6*, 384–387.

Kucharski, A. J.; Klepac, P.; Conlan, A. J. K.; Kissler, S. M.; Tang, M. L.; Fry, H.; Gog, J. R.; Edmunds, W. J.; CMMID COVID-19 Working Group. Effectiveness of Isolation, Testing, Contact Tracing, and Physical Distancing on Reducing Transmission of SARS-CoV-2 in Different Settings: A Mathematical Modelling Study. *Lancet Infect. Dis.* **2020,** *15*.

Kumar, P. K.; Kumar, M. R.; Kavita, K.; Singh, J.; Khan, R. Pharmacological Actions of Ocimum Sanctum–A Review Article. *IJAPBC* **2012,** *1*(3), 406–413.

Kumar, S.; Saxena, K.; Singh, U. N.; Saxena, R. Anti-inflammatory Action of Ginger: A Critical Review in Anemia of Inflammation and Its Future Aspects. *Int. J. Herb. Med.* **2013,** *1*(4), 16–20.

Kyo, E.; Uda, N.; Suzuki, A.; Kakimoto, M.; Ushijima, M.; Kasuga, S.; Itakura, Y. Immunomodulatory Effects of Aged Garlic Extract. *J. Nutri.* **2001,** *131*(3), 1075S–1079S.

Kyo, E.; Uda, N.; Suzuki, A.; Kakimoto, M.; Ushijima, M.; Kasuga, S.; Itakura, Y. Immunomodulatory Effects of Aged Garlic Extract. *J. Nutrition* **2001,** *131*(3), 1075S–1079S.

Lakshmi, T.; Krishnan, V.; Rajendran, R.; Madhusudhanan, N. Azadirachta Indica: A Herbal Panacea in Dentistry–An Update. *Pharm. Rev.* **2015,** *9*, 41–44.

Langner, E.; Greifenberg, S.; Gruenwald, J. Ginger: History and Use. *Adv. Ther.* **1998,** *15*, 25–30.

Lawson, L. D.; Ransom, D. K.; Hughes, B. G. Inhibition of Whole Blood Platelet-aggregation by Compounds in Garlic Clove Extracts and Commercial Garlic Products. *Thromb. Res.* **1992,** *65*, 141–156.

Ledford, H. Coronavirus Breakthrough: Dexamethasone is First Drug Shown to Save Lives. *Nature* **2020,** *582*(7813), 469.

Lemoine, M.; Nayagam, S.; Thursz, M. Viral Hepatitis in Resource-limited Countries and Access to Antiviral Therapies: Current and Future Challenges. *Future Virol.* **2013,** *8*(4), 371–380.

Mahajan, N.; Rawal, S.; Verma, M.; Poddar, M.; Alok, S. A Phytopharmacological Overview on *Ocimum* Species with Special Emphasis on *Ocimum Sanctum. Biomed. Prev. Nutr.* **2013,** *3*, 185–192.

Mahfuzul Hoque, M. D.; Bari, M. L.; Inatsu, Y.; Juneja, V. K.; Kawamoto, S. Antibacterial Activity of Guava (Psidium Guajava L.) and Neem (Azadirachta Indica A. Juss.): Extracts Against Foodborne Pathogens and Spoilage bacteria. *Foodborne Pathog. Dis.* **2007,** *4*, 481–488.

Mary-Lou, E. F.; Kronkright, D. P.; Norton, R. E. *The Conservation of Artifacts Made from Plant Materials*; Getty Publications, 1991; p 49. ISBN 978-0-89236-160-1.

Mascolo, N.; Jain, R.; Jain, S. C.; Capasso, F. Ethnopharmacologic Investigation of Ginger (*Zingiber Officinale*) *J. Ethnopharmacol.* **1989,** *27*(1–2), 129–140.

Mediratta, P. K.; Sharma, K. K.; Singh, S. Evaluation of Immunomodulatory Potential of *Ocimum Sanctum* Seed Oil and Its Possible Mechanism of Action. *J. Ethnopharmacol.* **2002,** *80*, 15–20.

Mediratta, P. K.; Sharma, K. K.; Singh, S. Evaluation of Immunomodulatory Potential of *Ocimum Sanctum* Seed Oil and Its Possible Mechanism of Action. *J. Ethnopharmacol.* **2002,** *80*, 15–20.

Miller, A. M.; Stella, N. CB2 Receptor-mediated Migration of Immune Cells: It Can Go Either Way. *Br. J. Pharmacol.* **2008,** *153*, 299–308.

Mishra, R. K.; Singh, S. K. Reversible Antifertility Effect of Aqueous Rhizome Extract of *Curcuma Longa* L. in Male Laboratory Mice. *Contraception* **2009,** *79*, 479–487.

Mohan, L.; Amberkar, M. V.; Kumari, M. Ocimum Sanctum Linn. (TULSI)-an Overview. *Int. J. Pharm. Sci. Rev. Res.* **2011,** *7*, 51–53.

Mohankumar, S.; McFarlane, J. R. An Aqueous Extract of *Curcuma Longa* (Turmeric) Rhizomes Stimulates Insulin Release and Mimics Insulin Action on Tissues Involved in Glucose Homeostasis *In Vitro*. *Phytother. Res.* **2011,** *25*, 396–401.

Molina, P. E.; Amedee, A.; Le Capitaine, N. J.; Zabaleta, J.; Mohan, M.; Winsauer, P.; Vande Stouwe, C. Cannabinoid Neuroimmune Modulation of SIV Disease. *J. Neuroimmune Pharmacol.* **2011,** *6*, 516–527.

Mondal, S.; Miranda, B. R. R. B.; Sushil, C. M. The Science Behind Sacredness of Tulsi (Ocimum Sanctum LINN.). *Ind. J. Physiol. Pharmacol.* **2009,** *53*(4), 291–306.

Mondal, S.; Mirdha, B. R.; Mahapatra, S. C. The Science Behind Sacredness of Tulsi (Ocimum Sanctum Linn.) *Indian J. Physiol. Pharmacol.* **2009,** *53*, 291–306.

Mondal, S.; Varma, S.; Bamola, V. D.; Naik, S. N.; Mirdha, B. R.; Padhi, M. M., et al. Double-blinded Randomized Controlled Trial for Immunomodulatory Effects of Tulsi (*Ocimum sanctum* Linn.): Leaf Extract on Healthy Volunteers. *J. Ethnopharmacol.* **2011,** *136*, 452–456.

Mondal, S.; Varma, S.; Bamola, V. D.; Naik, S. N.; Mirdha, B. R.; Padhi, M. M.; et al. Double-blinded Randomized Controlled Trial for Immunomodulatory Effects of Tulsi (Ocimum Sanctum Linn.): Leaf Extract on Healthy Volunteers. *J. Ethnopharmacol.* **2011,** *136*, 452–456.

Motawi, T. K.; Hamed, M. A.; Shabana, M. H.; Hashem, R. M.; ABoul-Naserm, A. F. *Zingiber Officinale* Acts as a Nutraceutic Agent Against Liver Fibrosis. *Nutr. Metab.* **2011,** *8*, 40–51.

Narayan, P. Neem-papaya Juice Passes Dengue Test, 2012. http://articles.timesofindia.indiatimes.com/2012-12-20/chennai/35933070_1_dengue-virus-dengue-cases-dengue-patients (accessed Sep 10, 2012).

National Academy of Science. *Neem, A Tree for Solving Global Problems[R]*; NAS: Washington, DC, 1992.

National Institutes of Health, U. S. Department of Health and Human Services. Ayurvedic Medicine-An Introduction. 2005. http://www.nccam.nih.gov/sites/nccam.nih.gov/files/D287_BKG.pdf

Neem Foundation. Mumbai: 2012. All About Neem. http://www.neemfoundation.org (accessed Sept 10, 2012).

Newman, Cragg, and Sander (2003); Butler 2004; Balunas and Kinghorn 2005; Gurib-Fakim 2006; Newman and Cragg 2007).

Newman, D. J.; Cragg, G. M. Natural Products as Sources of New Drugs Over the Last 25 Years. *J. Nat. Prod.* **2007,** *70*, 461–477.

Novartis Eyes Traditional Chinese Medicine. United Press International. http://www.upi.com/NewsTrack/view.php?StoryID=20061106-022125-5205r (accessed Aug 1, 2007).

nti-hyperlipidemic Effect of Triglize: A Polyherbal Formulation. *J. Pharmacol. Pharmacother.* **2010,** *2*, 118–122.

Nyika, A. Ethical and Regulatory Issues Surrounding African Traditional Medicine in the Context of HIV/AIDS. *Dev. World Bioeth.* **2006.**

Ogodo, A. C.; Ekeleme, U. G. In-vitro Antibacterial Activity of Garlic Cloves and Ginger Rhizomes on Food-borne Pathogens. *Int. J. Basic App. Sci.* **2013,** *2*(4), 387–392.

Pandey, G.; Madhuri, S. Pharmacological Activities of Ocimum Sanctum (Tulsi): A Review. *Int. J. Pharm. Sci. Rev. Res.* **2010,** *5*(1), 61–66.

Parasuraman, S.; Kumar, E. P.; Kumar, A.; Emerson, S. F. A

Pattanayak, P.; Behera, P.; Das, D.; Panda, S. K. *Ocimum Sanctum* Linn. A Reservoir Plant for Therapeutic Applications: An Overview. *Pharmacogn. Rev.* **2010,** *4*, 95. DOI: 10.4103/0973-7847.65323.

Pattanayak, P.; Behera, P.; Das, D.; Panda, S. K. *Ocimum Sanctum* Linn. A Reservoir Plant for Therapeutic Applications: An Overview. *Pharmacogn. Rev.* **2010,** *4*, 95. DOI: 10.4103/0973-7847.65323.

Pattanayak, P.; Behera, P.; Das, D.; Panda, S. K. Ocimum Sanctum Linn. A Reservoir Plant for Therapeutic Applications: An Overview. *Pharmacogn. Rev.* **2010,** *4*, 95–105.

Pavaraj, M.; Balasubramanian, V.; Baskaran, S.; Ramasamy, P. Development of Immunity by Extract of Medicinal Plant *Ocimum Sanctum* on Common Carp Cyprinus Carpio (L.). *Res. J. Immunol.* **2011,** *4*, 12–18.

Pokladnikova, J.; Selke-Krulichova, I. Prevalence of Complementary and Alternative Medicine Use in the General Population in the Czech Republic. *Forsch Komplementmed.* **2016,** *23*, 22–28.

Pole, S. *Ayurvedic Medicine: The Principles of Traditional Practice*; Jessica Kingsley Publishers: London, 2013.

Prakash, P.; Gupta, N. Therapeutic Uses of *Ocimum Sanctum* Linn (Tulsi) with a Note on Eugenol and Its Pharmacological Actions: A Short Review. *Indian J. Physiol. Pharmacol.* **2005,** *49* 125–131.

Puri, H. S. *Azadirachta Indica*. Harwood Academic Publishers, Neem The Divine Tree, Amsterdam, 1999; pp 1–3.

Rajamma, A. J.; Dubey, S.; Sateesha, S. B.; Tiwari, S. N.; Ghosh, S. K. Comparative Larvicidal Activity of Different Species of Ocimum Against Culex Quinquefasciatus. *Nat. Prod. Res.* **2011,** *25*, 1916–1922.

Rashrash, M.; Schommer, J. C.; Brown, L. M. Prevalence and Predictors of Herbal Medicine Use Among Adults in the United States. *J. Patient Exp.* **2017,** *4*, 108–113.

Ray, A.; Banerjee, B. D.; Sen, P. Modulation of Humoral and Cell Mediated Immune Responses by Azadirachta Indica (Neem) in Mice. *Indian J. Exp. Biol.* **1996,** *34*, 698–701.

Ribnicky, D. M.; Poulev, A.; Schmidt, B.; Cefalu, W. T.; Raskin, I. The Science of Botanical Supplements for Human Health: A View from the NIH Botanical Research Centers: Evaluation of Botanicals for Improving Human Health. *Am. J. Clin. Nutr.* **2008,** *87*, 472S–475S.

Richter, R. K. Herbal Medicine: Chaos in the Marketplace. Haworth Herbal Press: New York, 2003.

Rieder, S. A.; Chauhan, A.; Singh, U.; Nagarkatti, M.; Nagarkatti, P. Cannabinoid-induced Apoptosis in Immune Cells as a Pathway to Immunosuppression. *Immunobiology* **2010,** *215*, 598–605.

Sacchetti, G.; Maietti, S.; Muzzoli, M.; Scaglianti, M.; Manfredini, S.; Radice, M.; Bruni, R. Comparative Evaluation of 11 Essential Oils of Different Origin as Functional Antioxidants, Antiradicals and Antimicrobials in Foods. *Food Chem.* **2005,** *91*(4), 621–632.

Sadekar, R. D.; Kolte, A. Y.; Barmase, B. S.; Desai, V. F. Immunopotentiating Effects of Azadirachta Indica (Neem) Dry Leaves Powder in Broilers: Naturally Infected with IBD Virus. *Indian J. Exp. Biol.* **1998,** *36*, 1151–1153.

Saha, S.; Galhardi, L. C.; Yamamoto, K. A.; Linhares, R. E.; Bandyopadhyay, S. S.; Sinha, S., et al. Water Extracted Polysaccharides from *Azadirachta Indica* Leaves: Structural Features, Chemical Modification and The Anti-bovine Herpesvirus Type 1 (BoHV-1) Activity. *Int. J. Biol. Macromol.* **2010,** *47*(5), 640–645.

Saini, A.; Sharma, S.; Chhibber, S. Induction of Resistance to Respiratory Tract Infection with Klebsiella Pneumoniae in Mice Fed on a Diet Supplemented with Tulsi (*Ocimum Sanctum*) and Clove (*Syzgiumaromaticum*) Oils. *J. Microbiol. Immunol. Infect.* **2009,** *42*, 107–113.

Sanctum, L. D. O. Tulsi: A Potent Medicinal Herb. *Webmed Central Pharmacol.* **2010,** *1*(11), 1–12.

SARS. *Clinical Trials on Treatment Using a Combination of Traditional Chinese Medicine and Western Medicine*; WHO: Geneva; 2003; pp 53–61.

Sashidhara, K. V. *Natural Products as Drugs*. http://publications.nigms.nih.gov/medbydesign/medbydesign.pdf

Selvam, R.; Subramanian, L.; Gayathri, R.; Angayarkanni, N. The Anti-oxidant Activity of Turmeric (*Curcuma Longa*). *J. Ethnopharmacol.* **1995,** *47*, 59–67.

Shokri, H. A Review on the Inhibitory Potential of Nigella Sativa Against Pathogenic and Toxigenic Fungi. *Avicenna J. Phytomed.* **2016,** *6*(1), 21–33.

Shrestha, D. K.; Sapkota, H.; Baidya, P.; Basnet, S. Antioxidant and Antibacterial Activities of *Allium Sativum* and Allium Cepa. *Bull. Pharm. Res.* **2016,** *6*, 50–55.

Singh, N.; Hoette, Y.; Miller, R. *Tulsi: The Mother Medicine of Nature*, 2nd ed; Lucknow: International Institute of Herbal Medicine, 2010; pp 28–47.

Singh, V.; Amdekar, S.; Verma, O. Ocimum Sanctum (tulsi): Bio-pharmacological Activities. *Webmed Central Pharmacol.* **2010,** *1*, WMC001046. DOI: 10.9754/journal.wmc.001046

Siswomihardjo, W.; Badawi, S. S.; Nishimura, M.; Hamada, T. The Difference of Antibacterial Effect of Neem Leaves and Stick Extracts. *Int. Chin. J. Dent.* **2007,** *7*, 27–29.

Srivastava, S.; Lal, V. K.; Pant, K. K. Polyherbal Formulations Based on Indian Medicinal Plants as Antidiabetic Phytotherapeutics. *Phytopharmacology* **2013,** *2*, 1–15.

Stall, A.; Seebeck, E. Chemical Investigations of Alliin, and the Specific Principle of Garlic. *Adv. Enzymol.* **1951,** *11*, 377–400.

Subapriya, R.; Nagini, S. Medicinal Properties of Neem Leaves: A Review. *Curr. Med. Chem. Anti. Cancer Agents* **2005,** *5*, 149–156.

Subramanian, L.; Selvam, R. Prevention of C4-induced Hepatotoxicity by Aqueous Extract of Turmeric. *Nutr. Res.* **1999,** *19*, 429–441.

Suleria, H. A. R.; Butt, M. S.; Khalid, N.; Sultan, S.; Raza, A.; Aleem, M.; Abbas, M. Garlic (Allium Sativum): Diet Based Therapy of 21st Century–A Review. *Asian Pac. J. Trop. Dis.* **2015,** *5*, 271–278.

Tagoe, D. N. A.; Nyarko, H. D.; Akpaka, R. A Comparison of Antifungal Properties of Onion (*Allium Cepa*), Ginger (*Zingiber Officinale*) and Garlic (*Allium Sativum*) against *Aspergillus Flavus*: *Aspergillus niger* and *Cladosporium Herbarum*. *Res. J. Med. Plants.* **2011,** *5*, 281–287.

The Ayurvedic Centre-Historical Uses of Ayurvedic Herbs. http://www.holheal.com/index.html (accessed Jun 22, 2013).

Theuretzbacher, U. Accelerating Resistance, Inadequate Antibacterial Drug Pipelines and International Responses. *Int. J. Antimicrob. Agents* **2012,** *39*(4), 295–299.

Thoh, M.; Kumar, P.; Nagarajaram, H. A.; Manna, S. K. Azadirachtin Interacts with the Tumor Necrosis Factor (TNF) Binding Domain of Its Receptors and Inhibits TNF-induced Biological Responses. *J. Biol. Chem.* **2010,** *285*(8), 5888–5895.

Thyagarajan, S. P.; Jayaram, S.; Gopalakrishnan, V.; Hari, R.; Jeyakumar, P.; Sripathi, M. S. Herbal Medicines for Liver Diseases in India. *J. Gastroenterol. Hepatol.* **2002,** *17*(Suppl. 3), S370–S376.

Tilburt, J. C.; Kaptchuk, T. J. J. Herbal Medicine Research and Global Health: An Ethical Analysis. *Bull. World Health Organ.* **2008,** *86*(8), 594–599.

Tiwari, V.; Darmani, N. A.; Yue, B. Y.; Shukla, D. *In Vitro* Antiviral Activity of Neem (*Azadirachta Indica* L.) Bark Extract Against Herpes Simplex Virus Type-1 Infection. *Phytother. Res.* **2010,** *24*(8), 1132–1140.

Tomei, L.; Altamura, S.; Paonessa, G.; De Francesco, R.; Migliaccio, G. HCV Antiviral Resistance: The Impact of In Vitro Studies on the Development of Antiviral Agents Targeting the Viral NS5B Polymerase. *Antivir. Chem. Chemother.* **2005,** *16*(4), 225–245.

Tripathi, A. K.; Rajora, V. S.; Gupta, D. K.; Shukla, S. K. Immunomodulatory Activity of *Ocimum Sanctum* and Its Influence on Cyclophosphamide Induced Immunosuppression. *Indian J. Anim. Sci.* **2008,** *78*, 33–36.

United Nations Environment Programme. *Neem: The UN's Tree of the 21st Century*. United Nations Environment Programme: Nairobi 2012; http://www.unep.org/wed/tree-a-day/neem.asp

University of Maryland Medical Center, Author, 2013. http://umm.edu/health/medical/altmed/treatment/herbal-medicine#ixzz2kkQZ5fJX.

Upadhyay, S. N.; Dhawan, S.; Garg, S.; Talwar, G. P. Immunomodulatory Effects of Neem (Azadirachta Indica) Oil. *Int. J. Immunopharmacol.* **1992,** *14*, 1187–1193.

Upma, A.; Ashok, K.; Pankaj, K.; Tarun, K. The Nature's Gift to Mankind: Neem. *IRJP* **2011,** *2*(10), 13–15.

Van der Hoek, L. Human Coronaviruses: What Do They Cause. *Antivir. Ther.* **2007,** *12*, 651–658.

Vasudevan, P.; Kashyap, S.; Sharma, S. Bioactive Botanicals from Basil (*Ocimum sp.*). *J. Sci. Ind. Res. (C)* **1999,** *58*, 332–338.

Ventola, L. C. The Antibiotic Resistance Crisis: Causes and Threats. *Pharm. Therap.* **2015,** *40*(4), 277–283.

Vuorelaa, P.; Leinonenb, M.; Saikkuc, P.; Tammelaa, P.; Rauhad, J. P.; Wennberge, T.; Vuorela, H. Natural Products in the Process of Finding New Drug Candidates. *Curr. Med. Chem.* **2004,** *11*, 1375–1389.

White, B. Ginger: An Overview. *Am. Fam. Physician* **2007,** *75*(11), 1689–1691.

WHO Traditional Medicine Strategy 2002–2005. WHO: Geneva; 2002.

Willcox, M. L.; Bodeker, G. Traditional Herbal Medicines for Malaria. *BMJ* **2004,** *329*, 1156–1159.

World Health Organization (WHO). General Guidelines for Methodologies on Research and Evaluation of Traditional Medicines, 2001.

World Health Organization (WHO). General Guidelines for Methodologies on Research and Evaluation of Traditional Medicines. 2001.

World Health Organization. General Guidelines for Methodologies on Research and Evaluation of Traditional Medicine. World Health Organization: Geneva, 2000b; WHO/EDM/TRM/2000.1.

World Health Organization. http://www.who.int (accessed Sep 18, 2013).

World Health Organization. *Traditional Medicine Fact Sheet No 134*. 2017. http://www.siav-itvas.org/images/stories/doc/.../WHO_Traditional_medicine_2008.pdf/

Worthen, D. R.; Ghosheh, O. A.; Crooks, P. A. The In Vitro Anti-tumor Activity of Some Crude and Purified Components of Blackseed, *Nigella sativa* L. *Anticancer Res.* **1998,** *18*, 1527–1532.

Wu, C.; Wang, C.; Tsai, M.; Huang, W.; Kennedy, J. Trend and Pattern of Herb and Supplement Use in the United States: Results from the 2002, 2007, and 2012 National Health Interview Surveys. *Evid. Based Complement Altern. Med.* **2014,** 872320.

Xu, J.; Song, X.; Yin, Z. Q.; Cheng, A. C.; Jia, R. Y.; Deng, Y. X., et al. Antiviral Activity and Mode of Action of Extracts from Need Seed Kernel Against Duck Plague Virus *In Vitro*. *Poult. Sci.* **2012,** *91*(11), 2802–2807.

Xu, J.; Song, X.; Yin, Z. Q.; Cheng, A. C.; Jia, R. Y.; Deng, Y. X.; Ye, K. C.; Shi, C. F.; Lv, C.; Zhang, W. Antiviral Activity and Mode of Action of Extracts from Neem Seed Kernel Against Duck Plague Virus *In Vitro*. *Poult. Sci.* **2012,** *91*(11), 2802–2807.

Yang, A. P.; Liu, J. P.; Tao, W. Q.; Li, H. M. The Diagnostic and Predictive Role of NLR, d-NLR and PLR in COVID-19 Patients. *Int. Immunopharmacol.* **2020,** *84*, 106504.

Yu, Z. F.; Kong, L. D.; Chen, Y. Antidepressant Activity of Aqueous Extracts of *Curcuma Longa* in Mice. *J. Ethnopharmacol.* **2002,** *83*, 161–165.

Yue, G. G.; Chan, B. C.; Hon, P. M.; Kennelly, E. J.; Yeung, S. K.; Cassileth, B. R.; et al. Immunostimulatory Activities of Polysaccharide Extract Isolated from *Curcuma Longa*. *Int. J. Biol. Macromol.* **2010,** *47*, 342–347.

Zamiska, N. On the Trail of Ancient Cures. *Wall St. J.* **2006,** *November 15*, B1, B12.

Zaoui, A.; Cherrah, Y.; Lacaille-Dubois, M. A.; Settaf, A.; Amarouch, H.; Hassar, M. Diuretic and Hypotensive Effects of *Nigella Sativa* in the Spontaneously Hypertensive Rat. *Therapie* **2000,** *55*, 379–382.

Zarogoulidis, P.; Papanas, N.; Kioumis, I.; Chatzaki, E.; Maltezos, E.; Zarogoulidis, K. Macrolides: From In Vitro Anti-inflammatory and Immunomodulatory Properties to Clinical Practice in Respiratory Diseases. *Eur. J. Clin. Pharmacol.* **2012,** *68*(5), 479–503.

Zaslawski, C.; Davis, S. The Ethics of Complementary and Alternative Medicine Research: A Case Study of Traditional Chinese Medicine at the University of Technology, Sydney. *Monash Bioeth. Rev.* **2005,** *24*, 52–60.

Zhang, Y. Q.; Xu, J.; Yin, Z. Q.; Jia, R. Y.; Lu, Y.; Yang, F., et al. Isolation and Identification of the Antibacterial Active Compound from Petroleum Ether Extract of Neem Oil. *Fitoterapia* **2010,** *81*(7), 747–750.

Zhong, P.; Yu, Q.; Zhong, Y.; Jiao, X.; Ren, Y.; Yang, L., et al. Antibacterial Activity of 9-octadecanoic Acid-hexadecanoic Acid-tetrahydrofuran-3,4-diyl Ester from Neem Oil. *Agr. Sci. China* **2010,** *9*(8), 1236–1240.

Zhu, F. C.; Li, Y. H.; Guan, X. H.; Hou, L. H.; Wang, W. J.; Li, J. X.; Wu, S. P.; Wang, B. S.; Wang, Z.; Wang, L.; Jia, S. Y.; Jiang, H. D.; Wang, L.; Jiang, T.; Hu, Y.; Gou, J. B.; Xu, S. B.; Xu, J. J.; Wang, X. W.; Wang, W.; Chen, W. Safety, Tolerability, and Immunogenicity of a Recombinant Adenovirus Type-5 Vectored COVID-19 Vaccine: A Dose-escalation, Open-label, Non-randomised, First-in-human Trial. *Lancet* **2020,** *395*(10240), 1845–1854.

Zorofchian Moghadamtousi, S.; Hajrezaei, M.; Abdul Kadir, H.; Zandi, K. *Loranthus Micranthus* Linn: Biological Activities and Phytochemistry. *Evid. Based Complement. Alternat. Med.* **2013,** 9 pages. 273712.

CHAPTER 4

COVID-19 Pandemic: Role of Ayurveda for Prevention and Treatment

BHUSHAN R. RANE[1], TEJAS S. TELANGE[1], PRANIT S. WAGHCHAURE[1], RAJ K. KESERVANI[2], and ASHISH S. JAIN[1]

[1]*Department of Pharmaceutics, Shri D. D. Vispute College of Pharmacy & Research Center, Panvel, Maharashtra, India*

[2]*Faculty of B. Pharmacy, CSM Group of Institutions, Prayagraj, Uttar Pradesh, India*

ABSTRACT

The coronavirus disease 2019 (COVID-19) is a relatively new infectious disease characterized by atypical pneumonia and caused by severe acute respiratory syndrome coronavirus-2 (SARS-CoV-2). The virus is highly contagious among people and has produced a worldwide pandemic that led to a dramatic loss of human life worldwide. Fever, sore throat, tiredness, cough, and dyspnea are common symptoms of COVID-19, especially when paired with recent exposure. Supportive care measures like ventilation oxygenation, supplemental oxygen therapy, and fluid control are still the gold standard. Only in the setting of randomized clinical trials can antiviral be demonstrated to be safe and efficacious. Several drugs are now being tested, including chloroquine, hydroxychloroquine, favipiravir, monoclonal antibodies, angiotensin-2 receptor antagonists, antisense RNA, and corticosteroids. Along with this modern western medicine treatment, "Ayurvedic" medicine is getting prominence as an immunity booster and a way to keep the disease from progressing to symptomatic

COVID-19 and Immunomodulation with Special Emphasis on Nutraceutical and Herbal Formulation.
Rajesh K. Kesharwani & Raj K. Keservani (Eds)

and severe stages. The goal of this article is to summarize the most recent research discoveries and to cover key aspects of SARS-CoV-2 genetics, pathophysiology, and the host-immune response. Other research provides information on how to manage the outbreak and expand our understanding of this emerging infectious illness, along with current recommendations for diagnosis, prevention, and treatment of this pandemic.

4.1 INTRODUCTION

The current worldwide pandemic, coronavirus disease 2019 (COVID-19), is an infectious disease caused by the severe acute respiratory syndrome coronavirus 2 (SARS-CoV-2) and has spread widely over the world. A new beta coronavirus was discovered as the pathogen (2019-n-CoV) (Rathore and Ghosh, 2020). China was made aware of cases of "viral pneumonia" in Wuhan, the People's Republic of China, on December 31, 2019. This necessitated an exhalation. This broke out in a seafood wholesale market in Wuhan, China's Huanan seafood wholesale market (Holshue et al., 2020). Diseases spread uncontrollably from Wuhan to adjacent provinces (Hubei, Zhejiang, Henan, Guangdong, Hunan, etc.) and cities (Beijing and Shanghai) (Wu et al., 2020). Furthermore, the disease has now spread around the world, resulting in a pandemic.

During the initial outbreak of 2019-n-CoV in China, the virus and disease were typically referred to as "Wuhan coronavirus" and "Wuhan pneumonia," accordingly. COVID-19 (CO for corona, VI for the virus, D for disease, and 19 for the year the outbreak was first discovered) and SARS-CoV-2 were officially named by the World Health Organization (WHO) on February 11, 2020 (The New York Times, 2021; Eurosurveillance, 2020). With about 220 countries and territories, 2019-n-CoV has affected a large number of people around the world (Islam et al., 2020).

The respiratory system and other body system organs are particularly affected by the SARS-CoV-2 virus. People get infected when they breathe, talk, cough, or sneeze into air that has been contaminated with droplets and minute airborne particles (Centers for Disease Control and Prevention, 2021; Greenhalgh et al., 2021). Infectivity can occur as early as 3 days prior to the onset of symptoms. More than 208,968,322 cases and 3422,527 deaths had been documented globally as of August 11, 2021, with numbers rapidly increasing in several nations. Visit the WHO website for the most up-to-date information on COVID-19 (https://www.who.int/emergencies/diseases/novel-coronavirus-2019) (World Health Organization, 2021).

4.2 HISTORY AND BACKGROUND

A hospital in Wuhan, Huanan Province, noticed numerous atypical cases of pneumonia in December 2019 (Zhou et al., 2020). Dry cough, dyspnea, and bilateral lung infiltrates were the most frequently encountered symptoms among these patients. The coronavirus cases were promptly reported to the WHO's China field offices. On December 31, 2019, a large number of cases were recorded, and investigations revealed that the disease originated in the Huanan seafood market, a wet market. The market sold a wide range of vertebrates and invertebrate' species, both wild and farm raised, and was declared closed on January 1, 2020 (Wu et al., 2020). The pathogen responsible for the peculiar pneumonia was identified as the new coronavirus by Chinese researchers on January 7, 2020. China registers the first death on January 11, 2020, and a day later shares the genetic sequence of the unique coronavirus with the rest of the world, which might be extremely helpful in developing and constructing a diagnostic tool for the novel coronavirus. The first case of the novel coronavirus was discovered in Thailand on January 13, 2020, followed by a burst of cases in the United States on January 20, 2020 (Holshue et al., 2020), and a swift detection in Europe on January 24, 2020, with the identification of the first three cases (Spiteri et al., 2020). By the end of January 2020, coronavirus had been discovered to have originated from wild bats and to belong to the same family as SARS; thus, this coronavirus is known as SARS-CoV-2. By January 30, 2020, the WHO will have declared coronavirus a global public health emergency. The first fatality outside of China occurred on February 2, 2020, in the Philippines (The New York Times, 2021). On February 11, 2020, WHO declared that the atypical pneumonia disease's official name would be COVID-19 and that the cause would be SARS-CoV-2 (World Health Organization, 2020). The first death in Europe occurred in France on February 15, 2020 (Spiteri et al., 2020), followed by an outbreak in Iran on February 19, 2020, and on March 11, 2020, COVID-19 has proclaimed a global pandemic, with coronavirus cases continuing to rise since then.

4.3 ETIOLOGY

Coronaviruses are enclosed, positive-sense, single-stranded RNA viruses with a genomic size of 26–32 kb that belong to the coronaviridae family's orthocoronavirinae subfamily (Cascella et al., 2020; Chan et al., 2013). Based on their genetic architecture, these are further split into four genera: α, β, γ, and δ (Yuki et al., 2020). Only mammals are infected by α and β coronaviruses (Rabi et al., 2020). Human coronaviruses, such as 229E and NL63, are responsible for the common cold and croup and are categorized as coronaviruses. Within coronaviruses, severe acute respiratory syndrome coronavirus (SARS-CoV), Middle East respiratory syndrome coronavirus, and SARS-CoV-2 are mentioned. Fever, cough, and respiratory problems are common symptoms of beta-coronaviruses that have produced epidemics in humans. Embecovirus (lineage-A), serbecovirus (lineage-B), merbecovirus (lineage-C), and nobecovirus (lineage-D) are the four lineages recognized within the genus *Betacoronavirus*. SARS-CoV-2 is designated as a serbecovirus (lineages-B). "Severe Acute Respiratory Syndrome" or "SARS" was the first coronavirus to cause serious sickness, and it was initially detected at the end of February 2003 in Foshan, China. The second was the Middle East respiratory disease caused by a coronavirus, which was discovered in Saudi Arabia in 2012. Civet cats and dromedary camels, respectively, transmitted both to humans (Wiersinga et al., 2020; Zhong et al., 2003; Zaki et al., 2012). The genome of the novel beta coronavirus (2019-n-CoV) had a nucleotide identity of 89% with bat SARS-like-CoVZXC21 and 82% with human SARS-CoV. In a conclusion, the novel coronavirus (2019-n-CoV) was dubbed SARS-CoV-2 (Chen et al., 2020). "SARS-CoV-2" most likely arose from a strain seen in bats, according to genomic analysis, which demonstrated a significant degree of similarity between "SARS-CoV-2 and RaTG13" of bats (*Rhinolophus affinis*) (Chen et al., 2020; Andersen et al., 2020).

4.4 PATHOPHYSIOLOGY

The SARS-CoV-2, a beta coronavirus with a characteristic "crown-like" shape seen in electron micrographs, is the cause of COVID-19. SARS-CoV-2 has a diameter of 60–140 nm (Gosain et al., 2020) and is made up of single-stranded positive RNA that is encased and protected by a lipid bilayer and membrane proteins that contain four structural proteins: spike (S), membrane (M), envelop (E), and nucleocapsid (N) (Gavriatopoulou et al., 2020). The spike protein is made up of two subunits: S1 connects to the host's cell receptor, whereas S2 attaches to the viral body and plays a key role in viral body fusion into host cells (Parasher, 2020). The virus mostly affects the respiratory system and is spread through contact droplets and fomites from an infectious individual who is symptomatic or asymptomatic. The "incubation period," or the interval between infection and onset of symptoms, is between 2 and 14 days (Harrison et al., 2020). The coronavirus slowly and gradually triggers a response within the lungs during the incubation phase.

The alveoli, also known as "air sacs" or "air spaces," are found in the lungs. The alveoli, which are hollow cup-shaped cavities and the main functional unit of the lungs that forms the lungs physiology, are the work-horses of the lungs. The alveolar membrane is where oxygen and carbon dioxide are exchanged and where we breathe in oxygen and exhale carbon dioxide. Three major alveolar cells make up the alveoli wall. There are two kinds of "pneumocytes," as well as a massive "phagocytic cell" known as an "alveolar macrophage." Type-1 cells also referred to as "type-1 pneumocytes" or "type-1 alveolar cells" are the cells that make up the alveoli structure. Type-2 cells, also described as "type-2 pneumocytes" or "type-2 alveolar cells," create pulmonary surfactant, which cushions the inner lining of the alveoli, lowers surface tension, keeps alveoli open, and allows for oxygen and carbon dioxide exchange. They also differentiate to restore damaged type-1 cells. SARS-CoV-2 assaults alveolar epithelial cells, which are predominantly found on type-2 pneumocytes and are only present in the alveoli, causing respiratory symptoms.

4.4.1 MECHANISM

The coronavirus utilizes "surface proteins" termed spike proteins to target and bind to the angiotensin-converting enzyme-2 (ACE-2) receptor and enzyme on the surface of type-2 alveolar cells. Spike protein-derived cell invasion was thought to rely on both ACE-2 and the host cellular transmembrane protease serine precursor-2 (Li et al., 2020). The ACE-2 receptor is essential for viral entry into the host cells. These receptors are found on a variety of cell types, primarily nasal, and bronchial epithelial cells, and are predominately found on type-2 alveolar cells in organs such as the lungs, heart, small intestine, large intestine, and kidneys (Wiersinga et al., 2020; Shi et al., 2020). SARS-CoV-2 enters by endocytosis or direct fusion of the viral envelope with the host membrane (Parasher, 2020). Once within the host cell, the virus particles become uncoated, and the virus's genome enters the cytoplasm. Because coronaviruses have positive single-strand (+ss) RNA, they can synthesize their proteins and fresh viral genome directly in the cytoplasm by targeting the host ribosomes. The viral genome will interact with an enzyme called "RNA-dependent RNA polymerase" (RdRP), which enters the nucleus through the importin channel and then replicates to generate multiple single-stranded (ss) viral RNAs. Ribosomes will translate viral RNA into proteins, which will be used to produce RNA polymerase. RNA polymerase will then read the virus's positive strand of RNA to create a negative RNA strand. RNA polymerase will use the negative strand to generate a positive RNA strand and other tiny positive RNA strands (Yang and Shen, 2020). These short RNA strands will be scanned by the host's ribosome in the endoplasmic reticulum (ER) to assist in the formation of the virus's structural components. The ER will deliver these auxiliary and structural proteins to the Golgi apparatus, where they will be neatly wrapped around the positive RNA strand to form a new virus or viral bodies (Harrison et al., 2020). Exocytosis allows these young new viruses or offspring viruses to be discharged from the host cells (Yang and Shen, 2020). The macrophages will now recognize these new viral particles as antigens.

4.4.2 HOST RESPONSE

While the virus replicates in alveolar cells, it also destroys them and most likely triggers an inflammatory response. Injured alveolar cells release interferons, cytokines, and intracellular components such as DAMPS. Interferon acts in a paracrine manner that has a variety of effects on the cells around it, preparing them to defend against viral infection. The major role is to induce protection against viruses and non-infected cells in the surrounding area. The alveolar macrophages detect cell injury through the alveolar cells' "Damage associated molecular patterns." Injured alveolar cells also emit cytokines, which they respond to. This induces alveolar macrophages to release cytokines such tumor necrosis factor (TNF), interleukin-1 (IL-1), interleukin-6 (IL-6), and interleukin-8 (IL-8) as well as chemokines like "Granulocyte-Colony Stimulating Factor" and

"Monocyte Chemoattractant Protein-1" (Parasher, 2020; Yao et al., 2021). The inflammatory process in the lung parenchyma stimulates the nerve endings that cause the cough reflex to activate. Early on, these individuals usually have a dry cough.

The TNF, IL-1, and IL-6 are proinflammatory cytokines produced primarily by activated macrophages with increased vascular permeability while also increasing adhesion molecule expression. More immune cells, such as neutrophils and monocytes, can be recruited as a consequence of this (Cascella et al., 2020). They will bind to these adhesion proteins and travel to the injured area. T cells and other chemokines will attract neutrophils, while IL-8 will attract monocytes (Xu et al., 2020). Increased vascular permeability promotes fluid leakage into the interstitial, resulting in interstitial edema, and then into the alveoli, resulting in pulmonary edema, as well as dyspnea and decreased oxygenation, resulting in hypoxemia (low oxygen levels in the blood) (Azer, 2020). White blood cell (WBC) counts in serum rise when the number of circulating macrophages and neutrophils rises (Yuki et al., 2020). Neutrophils begin devouring viruses and other debris in the area, which might be hazardous after a while since chemicals are released as a by-product, causing damage to the surrounding tissues. As a result, we have damaged alveolar cells all around, which means less surfactant is produced, prompting the alveoli to collapse and oxygenation to be compromised, resulting in hypoxemia (Chen et al., 2020). Other inflammatory mediators released by injured endothelium cells and WBC include arachidonic acid metabolites, "prostaglandins" (PGs), and "leukotrienes." These leukotrienes will now promote bronchi constriction, which will limit breathing and result in hypoxemia. The PGs, IL-1, IL-6, and TNF are all involved in the development of fever, which is a major characteristic of COVID-19. Chemoreceptors in the aortic arch and the brain are stimulated by low oxygen levels in the blood. The brain's cardiopulmonary center will be stimulated by the stimulated chemoreceptors, which will signal the lungs to breathe more to increase oxygen levels in the blood and the heart to beat faster to transport oxygen to all body organs. As a result, patients with hypoxemia are frequently tachypneic and tachycardic. Some people may be infected with a virus but not show symptoms because their immune system suppresses it, resulting in relatively minimal symptoms such as coughing, shortness of breath, and a low-grade temperature (between 99.5°F and 101°F) (Oran and Topol, 2021).

Lymphopenia, which occurs more commonly in severe coronavirus cases and almost invariably results in a drop in T-cell numbers, is a common observation in viral infection in general, which includes COVID-19. The "neutrophil-to-lymphocyte ratio," "monocyte-to-lymphocyte ratio," and cytokine levels all rose over time (Tavakolpour et al., 2020). In the course of viral infection, cytokines play a critical role in immunopathology. Immunological harm to the human body can be caused by uncontrolled and excessive immune responses (Ye et al., 2020). Patients with severe SARS-CoV-2 had significantly greater cytokine and chemokine levels than patients with mild-to-moderate SARS-CoV-2 (Coperchini et al., 2020). We have rapidly boosted levels of cytokines and chemokines that attract a large number of inflammatory cells, such as neutrophils and monocytes, resulting in an excessive infiltration of inflammatory cells into lung tissue and consequently lung injury (Ye et al., 2020). Increased amounts of proinflammatory cytokines (TNF, IL-6, IL-1) are produced as mononuclear macrophages accumulate (Coperchini et al., 2020). IL-6 is a powerful proinflammatory cytokine that was also generated during this phase and has a wide range of impacts. C-reactive protein (CRP) is tested in the blood and is an excellent marker of inflammation. It induces hepatocytes to generate acute-phase reactants such as CRP, fibrinogen, and hepcidin (Shi et al., 2020). ARDS is the most common cause of COVID-19. It is characterized by a damaged lung accumulation of fluid ventilation/perfusion mismatch and hypoxemia (Harrison et al., 2020; Shi et al., 2020). People with COVID-19 have varying degrees of severity; now, the majority of cases have a mild infection (80%), about 15% have severe disease with hypoxemia, dyspnea, and lung changes seen on imaging, and 5% are critically ill with respiratory failure from ARDS or multiorgan dysfunction (Wang and Ma, 2008), which involves the liver (such as liver derangement), and the heart can leak troponin. The cytokine storm promotes ARDS, or multiorgan dysfunction, and is a major contributor to COVID-19 aggravation or death.

4.5 SIGN AND SYMPTOMS FOR COVID-19

Fever, dry cough, and fatigue are the most common COVID-19 symptoms.

Other less common symptoms that may affect some patients include loss of taste or smell, conjunctivitis, nasal congestion (also known as red eyes) a scratchy throat, headache, muscle or joint pain, skin rash of various types, nausea or vomiting diarrhea, and dizziness or chills.

4.5.1 *SEVERE COVID-19 SYMPTOMS*

Severe COVID-19 symptoms include Difficulty breathing, appetite loss, and confusion, chest discomfort or pressure that persists, temperatures exceeding 38°C.

4.5.2 *SOME OF THE LESS PREVALENT SYMPTOMS*

Some of the less prevalent symptoms are as follows: irritability, confusion, reduced consciousness (often linked with seizures), anxiety, depression, and sleep difficulties are some of the less prevalent symptoms.

4.5.3 *MORE SEVERE AND INFREQUENT NEUROLOGICAL CONSEQUENCES*

More severe and infrequent neurological consequences are as follows: strokes, brain inflammation, disorientation, and nerve damage (Yuki et al., 2020; Parasher, 2020).

4.6 VARIANTS OF CORONAVIRUS

The SARS-CoV-2 has four dominant forms that are currently circulating around the world. The Greek alphabet should be used to designate the variants, according to the WHO.

Alpha (B.1.1.7) was first discovered in London and Kent and was formerly known as UK variation. Scientists estimate that these mutations could increase the virus's transmissibility by up to 70%, making it easier to spread. The alpha form has a mutation in the spike protein, which aids the virus in infecting its host.

Beta (B.1.351), formerly known as the South Africa variety, was first discovered in South Africa and Nigeria.

Gamma (P.1), also known as the Brazil variety, was initially discovered in Brazil. The gamma version of the virus appears to be more infectious than earlier strains.

Delta (B.1.617.2) is a recognized Indian variation that was initially discovered in India. The highly contagious form is producing more instances of COVID-19 in children and teenagers (World Health Organization, 2021; The Centers for Disease Control and Prevention, 2020).

4.7 DIAGNOSIS

4.7.1 MOLECULAR TEST

Molecular diagnostic tests look for virus components in samples taken from the upper respiratory tract (nasal- and oropharyngeal samples) and lower respiratory tract (expectorated sputum and bronchoalveolar lavage (only for mechanically ventilated patients) because they seem to stay positive for an extended period of time, molecular diagnostic tests look for virus components in samples taken from the upper respiratory tract (nasal- and oropharyngeal samples) and lower respiratory tract (expectorated sputum and bronchoalveolar lavage (only for mechanically ventilated patients). The obtained samples must be kept at 4°C until they are sent to the laboratory, where the genetic material is amplified using reverse polymerase chain reaction (RT-PCR) or real-time RT-PCR (Cascella et al., 2020). Now, from an existing viral RNA molecule, a double-stranded DNA molecule must be synthesized. On the amplified genetic material, the conserved portions of the SARS-CoV-2 genetic code are eventually detected. If the test is positive, it is recommended that the test be repeated for verification and that the evaluation be repeated to check for viral clearance. Because 53.3% of COVID-19-confirmed patients had positive oropharyngeal swabs, and 71% of patients were RT-PCR positive with sputum samples, the molecular test is insensitive and may not be very reliable (Fang et al., 2020).

4.7.2 SEROLOGY

The specificity and sensitivity of a serology or antibody test are both limited. Serology diagnosis aids in the detection of antibodies produced in response to infection. A blood sample is required for this test since antibodies take a few weeks to form and may remain in the blood for weeks or months after recovery. As a result, a positive test result simply confirms that a person has been exposed to the virus, not that they are infected. It should not be used to diagnose COVID-19. The specificity of the serology test appears to be greater than 99%, with a sensitivity of 96% (Cascella et al., 2020; Wiersinga et al., 2020). These tests are especially beneficial:

1. If a virus test is not available, a serology test together with the clinical picture may be used to make decisions.
2. Patients with late-stage disease complications and their doctors must make quick decisions (the viral test takes more time to get the results).
3. In certain patients, viral shedding is reduced, resulting in falsely negative RT-qPCR results. In serum, plasma, and whole blood, the serology test can identify "immunoglobulin M" and "immunoglobulin G" antibodies against SARS-CoV-2 (Loeffelholz and Tang, 2020).

4.7.3 LABORATORY EXAMINATIONS

- A normal or decreased WBC count and lymphopenia can be seen in many cases at the beginning of the disease, which is interestingly believed to be a terrible prognostic.
- Lactate dehydrogenase, CRP, creatine kinase, liver enzymes, aspartate aminotransferase, and alanine aminotransferase levels are all elevated.
- Some patients have an increased "neutrophil-to-lymphocyte ratio." The inflammatory storm can be expressed by the "platelet-to-lymphocyte ratio."
- In a critical stage, increased "D-dimer" levels persist in blood cells, and a rapid multiorgan imbalance (high amylase, coagulation problems, etc.) is discovered (Cascella et al., 2020; Parasher, 2020).
- In severe cases, coagulation abnormalities might be seen, as evidenced by an increase in prothrombin time and the international normalized ratio (Gosain et al., 2020).

4.7.4 IMAGING

4.7.4.1 CHEST X-RAY EXAMINATION

Within the diagnostic procedure, management, and follow-up, radiological imaging plays a critical role. The "chest radiograph" is frequently uncertain and has limited sensitivity in detecting early lung alterations in the early stages of the disease, and it can be completely negative. The chest X-ray examination usually shows bilateral multifocal alveolar opacities, which tend to meet up to the entire opacity of the lung as the infection develops in the more advanced or critical phases of illness. Pleural effusion is a possibility (Cascella et al., 2020).

4.7.4.2 CHEST-COMPUTED TOMOGRAPHY

Even at the earliest stages of sickness, chest-computed tomography (CT), particularly high-resolution CT, was the method of choice in the research of COVID-19 pneumonia. Multifocal bilateral "ground or ground glass" (GG) areas with patchy distribution, generally peripheral/subpleural, combined with increasing involvement of the posterior regions and lower lobes, are the most typical results. Some of the patients have the "reversed halo sign," which is defined as a central area of patchy opacities surrounded by a peripheral ring with consolidation. Cavitations, calcifications, lymph-adenopathies, and pleural effusion are among the other findings (Cascella et al., 2020; Buda et al., 2020).

4.7.4.3 LUNG ULTRASOUND

COVID-19 infections have characteristics of interstitial pneumonia, such as an irregular pleural line, B-lines (multifocal, discrete, or confluent), small (centomeric) consolidations, both nontranslobar and translobar consolidations, and a multilobar distribution of abnormalities, which can be seen on ultrasound. The pleural cavity's fluid is scant and occurs in small amounts (Cascella et al., 2020; Buda et al., 2020; Peng et al., 2020). The ultrasonography results were as follows:

- Thickened/Irregular pleural line,
- B-line at the times of confluent,
- Using an air bronchogram to consolidate,
- Consolidations of the sub-pleura,
- Pleural consolidation with localized pleural fibrosis.

At the early and mild phases of infection, ultrasonography abnormalities on the lungs may be apparent. As the disease progresses, the number of B-lines in the patient increases, resulting in the interstitial syndrome, which is followed by the alveolar–interstitial syndrome, and finally the white lung (Peng et al., 2020). In patients with COVID-19, the posterior chest zones are frequently contaminated. The more B-line artifacts are seen, the more interstitial tissue is impacted.

4.8 TREATMENTS

The number of new confirmed and suspected COVID-19 cases has been decreasing globally as a result of government actions, control measures, and best practices for supportive management, as well as changes in personal behavior (such as social isolation, sanitization, and mask use). The enormous outbreak that spread across the globe is still a huge issue for clinicians, and the risk of transmission has not been eliminated. Supportive care treatments such as invasive mechanical ventilation oxygenation, supplemental oxygen therapy, and hydration control are still the global standard. Various clinical trials are attempting to identify the most effective treatment or combination against this pandemic disease, and patients are highly encouraged to enroll in ongoing trials. Darunavir, favipiravir, nafamostat mesylate, and other therapeutic drugs are currently employed. In Table 4.1, monoclonal antibodies, corticosteroids, anticoagulants, angiotensin 2 receptor antagonists, and antibacterials are assessed.

Ayurveda is a traditional Indian medicine system that is one of the world's oldest holistic healing systems. The old Ayurvedic scriptures, "Charaka Samhita" and "Sushruta Samhita," address epidemic management and define immunity as the ability to avoid sickness and stop it in its tracks. The COVID-19 has triggered a global health emergency of unprecedented proportions. According to the current knowledge of COVID-19, a healthy immune system is essential for illness prevention and protection.

TABLE 4.1 Strategies for COVID-19 by Conventional Means

Sr. no.	Drug used	Mechanism	Dose	Side effects	Contraindications	Reference
1	**Antiviral**					
	1. Darunavir (Prezista)	Protease inhibitor: inhibiting gag-pol polyprotein cleavage	800 mg daily	Nausea, vomiting, diarrhea, stomach pain, headache, rash	Coadministration with CYP3A highly dependent drugs is associated with serious and/or life-threatening events	Khan et al., 2021; Costanzo et al., 2020; Riva et al., 2020
	2. Favipiravir (Avigan)	RdRp inhibitor	1600 mg twice daily on day 1 and 600 mg twice daily on days 2–14	Decreased RBC production, increases in liver function parameters	Using in women who might be or are pregnant	Du and Chen, 2020; Chen et al., 2020; Shrestha et al., 2020
	3. Remdesivir (Veklury)	RdRp inhibitor	200 mg/dose	Swelling, bruising, or bleeding around the IV needle, rash, diarrhea, renal impairment, hypotension, and increased hepatic enzymes	Hypersensitivity to remdesivir or any component of the formulation	Khanal, 2020; Zhang and Zhou, 2020; Wang et al., 2020
	4. Ribavirin (Virazole)	Viral protein synthesis inhibitor	6 g over 12–18 h daily, Oral inhalation	Anxiety, cough or hoarseness, diarrhea, sleeplessness, headache, vomiting, nausea, lack of appetite	Hypersensitivity to ribavirin or any component of the formulation; pregnant women or may become pregnant	Khalili et al., 2020; Elfiky et al., 2020; Tong et al., 2020

TABLE 4.1 *(Continued)*

Sr. no.	Drug used	Mechanism	Dose	Side effects	Contraindications	Reference
	5. Nafamostat mesylate	Serine protease inhibitor	0.1–0.2 mg/kg/h of mixed with 5% DW	Nausea, vomiting, sweating, chest discomfort agranulocytosis, hyperkalemia	Heparin	Hempel et al., 2020; Hoffmann et al., 2020; Jang and Rhee, 2020
	6. Lopinavir/Ritonavir (Kaletra/Norvir)	Protease inhibitor, CYP4503A inhibitor	400 mg/100 mg; or 200 mg/50 mg	Headache, stomach pain or Diarrhea, chest pain, or pressure. Dizziness or passing out	Hypersensitivity to lopinavir, ritonavir, pregnancy; hepatic, or renal failure; coadministration with disulfiram or metronidazole	Uzunova et al., 2020; Cao et al., 2020
	7. Umifenovir (Arbidol)	Hemagglutinin inhibitor	200 mg three times daily	Limited allergic reactions	Increased sensitivity to the medication in children under 2two years	Haviernik et al., 2018; Lian et al., 2019
2	**Antibacterial**					
	1. Azithromycin (Zithromax)	RNA-dependent protein synthesis inhibitor	500 mg on day 1 followed by 250 mg once daily	Stomach pain, diarrhea, nausea, vomiting, shortness of breath, sudden dizziness	Hypersensitivity to azithromycin. History of cholestatic jaundice/ hepatic dysfunction associated with prior azithromycin use	Parnham et al., 2014; Gautret et al., 2020

TABLE 4.1 *(Continued)*

Sr. no.	Drug used	Mechanism	Dose	Side effects	Contraindications	Reference
3	**Antimalerial**					
	1. Chloroquine (Aralen)	Lysosome inhibitor	600 mg base once on day 1 followed by 300 mg base once daily for a total treatment duration	Nausea, vomiting, diarrhea, headache, hair loss, increased sensitivity to light	Hypersensitivity to chloroquine, the presence of retinal or visual field changes of any etiology (when used for indications other than acute malaria)	Vincent et al., 2005; Wang et al., 2020
	2. Hydroxychloroquine (Plaquenil)	Lysosome inhibitor	800 mg once on day 1, followed by 400 mg/day as a single dose or in two divided doses	Headache, dizziness, nausea, vomiting, stomach pain, weight loss, feeling irritated, skin rash, hair loss	Known hypersensitivity to HCQ, 4-aminoquinoline derivatives, or any component of the formulation	Liu et al., 2020; Chen et al., 2020; Egeli et al., 2021
4	**Immunomodulatory agent**					
	1. Thalidomide (Thalomid)	TNF-α suppressor	100 mg/day	Drowsiness, dizziness, and rash	Hypersensitivity to thalidomide or any component of the formulation, pregnancy	Khalil et al., 2020; Franks et al., 2004; Chen et al., 2020
5	**Monoclonal antibody**					
	1. Bevacizumab	Anti-VEGF	7.5 or 15 mg/kg IV	Dry mouth, cough, voice changes, loss of appetite, diarrhea, nausea, vomiting, constipation	Hypersensitivity in severe cardiac disease, thrombosis, hemorrhage, stroke, hemoptysis, or colon Perforation	Garcia et al., 2020; Chen et al., 2021

TABLE 4.1 *(Continued)*

Sr. no.	Drug used	Mechanism	Dose	Side effects	Contraindications	Reference
	2. Tocilizumab (Actemra)	Interleukin inhibitor	8 mg/kg, maximum (800 mg/dose)	Headache, dizziness, upper abdominal pain, mouth ulcers, neutropenia, thrombocytopenia, increased liver enzymes, increased total cholesterol and triglycerides	Known hypersensitivity to Tocilizumab or any component of the formulation	Zhang et al., 2020; Xu et al., 2020
	3. Sarilumab	IL-6 receptor inhibitor	200–400 mg/IV/daily	Neutropenia, increased ALT, injection site redness, upper respiratory infections, nasal congestion, and runny nose	Active tuberculosis, inactive tuberculosis, opportunistic fungal infection	Della-Torre et al., 2020; Lescure et al., 2021
6	**Interleukin antagonist**					
	1. Anakinra	Recombinant IL-1 receptor antagonist	2 mg/kg/day (max: 100 mg/day) or 4 mg/kg/day (max: 200 mg/day)	Redness, swelling, bruising, or pain at the site of injection	*E. coli* protein hypersensitivity or hypersensitivity to Anakinra or any components of the product	Somagutta et al., 2021; O'Horo, 2020

TABLE 4.1 *(Continued)*

Sr. no.	Drug used	Mechanism	Dose	Side effects	Contraindications	Reference
7	**Biological response modifier**					
	1. Interferons (α, β, λ)	Hindering the viral replication, the viral load reduction	The EC50 for IFN-α and IFN-β in vitro: 1.35 IU/ml and 0.76 IU/ml, respectively	**INF-α**: Cardiac arrhythmias, anorexia, seizures, retinopathy, numbness, palpitation, paresthesia, and dizziness **INF-β**: Sinus tachycardia, neutropenia, hypothyroidism, depression, pancytopenia, hyperthyroidism **INF-λ:** Bronchospasm, pancreatitis, hyponatremia, interstitial pneumonitis	**INF-α:** Anemia, depression, diabetes mellitus, hypertension, hyperthyroidism, thrombocytopenia, retinopathy, leukopenia, seizures, coronary artery disease, autoimmune hepatitis **INF-β**: Depression, lactation **INF-λ:** Hypersensitivity	Sallard et al., 2020; Meng et al., 2020; Mantlo et al., 2020
8	**Angiotensin II receptor antagonists**					
	1. Losartan (Cozaar)	Angiotensin II receptor blockade	15 mg/kg	Dry cough, cramps, pain in legs or back, stomach pain, diarrhea, headache, dizziness; tired feeling; insomnia	Hypersensitivity to losartan or any component of the formulation	Li et al., 2020; Kuba et al., 2005

TABLE 4.1 *(Continued)*

Sr. no.	Drug used	Mechanism	Dose	Side effects	Contraindications	Reference
9	**Adrenal cortex hormones**					
	1. Corticosteroids	Anti-inflammation and antifibrotic agent	Dexamethasone 6 mg/day oral/ IV or equivalent total daily doses of alternative glucocorticoids	Fluid retention or swelling of feet and legs, high blood pressure, increase blood sugar levels, increased risk of infection	Hypersensitivity to active ingredient or any component of the formulation, uncontrolled active infection	Nasim et al., 2020; Munch et al., 2021; Sterne et al., 2020
10	**Anthelmintic**					
	1. Ivermectin (Stromectol)	IMP α/β1-mediated nuclear import inhibitor	600 μg/kg once daily	Headache, muscle aches; dizziness; nausea, diarrhea; mild skin rash	Hypersensitivity to ivermectin or any component of the formulation	Patrì and Fabbrocini, 2020; Chowdhury et al., 2021; Gupta et al., 2020
11	**Anticoagulant**					
	1. Heparin (LMWH)	Antithrombin	LMWH 0.4–0.6 mg/kg two times daily	Bruising, bleeding, irritation, pain, redness	Hypersensitivity, past or present heparin-induced thrombocytopenia and active bleeding	Gozzo et al., 2020; Patell et al., 2020

Ayurvedic medicine, in addition to current treatment medicines such as favipiravir, hydroxychloroquine, monoclonal antibodies, corticosteroids, and anticoagulants, serves as immune boosters and prevents disease progression to symptomatic and severe states. Various Ayurvedic medicines are mentioned in Table 4.2.

4.8.1 GENERAL AND PHYSICAL MEASURES

Gargle with a pinch of turmeric and salt in warm water. Gargling can also be done using water heated with Triphala (dry fruits of *Emblica officinalis*, *Terminalia chebula*, and *Terminalia bellerica*) or Yashtimadhu (*Glycyrrhiza glabra*).

Once or twice a day, nasal installation/application medicinal oil (Anu taila or Shadbindu Taila) or plain oil (sesame or coconut) or nasal application of cow's ghee (Goghrita), especially before going out and returning home.

Once a day, inhale steam from ajwain (*Trachyspermum ammi*), Pudina (*Mentha spicata*), or eucalyptus oil.

Moderate physical exercise and 6–8 h of sleep are advisable.

4.8.2 DIETARY MEASURES

For drinking, use warm water or water that has been boiled with herbs such as ginger (*Zingiber oficinale*), coriander (*Coriandrum sativum*), basil (*Ocimum sanctum/Ocimum basilicum*), cumin (*Cuminum cyminum*) seeds, and so on.

Once a night, drink Golden Milk (half a teaspoon haldi [*Curcuma longa*] powder in 150 ml hot milk). If you have indigestion, stay away from it.

For prophylactic treatment, it is recommended to take 500 mg extract or 1–3 g powder of Ashwagandha (*Withania somnifera*) and Guduchi Ghana vati (*Tinospora cordifolia*) twice daily with warm water for 15 days or 1 month, or as instructed by an Ayurvedic physician. Guduchi (*T. cordifolia*) + Pippali (*Piper longum*), 375 mg twice daily with warm water for 15 days for asymptomatic conditions. Ayurvedic medicines can also be taken with honey, milk, ghee, or warm water under the supervision of an Ayurvedic physician (Ministry of Ayush Govt. of India, 2020).

TABLE 4.2 Useful Preventive Measures Against COVID-19 by "Ayurvedic" Medicines.

Ayurvedic medicines	Phytoconstituents	Category
1. *Tinospora cordifolia* (guduchi or giloy)	Diterpenoid lactones, steroids, glycosides aliphatic compounds, polysaccharides tinosporin, tinosporide, and cordifolide	Antioxidant, phagocytic activities, antipyretic action as well as immunomodulatory properties (Subhrajyoti, 2020; Srivastava and Singh, 2021)
2. *Emblica officinalis* (amalaki or Indian gooseberry)	Vitamin C, hydrolysable tannins, Ellagic acid, linolic acid, etc.	Cytoprotective, anti-inflammatory, antimicrobial, antioxidant, and immunomodulator activities (Chauhan et al., 2020)
3. *Withania somnifera* (aswagandha or Indian ginseng)	Withaferin A, with anolide-D, withanosides, with anones, sitoindosides, anaferine, isopelletierine	Anti-inflammatory, antidepressant, antioxidant, and immunomodulatory activities (Jain and Mathur, 2020)
4. *Piper longum* (pippali or long pepper)	Piperine, piplartine, pellitorine, caryophyllene	Antitumor, immunomodulatory, antifungal, antimicrobial, anti-inflammatory, antiobesity, cardioprotective, antioxidant, hepatoprotective, antidepressant, and antiamoebic (Subramaniam et al., 2021)
5. *Terminalia chebula* (haritaki or harad)	Chebulinic acid, chebulagic acid, punicalagin, punicalin, chebulic acid, gallic acid, ellagic acid, corilagin, chebumeinin A and chebumeinin B, chebulagic acid (CHLA), chebulinic acids (CHILI), punicalagin (PUG), and punicalin (PUN)	Antiviral, antibacterial, antifungal, antiprotozoal, anti-inflammatory, antimutagenic, anticancer, anti-oxidant, antidiabetic immunomodulatory, antipyretic, analgesic (Hussain et al., 2020)
6. *Allium sativum* (lahasun or garlic)	Alliin, vitamins (folic acid, niacin, Riboflavin, thiamine, vitamin C), allicin, allisatin, (*E*)-ajoene, (*Z*)-ajoene, allixin, γ-glutamyl-S-2-propenyl cysteine, diallyl disulfide, methyl allyl disulfide, *S*-allyl-cysteine, 1,2-vinyldiithin	Anti-inflammatory, antimicrobial activity, anticancer, antiviral (Chakraborty and Majumder, 2020)

TABLE 4.2 *(Continued)*

Ayurvedic medicines	Phytoconstituents	Category
7. *Curcuma longa* (haridra or haldi)	Curcumene, curcumenone, curcone, eugenol, curcumins	Antibacterial, anti-inflammatory, antiviral, and antioxidant properties (Chauhan et al., 2020; V A, 2020)
8. *Zingiber officinale* (sunthi or ginger)	α- and β-Zingiberenes, zingiberol, zingerone, gingerol, α-curcumene	Anti-inflammatory, anticholinergic, antihistaminic, antioxidant (Singh et al., 2021)
9. *Azadirachta indica* (neem or Margosa)	Limonoids are azadirachtin, 3-deacetyl-3-cinnamoylazadirachtin, Itigloyl-3-acetyl-II-methoxyazadirachtin, 22, 23-dihydro-23-β-methoxyazadirachtin, nimbanal, 3-tigloylazadirachtol, 3-acetyl-salanno V nimbidio Vmargocin, margocinin, margocilin, and terpenoids are isoazadirolide, 6 nimbocinolide, nimbonone, nibonolone, methyl grevillate, and margosinone	Anti-inflammatory, antimicrobial, antitumor, antifungal, and immunostimulant activity (Mafara and Bakura, 2021)
10. *Moringa pterygosperma* (Sigru or Sahijana)	Sterols, moringine, moringinine, pteregospermine	Antimicrobial, antioxidant, anti-inflammatory, and antiviral activities (Subrajyoti, 2020)
11. *Glycyrrhiza glabra* (yashtimadhu or liquorice)	Glycyrrhizin (also known as glycyrrhizic acid/glycyrrhizinic acid), hispaglabridin, isoliquiritigenin, isoliquiritin, licochalcone A, liquiritigenin, liquiritin, liquiritin apioside, prenyllicoflavone A, salicyclic acid, shinflavanone, shinpterocarpin, sitosterol, stigmasterol, syringic acid, transferulic	Anti-inflammatory, antipyretic, and antioxidant (Maurya and Sharma, 2020)
12. *Mangifera indica* (amra or mango)	Mangiferin, quercetin, gallic acid	Antiviral as well as anti-influenzal activities (Kumari et al., 2021)

TABLE 4.2 *(Continued)*

Ayurvedic medicines	Phytoconstituents	Category
13. *Ocimum sanctum* (tulasi or holy basil)	Monoterpenoids (carvone, cineole, fenchone, geraniol, linalool, myrcene, and thujone), sesquiterpenoids (caryophyllene and farnesol), triterpenoid (ursolic acid), and flavonoid (apigenin)	Antibacterial, antifungal, adaptogenic, antiviral, and immunomodulatory activities (Subrajyoti, 2020; Singh et al., 2021)
14. *Centella asiatica* (mandukaparni or gotukola)	Asiatic acid, centric acid, centellic acid, carotene, betulinic acid, thankunic acid, and isothankunic acid	Antioxidative, anti-inflammatory, and effective drug for neurodegenerative disease, analgesic, and immunomodulatory (Kumari et al., 2021)
15. *Terminalia bellerica* (vibhitaki or bahed)	Chebulagic acid, ellagic acid, gallic acid, mannitol	Antispasmodic, antihistaminic, antibacterial, antiviral, and antioxidant property (Subrajyoti, 2020)
16. *Albizia lebbek* (sirisa or siris)	Albigenin, albiziagenin, lebbecacidin, myricitrin	Anti-inflammatory, antihistamine, antioxidant, and anticancer activities (Kumari et al., 2021)
17. *Cinnamomum cassia* (cinnamon)	Cinnamaldehyde (60.41%) and eugenol (3.19%)	Antimicrobial, antiviral, antifungal, antioxidant, antihypertensive, antidiabetic, antitumor, gastroprotective, and immunomodulatory effects (Singh et al., 2021)
18. *Syzygium aromaticum* (clove)	Eugenol, eugenilinhydroxicinamic acids, hidroxibenzoic acids, and hidroxiphenylpropens	Antibacterial, antifungal, antioxidant, and anticarcinogenic (Subrajyoti, 2020; Singh et al., 2021)
19. *Piper nigrum* (black pepper)	Amide alkaloid piperine (1-peperoyl piperidine)	Antihypertensive, anti-Alzheimer's, antidepressant, antiplatelets, anti-inflammatory, antioxidant, antipyretic, antitumor, antiasthmatic, analgesic, antimicrobial (Singh et al., 2021)

4.9 PREVENTIONS

The WHO and other organizations have recommended the following broad advice to avoid infection and slow the spread of COVID-19.

The current technique for breaking the corona chain and limiting the transmission of infections is to take preventive actions. Preventive techniques are primarily focused on patient isolation and infection control, which includes proper steps to be taken during diagnosis and clinical care of an infected patient.

- Avoid close contact with people who have acute respiratory illnesses.
- Wash your hands frequently with soap and water or an alcohol-based hand rub or sanitizer, especially after coming into contact with sick persons or their environment.
- Keep at least 1 m apart from those who are coughing or sneezing. Immunocompromised people should avoid going to public gatherings.
- After engaging with a potentially contaminated environment, avoid touching your face, eyes, or mouth.
- Cover your mouth and nose when coughing or sneezing; if you are sick, stay at home.
- Practice physical separation by avoiding needless travel and staying away from large groups of people, as well as refraining from smoking and other behaviors that damage the lungs.
- Healthcare professionals treating infected patients should wear personal protective equipment (PPE) such as N95 or FFP3 masks, eye protection, gowns, and gloves to prevent the deadly disease from spreading (World Health Organization, 2021).

KEYWORDS

- coronavirus
- severe acute respiratory syndrome coronavirus-2 (SARS-CoV-2)
- acute respiratory syndrome (ARDS)
- pneumonia
- Ayurveda
- therapeutics
- pandemic

REFERENCES

Andersen, K.; Rambaut, A.; Lipkin, W.; Holmes, E.; Garry, R. The Proximal Origin of SARS-CoV-2. *Nat. Med.* **2020,** *26*(4), 450–452.

Ayush.gov.in. 2021. https://www.ayush.gov.in/docs/Guidelines%20for%20AYURVEDA%20Practitioners%20for%20Home%20Quarantine%20COVID%2019%20Patients.pdf (accessed Sep 2, 2021).

Azer, S. COVID-19: Pathophysiology, Diagnosis, Complications and Investigational Therapeutics. *New Microbes New Infect.* **2020,** *37*, 100738.

Buda, N.; Segura-Grau, E.; Cylwik, J.; Wełnicki, M. Lung Ultrasound in the Diagnosis of COVID-19 Infection - A Case Series and Review of the Literature. *Adv. Med. Sci.* **2020,** *65*(2), 378–385.

Cao, B.; Wang, Y.; Wen, D.; Liu, W.; Wang, J.; Fan, G.; Ruan, L.; Song, B.; Cai, Y.; Wei, M.; Li, X. A Trial of Lopinavir–ritonavir in Adults Hospitalized with Severe COVID-19. *N. Engl. J. Med.* **2020.**

Cascella, M.; Rajnik, M.; Cuomo, A. et al. Features, Evaluation and Treatment Coronavirus (COVID-19). Stat Pearls [Internet]. Treasure Island (FL): Stat Pearls Publishing, 2020.

Centers for Disease Control and Prevention. *Disease of the Week - COVID-19*. 2021. https://www.cdc.gov/dotw/COVID-19/index.html (accessed Aug 31, 2021).

Chakraborty, D.; Majumder, A. Garlic (Lahsun)–an Immunity Booster Against SARS-CoV-2. *Biotica Res. Today* **2020,** *2*(8), 755–757.

Chan, J.; To, K.; Tse, H.; Jin, D.; Yuen, K. Interspecies Transmission and Emergence of Novel Viruses: Lessons from Bats and Birds. *Trends Microbiol.* **2013,** *21*(10), 544–555.

Chauhan, V. P.; Dutt, B.; Vyas, M.; Gupta, S. K. Effect of Immune-modulators (RasayanaDravya) in Janapadodhwansa WSR to COVID-19. *J. Ayu. Herb.* **2020,** *6*(1), 26–29.

Chen, C.; Huang, J.; Cheng, Z.; Wu, J.; Chen, S.; Zhang, Y.; Chen, B.; Lu, M.; Luo, Y.; Zhang, J.; Yin, P. Favipiravir versus Arbidol for COVID-19: A Randomized Clinical Trial. *Med. Rxiv*. **2020.**

Chen, C.; Qi, F.; Shi, K.; Li, Y.; Li, J.; Chen, Y. et al. Thalidomide Combined with Low-dose Short-term Glucocorticoid in the Treatment of Critical Coronavirus Disease 2019. *Clin. Transl. Med.* **2020,** *10*(2).

Chen, H. X.; Chen, Z. H.; Shen, H. H. [Structure of SARS-CoV-2 and treatment of COVID-19]. *Sheng Li Xue Bao*. **2020,** *72*(5), 617–630.

Chen, Y.; Zhou, Y. W.; Cheng, K.; Li, Z. P.; Luo, D. Y.; Qiu, M.; Li, Q.; Wang, X.; Shen, Y. L.; Cao, D.; Yang, Y. Bevacizumab Combined with S-1 and Raltitrexed for Patients with Metastatic Colorectal Cancer Refractory to Standard Therapies: A Phase II Study. *The Oncologist* **2021.**

Chen, Z.; Hu, J.; Zhang, Z.; Jiang, S.; Han, S.; Yan, D.; Zhuang, R.; Hu, B.; Zhang, Z. Efficacy of Hydroxychloroquine in Patients with COVID-19: Results of a Randomized Clinical Trial. *Medrxiv* **2020.**

Chen, N.; Zhou, M.; Dong, X.; Qu, J.; Gong, F.; Han, Y.; Qiu, Y.; Wang, J.; Liu, Y.; Wei, Y.; Xia, J.; Yu, T.; Zhang, X.; Zhang, L. Epidemiological and Clinical Characteristics of 99 Cases of 2019 Novel Coronavirus Pneumonia in Wuhan, China: A Descriptive Study. *Lancet* **2020,** *395*(10223), 507–513.

Chowdhury, A. T.; Shahbaz, M.; Karim, M. R.; Islam, J.; Guo, D.; He, S. A Randomized Trial of Ivermectin-Doxycycline and Hydroxychloroquine-Azithromycin Therapy on COVID19 Patients.

Coperchini, F.; Chiovato, L.; Croce, L.; Magri, F.; Rotondi, M. The Cytokine Storm in COVID-19: An Overview of the Involvement of the Chemokine/Chemokine-receptor System. *Cytokine Growth Factor Rev.* **2020,** *53*, 25–32.

Costanzo, M.; De Giglio, M. A.; Roviello, G. N. SARS-CoV-2: Recent Reports on Antiviral Therapies based on Lopinavir/Ritonavir, Darunavir/Umifenovir, Hydroxychloroquine, Remdesivir, Favipiravir and other Drugs for the Treatment of the New Coronavirus. *Curr. Med. Chem.* **2020,** *27*(27), 4536–4541.

Della-Torre, E.; Campochiaro, C.; Cavalli, G.; De Luca, G.; Napolitano, A.; La Marca, S.; Boffini, N.; Da Prat, V.; Di Terlizzi, G.; Lanzillotta, M.; Querini, P. R. Interleukin-6 Blockade with Sarilumab in Severe COVID-19 Pneumonia with Systemic Hyperinflammation: An Open-label Cohort Study. *Ann. Rheum. Dis.* **2020,** *79*(10), 1277–1285.

Du, Y. X.; Chen, X. P. Favipiravir: Pharmacokinetics and Concerns about Clinical Trials for 2019-nCoV Infection. *Clin. Pharm. Therap.* **2020,** *108*(2), 242–247.

Egeli, B. H.; Sparks, J. A.; Kim, A. H.; Liew, J. W. Hydroxychloroquine for the Treatment of COVID-19 and Its Potential Cardiovascular Toxicity: Hero or Villain? *Best Pract. Res. Clin. Rheumatol.* **2021,** 101658.

Elfiky, A. A. Ribavirin, Remdesivir, Sofosbuvir, Galidesivir, and Tenofovir against SARS-CoV-2 RNA Dependent RNA Polymerase (RdRp): A Molecular Docking Study. *Life Sci.* **2020,** *253*, 117592.

Eurosurveillance. Updated Rapid Risk Assessment from ECDC on the Novel Coronavirus Disease 2019 (COVID-19) Pandemic: Increased Transmission in the EU/EEA and the UK. **2020,** *25*(10).

Fang, Y.; Zhang, H.; Xie, J.; Lin, M.; Ying, L.; Pang, P.; Ji, W. Sensitivity of Chest CT for COVID-19: Comparison to RT-PCR. *Radiology* **2020,** *296*(2), E115–E117.

Franks, M. E.; Macpherson, G. R.; Figg, W. D. Thalidomide. *Lancet* **2004,** *363*(9423), 1802–1811.

Garcia, J.; Hurwitz, H. I.; Sandler, A. B.; Miles, D.; Coleman, R. L.; Deurloo, R.; Chinot, O. L. Bevacizumab (Avastin®) in Cancer Treatment: A Review of 15 years of Clinical Experience and Future Outlook. *Cancer Treat. Rev.* **2020,** *86*, 102017.

Gautret, P.; Lagier, J. C.; Parola, P.; Meddeb, L.; Sevestre, J.; Mailhe, M.; Doudier, B.; Aubry, C.; Amrane, S.; Seng, P.; Hocquart, M. Clinical and Microbiological Effect of a Combination of Hydroxychloroquine and Azithromycin in 80 COVID-19 Patients with at Least a Six-day Follow Up: A Pilot Observational Study. *Travel Med. Infect. Dis.* **2020,** *34*, 101663.

Gavriatopoulou, M.; Ntanasis-Stathopoulos, I.; Korompoki, E.; Fotiou, D.; Migkou, M.; Tzanninis, I.; Psaltopoulou, T.; Kastritis, E.; Terpos, E.; Dimopoulos, M. Emerging Treatment Strategies for COVID-19 Infection. *Clin. Exp. Med.* **2020,** *21*(2), 167–179.

Gosain, R.; Abdou, Y.; Singh, A.; Rana, N.; Puzanov, I.; Ernstoff, M. COVID-19 and Cancer: A Comprehensive Review. *Curr. Oncol. Rep.* **2020,** *22*(5).

Gozzo, L.; Viale, P.; Longo, L.; Vitale, D. C.; Drago, F. The Potential Role of Heparin in Patients with COVID-19: Beyond the Anticoagulant Effect. A Review. *Front. Pharmacol.* **2020,** *11*.

Greenhalgh, T.; Jimenez, J.; Prather, K.; Tufekci, Z.; Fisman, D.; Schooley, R. Ten Scientific Reasons in Support of Airborne Transmission of SARS-CoV-2. *Lancet* **2021,** *397*(10285), 1603–1605.

Gupta, D.; Sahoo, A. K.; Singh, A. Ivermectin: Potential Candidate for the Treatment of COVID-19. *Braz. J. Infect. Dis.* **2020,** *24*(4), 369–371.

Harrison, A.; Lin, T.; Wang, P. Mechanisms of SARS-CoV-2 Transmission and Pathogenesis. *Trends Immunol.* **2020,** *41*(12), 1100–1115.

Haviernik, J.; Štefánik, M.; Fojtíková, M.; Kali, S.; Tordo, N.; Rudolf, I.; Hubálek, Z.; Eyer, L.; Ruzek, D. Arbidol (Umifenovir): A Broad-spectrum Antiviral Drug that Inhibits Medically Important Arthropod-borne Flaviviruses. *Viruses* **2018,** *10*(4), 184.

Hempel, T.; Raich, L.; Olsson, S.; Azouz, N. P.; Klingler, A. M.; Rothenberg, M. E.; Noé, F. Molecular Mechanism of SARS-CoV-2 Cell Entry Inhibition via TMPRSS2 by Camostat and Nafamostat Mesylate. *BioRxiv*. **2020.**

Hoffmann, M.; Schroeder, S.; Kleine-Weber, H.; Müller, M. A.; Drosten, C.; Pöhlmann, S. Nafamostat Mesylate Blocks Activation of SARS-CoV-2: New Treatment Option for COVID-19. *Antimicrob. Agents Chemother.* **2020,** *64*(6), e00754–e00820.

Holshue, M. L.; DeBolt, C.; Lindquist, S.; Lofy, K. H.; Wiesman, J.; Bruce, H.; Pillai, S. K. First Case of 2019 Novel Coronavirus in the United States. *N. Engl. J. Med.* **2020.**

Hussain, I.; Amjad, N.; Khan, B. A.; Awan, S. B.; Hussain, N.; Rashid, S. A. Broad Antimicrobial Effects of Terminalia Chebula: A Useful Candidate for its Clinical Studies Verses SARS-CoV-2. **2020.**

Islam, M.; Alam, S.; Kundu, S.; Hossan, T.; Kamal, M.; Cavestro, C. Prevalence of Headache in Patients with Coronavirus Disease 2019 (COVID-19): A Systematic Review and Meta-Analysis of 14,275 Patients. *Front. Neurol.* **2020,** *11*.

Jain, R.; Mathur, K. An Insight to Curative Effects of Ashwagandha (*Withaniasomnifera*), An Ayurveda Herb. *J. Med. Plants* **2020,** *8*, 227–235.

Jang, S.; Rhee, J. Y. Three Cases of Treatment with Nafamostat in Elderly Patients with COVID-19 Pneumonia Who Need Oxygen Therapy. *Int. J. Infect. Dis.* **2020,** *96,* 500–502.

Khalil, A.; Kamar, A.; Nemer, G. Thalidomide-revisited: Are COVID-19 Patients Going to be the Latest Victims of Yet Another Theoretical Drug-repurposing? *Front. Immunol.* **2020,** *11,* 1248.

Khalili, J. S.; Zhu, H.; Mak, N. S.; Yan, Y.; Zhu, Y. Novel Coronavirus Treatment with Ribavirin: Groundwork for an Evaluation Concerning COVID-19. *J. Med. Virol.* **2020,** *92*(7), 740–746.

Khan, S. A.; Zia, K.; Ashraf, S.; Uddin, R.; Ul-Haq, Z. Identification of Chymotrypsin-like Protease Inhibitors of SARS-CoV-2 via Integrated Computational Approach. *J. Biomol. Struct. Dyn.* **2021,** *39*(7), 2607–2616.

Khanal, P. Remdesivir for COVID-19 Treatment: Mechanism of Action, Synthesis, and Clinical Trials. *J Pharm Pharm Sci.* **2020.**

Kuba, K.; Imai, Y.; Rao, S.; Gao, H.; Guo, F.; Guan, B.; Huan, Y.; Yang, P.; Zhang, Y.; Deng, W.; Bao, L. A Crucial Role of Angiotensin Converting Enzyme 2 (ACE2) in SARS Coronavirus–induced Lung Injury. *Nat. Med.* **2005,** *11*(8), 875–879.

Kumari, R.; Venaik, A.; Hasibuzzaman, M. A.; Azure, S. A.; Ojha, R. P.; Sahi, A. K. Repurposing of the Herbals Immune-Boosters in the Prevention and Management of COVID-19: A Review. *J. Pure Appl. Microbiol.* **2021,** *15*(1), 1–9.

Lescure, F. X.; Honda, H.; Fowler, R. A.; Lazar, J. S.; Shi, G.; Wung, P.; Patel, N.; Hagino, O.; Bazzalo, I. J.; Casas, M. M.; Nuñez, S. A. Sarilumab in Patients Admitted to Hospital with Severe or Critical COVID-19: A Randomised, Double-blind, Placebo-controlled, Phase 3 Trial. *Lancet Respir. Med.* **2021,** *9*(5), 522–532.

Li, G.; Hu, R.; Zhang, X. Antihypertensive Treatment with ACEI/ARB of Patients with COVID-19 Complicated by Hypertension. *Hypertens. Res.* **2020,** *43*(6), 588–590.

Li, H.; Zhou, Y.; Zhang, M.; Wang, H.; Zhao, Q.; Liu, J. Updated Approaches against SARS-CoV-2. *Antimicrob. Agents Chemother.* **2020,** *64*(6).

Lian, N.; Xie, H.; Lin, S.; Huang, J.; Zhao, J.; Lin, Q. Umifenovir Treatment is not Associated with Improved Outcomes in Patients with Coronavirus Disease 2019: A Retrospective Study. *Clin. Microbiol. Infect.* **2020,** *26*(7), 917–921.

Liu, J.; Cao, R.; Xu, M.; Wang, X.; Zhang, H.; Hu, H.; Li, Y.; Hu, Z.; Zhong, W.; Wang, M. Hydroxychloroquine, a Less Toxic Derivative of Chloroquine, is Effective in Inhibiting SARS-CoV-2 Infection in Vitro. *Cell Discov.* **2020,** *6*(1), 1–4.

Loeffelholz, M.; Tang, Y. Laboratory Diagnosis of Emerging Human Coronavirus Infections – The State of the Art. *Emerg. Microbes & Infect.* **2020,** *9*(1), 747–756.

Mafara, S. M.; Bakura, T. L. Multiple Potentials of Neem Tree (Azadirachta Indica); A Review. *Bakolori J. Gen. Stud.* **2021,** *11*(1), 1–2.

Mantlo, E.; Bukreyeva, N.; Maruyama, J.; Paessler, S.; Huang, C. Antiviral Activities of Type I Interferons to SARS-CoV-2 Infection. *Antiviral Res.* **2020,** *179,* 104811.

Maurya, D.; Sharma, D. Evaluation of Traditional Ayurvedic Kadha for Prevention and Management of the Novel Coronavirus (SARS-CoV-2) using in Silico Approach. *J. Biomol. Struct. Dyn.* **2020,** 1–16.

Meng, Z.; Wang, T.; Li, C.; Chen, X.; Li, L.; Qin, X.; Li, H.; Luo, J. An Experimental Trial of Recombinant Human Interferon Alpha Nasal Drops to Prevent Coronavirus Disease 2019 in Medical Staff in an Epidemic Area. *MedRxiv.* **2020.**

Munch, M. W.; Granholm, A.; Myatra, S. N.; Vijayaraghavan, B. K.; Cronhjort, M.; Wahlin, R. R.; Jakob, S. M.; Cioccari, L.; Kjaer, M. N.; Vesterlund, G. K.; Meyhoff, T. S. Higher vs Lower Doses of Dexamethasone in Patients with COVID-19 and Severe Hypoxia (COVID STEROID 2) Trial: Protocol and Statistical Analysis Plan. *Acta Anaesthesiol. Scand.* **2021.**

Nasim, S.; Kumar, S.; Azim, D.; Ashraf, Z.; Azeem, Q. Corticosteroid Use for 2019-nCoV Infection: A Double-edged Sword. Infect. *Control Hosp. Epidemiol.* **2020,** *41*(10), 1244–1245.

Nytimes.com. A Timeline of the Coronavirus Pandemic. 2021. https://www.nytimes.com/article/coronavirus-timeline.html (accessed Aug 31, 2021).

Nytimes.com. *Wuhan Coronavirus Looks Increasingly Like a Pandemic, Experts Say (Published 2020).* 2021, https://www.nytimes.com/2020/02/02/health/coronavirus-pandemic-china.html (accessed Aug 31, 2021).

O'Horo, J. C. *Anakinra*; Elsevier, 2020.

Oran, D.; Topol, E. The Proportion of SARS-CoV-2 Infections that are Asymptomatic. *Ann. Intern. Med.* **2021,** *174*(5), 655–662.

Parasher, A. COVID-19: Current Understanding of its Pathophysiology, Clinical Presentation and Treatment. *Postgrad. Med. J.* **2020,** *97*(1147), 312–320.

Parnham, M. J.; Haber, V. E.; Giamarellos-Bourboulis, E. J.; Perletti, G.; Verleden, G. M.; Vos, R. Azithromycin: Mechanisms of Action and their Relevance for Clinical Applications. *Pharmacol. Ther.* **2014,** *143*(2), 225–245.

Patell, R.; Midha, S.; Kimani, S.; Martin, R.; Neparidze, N.; Jaglal, M.; Freed, J.; Key, N. S. Variability in Institutional Guidance for COVID-19-associated Coagulopathy in the United States. *J. Thromb. Haemost.* **2020,** *120*(12), 1725–1732.

Patrì, A.; Fabbrocini, G. Hydroxychloroquine and Ivermectin: A Synergistic Combination for COVID-19 Chemoprophylaxis and Treatment? *J. Am. Acad. Dermatol.* **2020,** *82*(6), e221.

Peng, Q.; Wang, X.; Zhang, L. Findings of Lung Ultrasonography of Novel Corona Virus Pneumonia During the 2019–2020 Epidemic. *Intensive Care Med.* **2020,** *46*(5), 849–850.

Rabi, F.; Al Zoubi, M.; Kasasbeh, G.; Salameh, D.; Al-Nasser, A. SARS-CoV-2 and Coronavirus Disease 2019: What We Know So Far. *Pathogens* **2020,** *9*(3), 231.

Rathore, J. S.; Ghosh, C. Severe Acute Respiratory Syndrome Coronavirus-2 (SARS-CoV-2), A Newly Emerged Pathogen: An Overview. *Pathog. Dis.* **2020.**

Riva, A.; Conti, F.; Bernacchia, D.; Pezzati, L.; Sollima, S.; Merli, S.; Siano, M.; Lupo, A.; Rusconi, S.; Cattaneo, D.; Gervasoni, C. Darunavir Does Not Prevent SARS-CoV-2 Infection in HIV Patients. *Pharmacol. Res.* **2020,** *157*, 104826.

Sallard, E.; Lescure, F. X.; Yazdanpanah, Y.; Mentre, F.; Peiffer-Smadja, N. Type 1 Interferons as a Potential Treatment Against COVID-19. *Antiviral Res.* **2020,** *178*, 104791.

Shi, Y.; Wang, G.; Cai, X.; Deng, J.; Zheng, L.; Zhu, H.; Zheng, M.; Yang, B.; Chen, Z. An Overview of COVID-19. *J. Zhejiang Univ. Sci. B* **2020,** *21*(5), 343–360.

Shi, Y.; Wang, Y.; Shao, C.; Huang, J.; Gan, J.; Huang, X.; Bucci, E.; Piacentini, M.; Ippolito, G.; Melino, G. COVID-19 Infection: The Perspectives on Immune Responses. *Cell Death Differ.* **2020,** *27*(5), 1451.

Shrestha, D. B.; Budhathoki, P.; Khadka, S.; Shah, P. B.; Pokharel, N.; Rashmi, P. Favipiravir versus other Antiviral or Standard of Care for COVID-19 Treatment: A Rapid Systematic Review and Meta-analysis. *Virol. J.* **2020**, *17*(1), 1–5.

Singh, N. A.; Kumar, P.; Kumar, N. Spices and Herbs: Potential Antiviral Preventives and Immunity Boosters during COVID-19. *Phytother. Res.* **2021,** *35*(5), 2745–2757.

Somagutta, M. K.; Pormento, M. K.; Hamid, P.; Hamdan, A.; Khan, M. A.; Desir, R.; Vijayan, R.; Shirke, S.; Jeyakumar, R.; Dogar, Z.; Makkar, S. S. The Safety and Efficacy of Anakinra, an Interleukin-1 Antagonist in Severe Cases of COVID-19: A Systematic Review and Meta-Analysis. *J. Infect. Chemother.* **2021,** *53*(2), 221.

Spiteri, G.; Fielding, J.; Diercke, M.; Campese, C.; Enouf, V.; Gaymard, A.; Bella, A.; Sognamiglio, P.; Sierra Moros, M.; Riutort, A.; Demina, Y.; Mahieu, R.; Broas, M.; Bengnér, M.; Buda, S.; Schilling, J.; Filleul, L.; Lepoutre, A.; Saura, C.; Mailles, A.; Levy-Bruhl, D.; Coignard, B.; Bernard-Stoecklin, S.; Behillil, S.; van der Werf, S.; Valette, M.; Lina, B.; Riccardo, F.; Nicastri, E.; Casas, I.; Larrauri, A.; Salom Castell, M.; Pozo, F.; Maksyutov, R.; Martin, C.; Van Ranst, M.; Bossuyt, N.; Siira, L.; Sane, J.; Tegmark-Wisell, K.; Palmérus, M.; Broberg, E.; Beauté, J.; Jorgensen, P.; Bundle, N.; Pereyaslov, D.; Adlhoch, C.; Pukkila, J.; Pebody, R.; Olsen, S.; Ciancio, B. First Cases of Coronavirus Disease 2019 (COVID-19) in the WHO European Region, 24 January to 21 February 2020, 2021.

Srivastava, A. K.; Singh, V. K. Tinospora Cordifolia (Giloy): A Magical Shrub. *Asian J. Adv. Med. Sci.* **2021,** 22–30.

Stacks.cdc.gov. New COVID-19 Variants. 2021. https://stacks.cdc.gov/view/cdc/100425 (accessed Sep 1, 2021).

Sterne, J. A.; Murthy, S.; Diaz, J. V.; Slutsky, A. S.; Villar, J.; Angus, D. C.; Annane, D.; Azevedo, L. C.; Berwanger, O.; Cavalcanti, A. B.; Dequin, P. F. Association between Administration of Systemic Corticosteroids and Mortality Among Critically Ill Patients with COVID-19: A Meta-analysis. *JAMA* **2020,** *324*(13), 1330–1341.

Subhrajyoti, C. Immunomodulatory Herbs of Ayurveda and COVID-19: A Review Article. *J. Ayurveda Integr. Med. Sci.* **2020,** *5*(2), 203–208.

Subramaniam, K.; Subramanian, S. K.; Bhargav, S.; Parameswari, R.; Praveena, R.; Ravikumar, R.; Yuvaraj, E.; Kumar, V. M. Review on Potential Antiviral and Immunomodulatory Properties of Piper Longum. *IOP Conf. Ser.: Mater. Sci. Eng.* **2021,** *1145*(1), 012099.

Tavakolpour, S.; Rakhshandehroo, T.; Wei, E.; Rashidian, M. Lymphopenia during the COVID-19 Infection: What it Shows and What can be Learned. *Immunol. Lett.* **2020,** *225*, 31–32.

Tong, S.; Su, Y.; Yu, Y.; Wu, C.; Chen, J.; Wang, S.; Jiang, J. Ribavirin Therapy for Severe COVID-19: A Retrospective Cohort Study. *Int. J. Antimicrob. Agents* **2020,** *56*(3), 106114.

Uzunova, K.; Filipova, E.; Pavlova, V.; Vekov, T. Insights into Antiviral Mechanisms of Remdesivir, Lopinavir/Ritonavir and Chloroquine/Hydroxychloroquine Affecting the New SARS-CoV-2. *Biomed. Pharmacother.* **2020,** 110668.

Anil Kumar, V.; Kamini, S.; Himasree, P. A. Possible Character of Classical Therapeutic Rhizome of Turmeric for the Prevention and the Executives of Novel Corona Virus. *J. Med. Pharm. Allied Sci.* **2020,** *9*(3), 2527–2535.

Vincent, M. J.; Bergeron, E.; Benjannet, S.; Erickson, B. R.; Rollin, P. E.; Ksiazek, T. G.; Seidah, N. G.; Nichol, S. T. Chloroquine is a Potent Inhibitor of SARS Coronavirus Infection and Spread. *Virol. J.* **2005,** *2*(1), 69.

Wang, M.; Cao, R.; Zhang, L.; Yang, X.; Liu, J.; Xu, M.; Shi, Z.; Hu, Z.; Zhong, W.; Xiao, G. Remdesivir and Chloroquine Effectively Inhibit the Recently Emerged Novel Coronavirus (2019-nCoV) in Vitro. *Cell Res.* **2020,** *30*(3), 269–271.

Wang, Y.; Zhou, F.; Zhang, D.; Zhao, J.; Du, R.; Hu, Y.; Cheng, Z.; Gao, L.; Jin, Y.; Luo, G.; Fu, S. Evaluation of the Efficacy and Safety of Intravenous Remdesivir in Adult Patients with Severe COVID-19: Study Protocol for a Phase 3 Randomized, Double-blind, Placebo-Controlled, Multicentre Trial. *Trials* **2020,** *21*, 1–1.

Wang, H.; Ma, S. The Cytokine Storm and Factors Determining the Sequence and Severity of Organ Dysfunction in Multiple Organ Dysfunction Syndrome. *Am. J. Emerg. Med.* **2008,** *26*(6), 711–715.

Who.int. Coronavirus Disease (COVID-19) – World Health Organization. 2021. https://www.who.int/emergencies/diseases/novel-coronavirus-2019 (accessed Aug 11, 2021).

Who.int. Naming the Coronavirus Disease (COVID-19) and the Virus that Causes it. 2021. https://www.who.int/emergencies/diseases/novel-coronavirus-2019/technical-guidance/naming-the-coronavirus-disease-(covid-2019)-and-the-virus-that-causes-it (accessed Aug 31, 2021)

Wiersinga, W.; Rhodes, A.; Cheng, A.; Peacock, S.; Prescott, H. Pathophysiology, Transmission, Diagnosis, and Treatment of Coronavirus Disease 2019 (COVID-19). *JAMA* **2020,** *324*(8), 782.

Wu, Y.; Chen, C.; Chan, Y. The Outbreak of COVID-19: An Overview. *J. Chin. Med. Assoc.* **2020,** *83*(3), 217–220.

Xu X.; Han M.; Li T.; Sun W.; Wang D.; Fu B.; Zhou Y.; Zheng X.; Yang Y.; Li X.; Zhang, X. Effective Treatment of Severe COVID-19 Patients with Tocilizumab. *Proc. Natl. Acad. Sci. U.S.A.* **2020,** *117*(20), 10970–10975.

Xu, Z.; Shi, L.; Wang, Y.; Zhang, J.; Huang, L.; Zhang, C.; Liu, S.; Zhao, P.; Liu, H.; Zhu, L.; Tai, Y.; Bai, C.; Gao, T.; Song, J.; Xia, P.; Dong, J.; Zhao, J.; Wang, F. Pathological Findings of COVID-19 Associated with Acute Respiratory Distress Syndrome. *Lancet Respir. Med.* **2020,** *8*(4), 420–422.

Yang, N.; Shen, H. Targeting the Endocytic Pathway and Autophagy Process as a Novel Therapeutic Strategy in COVID-19. *Int. J. Biol. Sci.* **2020,** *16*(10), 1724–1731.

Yao, T.; Lin, H.; Mao, J.; Huo, S.; Liu, G. CT Imaging Features of Patients Infected with 2019 Novel Coronavirus. *Mol. Biol.* **2021,** *2*(1), 5–11.

Ye, Q.; Wang, B.; Mao, J. The Pathogenesis and Treatment of the 'Cytokine Storm' in COVID-19. *J. Infect.* **2020,** *80*(6), 607–613.

Yuki, K.; Fujiogi, M.; Koutsogiannaki, S. COVID-19 Pathophysiology: A Review. *J. Clin. Immunol.* **2020,** *215*, 108427.

Zaki, A.; van Boheemen, S.; Bestebroer, T.; Osterhaus, A.; Fouchier, R. Isolation of a Novel Coronavirus from a Man with Pneumonia in Saudi Arabia. *N. Engl. J. Med.* **2012,** *367*(19), 1814–1820.

Zhang, C.; Wu, Z.; Li, J. W.; Zhao, H.; Wang, G. Q. Cytokine Release Syndrome in Severe COVID-19: Interleukin-6 Receptor Antagonist Tocilizumab may be the Key to Reduce Mortality. *Int. J. Antimicrob. Agents* **2020,** *55*(5), 105954.

Zhang, L.; Zhou, R. Binding Mechanism of Remdesivir to SARS-CoV-2 RNA Dependent RNA Polymerase.

Zhong, N.; Zheng, B.; Li, Y.; Poon, L.; Xie, Z.; Chan, K.; Li, P.; Tan, S.; Chang, Q.; Xie, J.; Liu, X.; Xu, J.; Li, D.; Yuen, K.; Peiris, J.; Guan, Y. Epidemiology and Cause of Severe Acute Respiratory Syndrome (SARS) in Guangdong, People's Republic of China, in February, 2003. *Lancet* **2003,** *362*(9393), 1353–1358.

Zhou, F.; Yu, T.; Du, R.; Fan, G.; Liu, Y.; Liu, Z.; Xiang, J.; Wang, Y.; Song, B.; Gu, X.; Guan, L.; Wei, Y.; Li, H.; Wu, X.; Xu, J.; Tu, S.; Zhang, Y.; Chen, H.; Cao, B. Clinical Course and Risk Factors for Mortality of Adult in Patients with COVID-19 in Wuhan, China: A Retrospective Cohort Study. *Lancet* **2020,** *395*(10229), 1054–1062.

CHAPTER 5

Developing Vaccine Against COVID-19 and Immune Response

URMILA JAROULIYA[1] and RAJ K. KESERVANI[2]

[1]*School of Studies in Biochemistry, Jiwaji University, Gwalior, Madhya Pradesh, India*

[2]*Faculty of B. Pharmacy, CSM Group of Institutions, Prayagraj, Uttar Pradesh, India*

ABSTRACT

Coronavirus disease infected the entire world and is usually named as severe acute respiratory syndrome coronavirus 2 (SARS-CoV-2), which causes coronavirus disease 2019 (COVID-19). It is a quite contagious and pathogenic that emerged in overdue 2019 and has brought on deadly respiratory disease, which threatens human health and public protection. It is extensively believed that prepandemic normality will in no way go back until a secure and effective vaccine approach will become available and a worldwide vaccination program is applied efficiently. Globally research work is going on and coordination has resulted in a rapid development of vaccine. In this chapter, we discuss the role of immune response towards viral infection and the available vaccines towards COVID-19 infection.

5.1 INTRODUCTION

Coronaviruses are members of own family of viruses which causes severe acute respiratory syndrome (SARS) and Middle East respiratory syndrome

COVID-19 and Immunomodulation with Special Emphasis on Nutraceutical and Herbal Formulation.
Rajesh K. Kesharwani & Raj K. Keservani (Eds)

(MERS). This coronavirus 2019 (COVID-19) pandemic is as a result of extreme acute respiratory syndrome coronavirus 2 (SARS-CoV-2). COVID-19 was first identified in Wuhan (China), having symptoms of excessive respiratory problems in sufferers. In March 2020, the world health organization (WHO) declared the COVID-19 outbreak of a deadly disease. Until 22 August 2021, the data of infected persons mentioned globally is now over than 211 million and the number of deaths is over than 4.4 million, consistent with facts recorded by means of the world health organization (WHO, 2021).

The COVID-19 virus primarily affects the respiratory tract, spreads via droplets of saliva or discharge from the nostril when an infected individual coughs or sneezes. The unusual signs are fever, coughing, and trouble in breathing, even as many have required hospitalization or ventilators (Guan et al., 2019; Chen et al., 2020; Bhatraju et al., 2020). Aside from breathing issues COVID-19 causes nonbreathing signs and symptoms which include anosmia, fatigue, muscle/body aches, sore throat, diarrhea, thromboembolic disorders, myocarditis, and vasculitis (Wang et al., 2019; Pan et al., 2020; Huang et al., 2020; Giacomelli et al., 2020; Zhou et al.,.2020; Song et al., 2020; Recalcati et al., 2020). The median incubation duration is 5.1 days (range 1–14 days). An appropriate interval during which a person with COVID-19 is infectious is unsure. As per the present-day evidence, the duration of infectivity begins 2 days previous before the onset of symptoms and declines unexpectedly within the first week of symptom onset (Lauer et al., 2020). If medical analysis for COVID-19 infection is not on time by the second week of infection, which is related to laboratory characteristics of an immune-mediated cytokine typhoon, it reasons enormous inflammation and dispersed intravascular coagulation, typically which causes viremia (a clinical situation in which viruses enter the bloodstream) (Zhou et al., 2020; Tang et al., 2020). It became evident early on that the pandemic should best be managed with effective vaccines. This led to fast vaccine development, with restricted perception that might represent defensive immunity. This chapter describes the immune system role towards coronavirus infection and the available vaccine for COVID-19.

5.2 MORPHOLOGY OF CORONAVIRUS

Coronavirus belongs to the family coronaviridae. Its debris were prepared with long single-stranded RNA molecule, tightly packed into the center of the particle, and enclosed via a defensive capsid that is a lattice of a continuous moiety of protein molecules known as coat or capsid proteins. In coronavirus, these proteins are known as nucleocapsid (N). The nucleocapsid (N) proteins are involved in packaging the RNA genome inside the virions and play an important role in pathogenicity as an interferon (IFN) inhibitor. The coronavirus center particle is further surrounded by an outer membrane envelope, product of lipids (fats) with proteins inserted. These membranes derive from the cells wherein the virus was finally assembled and are changed to comprise particular viral proteins, such as the spike (S) accountable for recognizing host cell receptors, membrane (M) liable for shaping the virions (infectious virus particle), and envelope (E) proteins responsible for virions assembly and release (Schoeman and Fielding, 2019; Alsaadi et al., 2019; Fehr and Perlman, 2015). Besides these, there are four main structural and accessory proteins which are species-specific. As soon as the viral genome enters the cytoplasm of the target cell, and given its RNA genome, it converts into polyproteins; these polyproteins are processed into nonstructural proteins (NSPs) to shape a replication–transcription complex (RTC) that is engaged in genome transcription and replication process (Alanagreh et al., 2020).

5.3 IMMUNE SYSTEM

Immunity is the defense system of our body that defends us from infectious ailment and removes unwanted substances. This discriminatory potential to remove foreign substances is carried out through a complex system of interacting cells known as the immune system. The immune system includes innate and adaptive immunity.

The innate immunity gives the primary line of protection towards infection (Kimbrell and Beutler, 2001). Phagocytic cells (macrophages and neutrophils), barriers including skin, and other antimicrobial compounds synthesized by the host all play essential roles in innate immunity (Medzhitov and Janeway, 2000). The phagocytic cells in association with degradative enzymes, antimicrobial peptides, and reactive oxygen species kill the trapped microorganisms. As well as, they release signaling molecules that turn on an inflammatory reaction and initiate the adaptive immune system.

In comparison, adaptive immunity does no longer come into play till there is an antigenic challenge to the organism; means adaptive immune response becomes active towards an antigen within 5–6 days after the preliminary exposure to that antigen. Because maximum organisms (e.g., bacteria, viruses, and fungi) are recognized as foreign, the capacity to identify and dispose of these materials offers safety from infectious illnesses. Immunity is normally specific to a single organism or group of intently associated organisms. An effective immune response includes two main types of cells, B lymphocytes and T lymphocytes.

5.3.1 B LYMPHOCYTES

B (bursal or bone marrow-derived) lymphocytes mature inside the bone marrow. An easy definition of B lymphocytes is a population of cells that exhibit clonally numerous cell surface immunoglobulin (Ig) receptors recognizing particular antigenic epitopes. This antigen-binding or B-cell receptor is a membrane-bound antibody molecule. The binding of the antigen to the antibody causes the cell to divide rapidly into memory B cells and effector B cells known as plasma cells. Memory B cells have an extended life span, despite the fact that plasma cells stay alive just for a few days. These secreted antibodies are the most important effector molecules of humoral immunity. When infectious agents (antigen) enter inside the body, B cell receptors (BCRs) present on B cell surface, bind to these particular antigens and turn on the production of the antibodies.

5.3.2 T LYMPHOCYTES

T lymphocytes develop within the bone marrow. Unlike B cells, which mature in the bone marrow, T cells migrate to the thymus gland to mature. Inside the thymus, T cells multiply and differentiate into helper, regulatory, or cytotoxic T cells or grow to be memory T cells. They may be then dispatched to peripheral tissues or circulate inside the blood or lymphatic system. As soon as they are stimulated via the suitable antigen, helper T (Th) cells secrete chemical messengers referred to as cytokines, which stimulate the differentiation of B cells into plasma cells (antibody-producing cells). Regulatory T cells act to govern immune reactions.

Cytotoxic T (Tc) cells, which are activated via numerous cytokines, bind to and kill infected cells and cancer cells.

T-cell receptors (TCRs) are located mostly at the cellular membrane. TCRs can recognize only antigen that is bound to cell membrane proteins known as major histocompatibility complex (MHC) molecules. There are two essential types of MHC molecules: Class I MHC molecules, which are expressed by using almost all nucleated cells of vertebrate species and Class II MHC molecules, expressed effectively through antigen-presenting cells. While a naive T cell (cell that is earlier not interacted with antigen) comes in contact with antigen blended with a MHC molecule on a cell, the T cell proliferates and differentiates into memory T cells and numerous effector T cells. The well-known two kinds of T cells are T helper (Th) and T cytotoxic (Tc) cells. Presence of CD4 or CD8 membrane glycoproteins on their surfaces differentiates them from each other. T cells showing CD4 usually present Th cells, whereas the ones representing CD8 present Tc cells. After a Th cell acknowledges and interacts with an antigen–MHC class II molecule complex, the cell is activated and secretes numerous growth factors recognized together as cytokines. The secreted cytokines play an essential function in activating B cells, Tc cells, macrophages, and numerous other cells that take part in invading the infected cells and hence activating the immune system. In case of SARS-CoV-2 infection, poor T cell response contributes to endurance and severity of infection, while at the same time a strong T cell response can be defensive against infection.

5.3.3 IMMUNE RESPONSE TO VIRAL INFECTION

Viruses are widely recognized for the stimulation of innate response and viral infections are not often lethal, despite the fact that they're quite cytolytic to individual cells. Mortality usually happens when viruses go through a prime antigenic exchange (e.g., influenza viruses), or when host immunity is vulnerable. Many viruses result in the production of interferons that can inhibit viral replication by inducing an antiviral response. Innate defense comes into play to restrict or inhibit preliminary infection, to defend cells from infection, or to cast off virus-infected cells, and arise nicely before the onset of adaptive immunity. The innate immune response to viral infection is generally via the induction of interferons (IFN-α and IFN-β) and the activation of NK (natural killer) cells.

Double-stranded RNA (dsRNA) produced all through the viral life cycle can result in the expression of IFN-α and IFN-β through the infected cell. IFN-α and IFN-β can result in an antiviral response or resistance to viral replication through binding to the IFN α/β receptor. As soon as bound, IFN-α and IFN-β activate the JAK-STAT pathway, which in turn induces the transcription of numerous genes that degrades viral RNA. Different genes activated through IFN-α/β binding to its receptor additionally make a contribution to the inhibition of viral replication. The binding of IFN-α and IFN-β to NK cells induces lytic activity, making them very effective in killing virally infected cells. The activity of NK cells is also significantly improved via IL-12, a cytokine that is produced very early in a response to viral infection. NK cells produce proinflammatory cytokines; they are able to kill infected cells and have interaction with Dendritic cells (DC), and are an essential factor of innate defense towards viruses. NK cells are also essential in resistance to mouse and human cytomegalovirus, HIV, influenza virus, and Ebola viruses (Lodoen and Lanier, 2006).

5.3.4 CORONAVIRUS AND IMMUNE RESPONSE

As within the above phase it was pointed out that normally how immune system works towards viral infection. In case of SARS-CoV-2 infection, it indicates that more than one viral structural and nonstructural protein antagonizes interferon responses and tries to damage the body's innate antiviral cytokine responses that is yet to be studied. Effective innate immune reaction against viral infection depends on the type I interferon responses and its downstream cascade that concludes in controlling viral replication and induction of strong adaptive immune response.

Innate immune cells that are engaged in antiviral reaction acknowledge the attack of the virus through pathogen-associated molecular patterns (PAMPs). In case of coronavirus, PAMPs are recognized through Toll-like receptors (TLR3 and TLR7), or by way of the endosomal RNA receptors and the cytosolic RNA sensor RIG-I/MDA5 (retinoic acid-inducible gene I/melanoma differentiation-associated protein 5). Binding of pathogen (virus) to TLR3 and TLR7 results in the activation of the downstream signaling cascade, i.e., NF-κB and IRF3 followed through their nuclear translocation. Within the nuclei, these transcription factors persuade expression of type I IFN and several other proinflammatory cytokines and at the entry site these preliminary responses include the primary line protection towards viral infection (de Wit et al., 2016). Binding of Type I IFN to IFN-associated cell receptors activates the JAK-STAT signaling pathway, in which JAK1 and TYK2 kinases phosphorylate STAT1 and STAT2. This phosphorylated STAT1/2 form a complex with IRF9, and together they pass into the nucleus to initiate the transcription of IFN-stimulated genes (ISGs) under the regulation of IFN-stimulated response element (ISRE) containing promoters (de Wit et al., 2016).

In SARS-CoV-2 infection, type I IFN is tormented by viral infection. Corona virus interferes with numerous signaling pathways which results in type I IFN production or the signaling downstream of IFNAR. This interfering approach is firmly related to the ailment severity (Channappanavar and Perlman, 2017). It interferes immediately or circuitously with downstream signaling pathways including ubiquitination, degradation of RNA sensor adaptor molecules (MAVS and TRAF3/6), and inhibiting IRF3 nuclear translocation (Kindler et al., 2016).

No specific antiviral remedy for COVID-19 is presently available, so treating this disease especially includes symptomatic treatment and oxygen therapy. It's far recommended to screen inflammatory elements and lymphocyte subsets throughout the infection.

5.3.5 HOW COVID-19 AFFECTS OUR BODY SYSTEMS

Coronaviruses frequently infect human lung cells via a receptor for an enzyme known as Angiotensin-converting Enzyme 2 (ACE2). Preliminary work on SARS-CoV-2 has proven that this virus basically targets airways and alveolar epithelial cells, vascular endothelial cells, and macrophages inside the lung, all of which express the ACE2 host target receptor utilized by SARS-CoV-2. In the first step of virus infection, entry of SARS-CoV-2 into the host cell is mediated via its spike through which the S-glycoprotein recognizes and binds to the ACE2 receptors which are found in human's epithelia of the lung and small intestine. The virus carries into the lung cells and its genetic material (RNA) is released into the cytoplasm, where the viral RNA molecules cascade the cellular mechanism to make lots of copies of the viral RNA and pass signals to the cells to synthesize hundreds of thousands of nucleocapsid, membrane, envelope, and spike proteins and assemble the new virus particles which bud out of the cell surface membrane. Thus, newly generated viral particles release from the cell and outspread the infection (Wrapp et al., 2020).

The other major issue in extreme COVID-19 is the abnormal immune response provoked through SARS-CoV-2. The infection is intently related to a reduction in circulating immune T-cells such as Th and Tc (CD4 and CD8) cells, apart from growth inflammatory markers. Inflammatory cytokines including IL-6 are liberated through the innate immune system in response to an infection. In some instances of COVID-19, cytokine manufacturing spirals out of control into a circumstance called a "cytokine typhoon." This triggers intense infection, inflicting immune cells to harm our own cells. In lots of instances, the cytokine typhoon causes extra damage than the original infection. Cytokine typhoon is one of the key triggers of acute respiratory distress syndrome (ARDS) in COVID-19 sufferers, and it is suspected to affect most of the other lifestyle-threatening symptoms related to COVID-19 (Gupta et al., 2020; AlSamman et al., 2020). Most people are recovered from COVID-19 because of sturdy immune response and the infection in the lungs is cleared. Even though, in a few sufferers, a dysfunctional immune response occurs, which triggers a cytokine typhoon that mediates enormous lung infection. Aside from lung inflammation, elevated levels of cytokine typhoon reasons myocardial harm and circulatory failure that becomes the cause for multiorgan failure (Ruan et al., 2020). Older people (the ones elderly over 60 years) and those with co-morbidities are much more likely to show increase in this kind of dysfunctional immune response that causes pathology and additionally fails to effectively eliminate the pathogen. The exact motives for this are doubtful, although one cause can be getting old, lung microenvironment inflicting altered dendritic cell maturation and migration to the lymphoid organs (Zhao et al., 2011) and thereby faulty T cell activation. In comparison, youngsters experiencing excessive viral load have a tendency to no longer increase worse health condition, which may be because of strong immune response.

5.4 VACCINE

Both innate and adaptive immune response provides protection against pathogens, however infectious diseases, that have plagued human populations all through history, still reason for the loss of life of thousands and thousands of people every year. Globally, such diseases remain the main reason of death, even though tremendous use of vaccines and drug remedy has significantly decreased mortality from infectious illnesses in developed nations. Vaccines are biological preparation that offers active adaptive immunity towards particular illnesses. The administration of vaccines is referred to as vaccination. The science of vaccine evolution and production is known as vaccinology. Vaccination is the best approach for safety towards infectious illnesses (Plotkin, 2003). The primary vaccine towards smallpox discovered by British physician Edward Jenner in 1796 (Siegrist, 2018) was derived from the benign cowpox virus, which provides immunity against small pox. Scientists are working on the other inhibitory pathways to inhibit the entry of SARS-CoV-2; one of the pathways toward SARS-CoV-2 therapeutical study is to restrict the host target ACE2 receptor. Presently, there are compounds that focus on these molecules that have been clinically accepted for different symptoms.

Vaccines generally include drugs that resemble the microorganisms liable for the disease and are frequently made from one of the killed or attenuated microorganisms, their toxins, or their surface proteins that's delivered via mouth, through injection, or by nasal spray. Later in life when we get infected, the immune system will apprehend them as foreign particles and damage them. Throughout in the process of immune response development, the body produces antibodies towards particular microorganisms and creates defense. Later when the individual encounters that microorganism, the antibody prevents it from causing disease or attenuates the severity of the disease, no matter the way that a vaccine is made. There are nonetheless numerous illnesses causing globally huge morbidity and mortality, for which no vaccines are available. Hundreds of thousands of humans globally die of diseases like malaria, tuberculosis, and AIDS every year without effective vaccination.

5.4.1 IMMUNIZATION

Immunity against infectious microorganisms can be obtained by using active or passive immunization. Active immunity refers to the procedure of disclosing the body to an antigen to generate an adaptive immune response or it can be produced through a person's personal immune system. Active immunity can be attained by means of natural infection with a microorganism, or it could be obtained artificially by means of administration of a vaccine. In active immunization, the immune system performs an active part in proliferation of antigen reactive T and B cells which results in formation of memory cells, and respond through differentiating into plasma cells that produce excessive amount of serum antibodies, which protect the person from the infectious diseases and this response takes days or even weeks to expand but may be long lasting, even lifelong.

Passive immunity refers to safety through antibody or antitoxin produced by using one organism and transferred to some other. It offers instantaneous safety towards infection, however that protection is not permanent. The antibodies will degrade within duration of weeks or months, and the recipient will be no longer protected. Passive immunization can provide instantaneous protection to vacationers or healthcare people who will quickly be exposed to an infectious organism and have short active immunity to it. But no longer it activates the immune system, no generation of memory response and the safety given by it, is transient.

5.4.2 TYPES OF VACCINES

Various types of vaccines are available in market to boost the immune system and to prevent several serious life-threatening diseases. Main four types of available vaccines are:

- live attenuated vaccines;
- inactivated vaccines;
- toxoid vaccines;
- subunit, recombinant, polysaccharide, and conjugate vaccines;
- Apart from above mentioned vaccines some other types of vaccines are:
- Viral vector vaccine;
- DNA vaccine;
- RNA or mRNA vaccine.

5.4.2.1 LIVE/ATTENUATED VACCINES

Live (attenuated) vaccines are derived from "wild" viruses or bacteria, that it does no longer cause severe ailment in human beings with an active immune system. These wild viruses or bacteria are attenuated (weakened) in a laboratory usually through repeated culturing. The immune response to a live (attenuated) vaccine is actually same to that produced via a natural infection; this is because the immune system does not differentiate among an infection with a weakened vaccine virus and with a wild virus. Attenuated vaccines have beneficial effects because of their potential for growth; such vaccines offer extended immune response resulting in elevated immunogenicity and production of memory cells. For this reason, a single dose of these vaccines is most effective instead of repeated boosters. But, a few percentages of recipients do not respond to the primary dose of an injected live (attenuated) vaccine (which includes oral polio vaccine, measles, mumps, and rubella [MMR]) and a second dose is suggested to offer an exceedingly high level of immunity within the population (Plotkin et al., 1969; Takahashi et al., 1975).

These type of viral vaccines are currently available and routinely recommended for MMR, varicella, rotavirus, influenza (intranasal), and chickenpox. Based on this, "Codagenix and Indian Immunologicals Ltd" are developing COVID-19 vaccine.

5.4.2.2 INACTIVATED VACCINES

Inactivated vaccines aren't live and cannot replicate. These vaccines can't be a reason for disease, even in an immune-deficient individual. In the preparation of this type of vaccine pathogen is inactivated through heat or by using chemical treatment. Inactivated antigens are much less stricken by circulating antibody than are live antigens, so they will be accepted when antibody is present inside the blood. This form of vaccines induces a predominantly humoral antibody response. They're less powerful than attenuated vaccines in inducing cell-mediated immunity. The immunity offered by inactivated vaccines is usually not as long-lasting as that acquired from live (attenuated) vaccines. Multiple doses are required to achieve ongoing immunity. Usually, the primary dose does not produce protective immunity. Defensive immune response develops after the second or third dose (e.g., polio, hepatitis A, and rabies vaccines) (American Academy of Pediatrics, 2018). Janssen, Sinopharm, Sputnik, Sinovac, Covaxin, Covivac, and Coviran are some COVID-19 vaccines available on this type (Table 5.1).

5.4.2.3 *TOXOID VACCINE*

This type of vaccines is manufactured from selected toxins which have been weakened and are capable of inducing a humoral immune response. Vaccination with the toxoid induces antitoxoid antibodies that are also capable of binding to the toxin and neutralizing its effects. Vaccines for tetanus and diphtheria are example of toxoid-based vaccines.

5.4.2.4 *SUBUNIT, RECOMBINANT, POLYSACCHARIDE, AND CONJUGATE VACCINES ARE BIOSYNTHETIC VACCINES*

In the production of biosynthetic vaccines, homogeneous pieces of the virus or bacteria are used. The hepatitis B vaccine is a precedent of this type of vaccine, because these vaccines use most effective particular pieces of the pathogens that display a complete strong immune response, which targets the primary part of the pathogen. This type of vaccine is given to everyone who desires them, including people having weakened immune system and long-term health problems. Subunit vaccines (e.g., influenza and pneumococcal vaccines) and recombinant vaccines (e.g., hepatitis B, human papillomavirus [HPV], and influenza) are the examples of this type (Different types of vaccines, 2019).

A subunit vaccine like live attenuated and inactivated vaccine do not contain pathogens, they only contain an antigenic part of the pathogen. This part is necessary to elicit a protective immune response. The antigens involved can be any molecule, such as proteins, peptides or polysaccharides. They are quite more secure as there is no genetic material and cannot replicate within the body. They have a tendency to induce a humoral antibody response in addition to cell-mediated response. For long term immunity these vaccines require more than one dose. Hepatitis B, human papillomavirus, and influenza vaccines (injected forms) are examples of subunit vaccines. Zifivax and MVC-COV1901 are COVID-19 subunit vaccines (Table 5.1).

A conjugate vaccine is used with a purpose to call an immune system response towards the weak antigen. In a conjugate vaccine, the vulnerable antigen is covalently attached to a strong antigen, thereby eliciting a more potent immunological response against the weak antigen. An antigen can be a polysaccharide that is connected to strong protein antigen. However, peptide/protein and protein/protein conjugates have additionally been evolved. These vaccines are used to shield towards: Human papilloma-virus (HPV), whooping cough, pneumococcal disease, and meningococcal ailment.

5.4.2.5 VIRAL VECTOR VACCINE

In viral vector vaccine, virus is used as a vector to deliver genetic material against a particular antigen into the recipient cells. Genetic material provided by viral vector no longer integrates into the person's cellular genome. This type of vaccine uses a modified version of one virus as a vector to deliver a genetic material into the cell coding an antigen for some other infectious agent. Viral vector vaccines do no longer cause infection either the virus is used as the vector or the source of the antigen. This vaccine allows an expression of antigen within the cell and results in a strong cytotoxic T cell response, along with humoral immunity (Ura et al., 2014; CDC, 2021). Vaxzevria and Covishield are COVID-19 viral vector vaccines (Table 5.1).

5.4.2.6 DNA VACCINES

DNA vaccine is a type of vaccine that induces a specific antigen-coding DNA sequence into the cells of an organism as a mechanism to induce an immune response. It consists of plasmid DNA encoding antigenic proteins which can be injected immediately intradermally to the recipient. Muscle cells absorb the DNA and the encoded protein antigen is expressed, leading to both a humoral antibody response and a cell-mediated response. These vaccines work through allowing the expression of the microbial antigen within host cells that take up the plasmid, functions by generating the desired antigen within the cells, with the benefit that this could facilitate presentation through the major histocompatibility complex. Therefore, the immune response is same to the antigen expressed by the pathogen. These DNA vaccines cause extended expression of the antigen, which generates huge immunological memory. Presently numerous DNA vaccines are under human trial for malaria, AIDS, influenza, and herpesvirus (Jaurigue et al., 2017). Zycov-D is a COVID-19 DNA vaccine (Table 5.1).

5.4.2.7 RIBONUCLEIC ACID (RNA) VACCINE OR MESSENGER RNA (MRNA) VACCINE

This type of vaccine uses a replica of a molecule known as messenger RNA (mRNA) to stimulate an immune response. The vaccine transfects molecules of synthetic mRNA into immune cells, inflicting the cells to construct foreign proteins, which might generally, had been produced by a pathogen (which causes virulent disease). These protein molecules stimulate an adaptive immune response which teaches the body to identify and damage the corresponding pathogenic cells (Park et al., 2021). The mRNA is introduced through a component of the RNA encapsulated in lipid nanoparticles which defends the RNA strands and assists their absorption into the cells. The advantages of RNA vaccines over conventional protein vaccines are ease of design, speed, low price of manufacturing, and the induction of both cell and humoral immunity (Pardi et al., 2018; PGH Foundation, 2020). Pfizer-BioNTech and Moderma (spikevax) are COVID-19 mRNA type vaccine (Table 5.1).

5.4.3 VACCINE DEVELOPMENT AGAINST CORONAVIRUS (COVID-19)

Numerous factors need to be kept in mind in developing a successful vaccine. Initially in the development of an immune response, vaccine designers need to understand the essential differences between activation of the humoral and the cell-mediated immunity. Another important factor is the development of immunologic memory. For an example, a vaccine that induces a defensive primary response may also fail to induce the formation of memory cells, alleviating the vaccine effect and leaving the host unprotected after the primary response.

Vaccine development requires huge amount of virus, frequently in animals or from tissue culture at large scale. The viruses are inactivated through radiation, heat, or chemical substances, or are derived from genetically weakened strains. Other processes in vaccine development include isolation of viral proteins like spike instead of purifying the whole virus. This is more secure and less complicated to scale up. However, the immune system response to the isolated protein is often no longer as strong as it is organized in lattice form of the intact virus particle. A latest

TABLE 5.1 COVID-19 Vaccines and Immune Response.

COVID-19 vaccine	Type of vaccine	Manufacturer	Immune response
Oxford–AstraZeneca (Vaxzevria, Covishield)	Viral vector vaccine	British University of Oxford, British-Swedish company AstraZeneca	Induce a cytotoxic T lymphocyte (CTL) response (Ura et al., 2014) and humoral response
Pfizer-BioNTech (comirnaty)	mRNA vaccine	German company BioNTech and American company Pfizer	Induces secretion of type I interferons (IFNs) to the extracellular matrix that favors Th1 responses over Th2 (Cagigi and Lore, 2021)
Moderna COVID-19 vaccine (spikevax)	mRNA vaccine	American company Moderna	Induces secretion of type I interferons (IFNs) to the extracellular matrix that favors Th1 responses over Th2
Janssen (Johnson & Johnson)	Inactivated viral vaccine	Janssen Group and Beijing Institute of Biological Products	Induces predominantly humoral response than cytotoxic T lymphocyte (CTL) response
Sinopharm BIBP	Inactivated viral vaccine	China National Pharmaceutical	Induces predominantly humoral response than cytotoxic T lymphocyte (CTL) response
Sputnik V (Gam-Covid-Vac)	Inactivated viral vaccine	Russian Gamaleya Research Institute of Epidemiology and Microbiology	Induces predominantly humoral response than cytotoxic T lymphocyte (CTL) response
Sinovac-CoronaVac	Inactivated viral vaccine	Chinese company Sinovac Biotech	Induces predominantly humoral response than cytotoxic T lymphocyte (CTL) response
Covaxin	Inactivated viral vaccine	Indian company Bharat Biotech and the Indian Council of Medical Research	Induces predominantly humoral response than cytotoxic T lymphocyte (CTL) response
Sinopharm WIBP	Inactivated virus vaccine	China National Pharmaceutical Group (Sinopharm)	Induces predominantly humoral response than cytotoxic T lymphocyte (CTL) response
EpiVacCorona	Peptide vaccine	Russian State Research Center of Virology and Biotechnology VECTOR	Induces CD8 cytotoxic T lymphocytes, CD4 T cell response, and also elicit an effective humoral response (Malonis et al., 2020)

TABLE 5.1 *(Continued)*

COVID-19 vaccine	Type of vaccine	Manufacturer	Immune response
Zifivax	Subunit vaccine	Chinese company Anhui Zhifei Longcom Biopharmaceutical	Elicits humoral and cell-mediated immune response
CoviVac	Inactivated virus vaccine	Chumakov Centre at the Russian Academy of Sciences	Induce a cytotoxic T lymphocyte (CTL) response
MVC-COV1901	Subunit vaccine	Medigen Vaccine Biologics and Dynavax Technologies	Elicits humoral and cell-mediated immune response
ZyCoV-D	DNA plasmid	Indian-based pharmaceutical company Cadila Healthcare	Induces cell-mediated and humoral immune response
COVIran Barekat	Inactivated virus vaccine	Shifa Pharmed Industrial Co. in Iran	Induces predominantly humoral response than cytotoxic T lymphocyte (CTL) response

approach includes injecting individuals with RNA or DNA (nucleic acids) encoding for viral proteins. These nucleic acids can be administered alone or through man-made vectors that help in delivering the material into the body. In any method, enough material is needed to inject reasonable doses into millions of human beings (Roper and Rehm, 2009).

Traditionally for the preparation of coronavirus vaccines lots of problems has to be faced. Coronavirus vaccines tested in animal models have been immunogenic but generally no longer shown effective success in preventing the disease (Edridge et al., 2020). Further, there is an issue that vaccination like natural coronaviral infection may not result in long-lived immunity and reinfection may be possible (Graham et al., 2013). Earlier use of coronavirus vaccines (SARS-CoV and MERS-CoV) showed protective effect in some animal models through T-helper 2 (Th-2) cell-mediated immunity (Tseng et al., 2012). Mice vaccinated with inactivated whole virus vaccines, a recombinant DNA spike protein vaccine or a virus-like particle vaccine evolved lung pathology which includes eosinophilic infiltration 2 days after being challenged with SARS-CoV, which were no longer visible within the lungs of challenged unvaccinated mice (Deming et al., 2006). Mice immunized with SARS-CoVN protein vaccine evolved severe pneumonia or lung eosinophilic infiltrate upon viral challenge, wherein as mice immunized with viral replicon particles expressing glycoprotein did not suggest that N protein antigen may be the antigen related to this immunopathology. Comparable more suitable immunopathology has been visible in mice vaccinated with inactivated MERS-CoV vaccine, while challenged with live virus (Agrawal et al., 2016).

To make SAR-CoV-2 vaccine possible, collection of essential facts for vaccine development and assessment has to be well defined. This includes locating target antigen(s), immunization course, correlated immune safety, animal models, scalability, production facility, target product profile (TPP), outbreak forecasting, and target population.

5.4.4 PREVENTIVE VACCINES: IS IT POSSIBLE?

It is very widely known that SAR-CoV-2 infection affected the entire world and the continuous efforts in the direction of developing an effective SAR-CoV-2 vaccine had been in progress in the whole world. Numerous research organizations had started SAR-CoV-2 vaccine development within a few weeks after the outbreak. The target for antigen selection and vaccine development are totally based on SARS-CoV-2 and MERS-CoV vaccine studies. A possible mechanism based on scientific studies showed that by interrupting the interaction between full-length spikes (S) or S1 which includes receptor-binding domain (RDB) might be taken into consideration as an excellent vaccine antigen because it can result in neutralizing antibodies that protect host cell attachment and infection (Al-Amri et al., 2017; Du et al., 2007, 2009). According to the modern-day technological advancement, mRNA and nucleic acid-based vaccine has been taken into consideration as promising vaccine technology against COVID-19 infections. Although, mRNA vaccine designs have stepped forward stability and protein translation efficiency in inducing strong immune responses (Pardi et al., 2018; Maruggi et al., 2019).

5.5 CONCLUSION

It is well known that the COVID-19 infection affected entire population globally and it is the challenging task for whole world. The fast spreading of this surprisingly contagious disease has posed the severest danger to worldwide health in this century. Earlier than clinically accepted vaccines, there is no better way to defend us from SARS-CoV-2 than personal preventive measures which includes social distancing, wearing mask, and public health measures, consisting of active testing, case tracing, and restrictions on social gatherings. Current information of this novel coronavirus is just like a tip of the iceberg. Research into the characteristics of SARS-CoV-2, its interaction with the host immune responses may also help in offering a clearer image of how the pathogen causes illnesses in a few people, while maximum infected humans only display slight or no signs in any respect. Similarly, it was observed that how immune system provides protection and the long-term immune memory from getting better. Additionally, researchers are involved in designing preventive and therapeutic approach for future outbreak of similar coronaviruses. This prognostic view can also help in designing an immune intercession or preventive vaccine for COVID-19 in the near future. Tackling this epidemic is an extended-time period activity, needs lots of efforts by each person.

KEYWORDS

- **SARS-CoV-2**
- **coronavirus 19 (COVID-19)**
- **immune response**
- **vaccines**

REFERENCES

Agrawal, A. S.; Tao, X.; Algaissi, A.; Garron, T.; Narayanan, K.; Peng, B. H.; Couch, R. B.; Tseng, C. T. Immunization with Inactivated Middle East Respiratory Syndrome Coronavirus Vaccine Leads to Lung Immunopathology on Challenge with Live Virus. *Hum. Vaccin. Immunother.* **2016,** *12*, 2351–6.

Al-Amri, S. S.; Abbas, A. T.; Siddiq, L. A.; Alghamdi, A.; Sanki, M. A.; Al-Muhanna, M. K.; Alhabbab, R. Y.; Azhar, E. I.; Li, X.; Hashem, A. M. Immunogenicity of Candidate MERS-CoV DNA Vaccines Based on the Spike Protein. *Sci. Rep.* **2017,** *7*, 44875.

Alanagreh, L.; Alzoughool, F.; Atoum, M. The Human Coronavirus Disease COVID-19: Its Origin, Characteristics, and Insights into Potential Drugs and Its Mechanisms. *Pathogens* **2020,** *9*, 331.

Alsaadi, J.; Entedar, A.; Ian, M. Jones. Membrane Binding Proteins of Coronaviruses. *Future Virol.* **2019,** *14*(4), 275–286.

AlSamman, M.; Caggiula, A.; Ganguli, S.; Misak, M.; Pourmand, A. Non-Respiratory Presentations of COVID-19, a Clinical Review. *Am. J. Emerg. Med.* **2020,** *38*, 2444–2454.

Bhatraju, P. K.; Ghassemieh, B. J.; Nichols, M.; Kim, R., et al. COVID-19 in Critically Ill Patients in the Seattleregion—Case Series. *N. Engl. J. Med.* **2020,** *382*, 2012–2022.

Cagigi, A.; Loré, K. Immune Responses Induced by mRNA Vaccination in Mice, Monkeys and Humans. *Vaccines* **2021,** *9*, 61.

Centers for Disease Control and Prevention (CDC). Understanding and Explaining Viral Vector COVID-19 Vaccines. Updated January 5, 2021. https://www.cdc.gov/vaccines/COVID-19/hcp/viral-vector-vaccine-basics.html (accessed Feb 4, 2021).

Channappanavar, R.; Perlman, S. Pathogenic Human Coronavirus Infections: Causes and Consequences of Cytokine Storm and Immunopathology. *Semin. Immunopathol.* **2017,** 39, 529–539.

Chen, N.; Zhou, M.; Dong, X.; Qu, J.; Gong, F.; Han, Y.; Qiu, Y.; Wang, J.; Liu, Y.; Wei, Y.; Xia, J.; Yu, T.; Zhang, X.; Zhang, L. Epidemiological and Clinical Characteristics of 99 Cases of 2019 Novel Coronavirus Pneumonia in Wuhan, China: A Descriptive Study. *Lancet* **2020,** *395*, 507–513.

Wrapp, D.; Wang, N.; Corbett, K. S.; Goldsmith, J. A.; Hsieh, C. L.; Abiona, O.; Graham, B. S.; McLellan, J. S. Cryo-EM Structure of the 2019-nCoV Spike in the Prefusion Conformation. *Science* **2020,** *367*, 1260–1263.

de Wit, E.; van Doremalen, N.; Falzarano, D.; Munster, V. J. SARS and MERS: Recent Insights into Emerging Coronaviruses. *Nat. Rev. Microbiol.* **2016,** *14*, 523–534.

Deming, D.; Sheahan, T.; Heise, M.; Yount, B.; Davis, N., et al. Vaccine Efficacy in Senescent Mice Challenged with Recombinant SARS-CoV Bearing Epidemic and Zoonotic Spike Variants. *PLoSMed.* **2006,** *3*, e525.

Different Types of Vaccines. History of Vaccines. 2019. www.historyofvaccines.org.

Du, L.; He, Y.; Zhou, Y.; Liu, S.; Zheng, B. J.; Jiang, S. The Spike Protein of SARS-CoV a Target for Vaccine and Therapeutic Development. *Nat. Rev. Microbiol.* **2009,** *7*, 226–36.

Du, L.; Zhao, G.; He, Y.; Guo, Y.; Zheng, B. J.; Jiang, S., et al. Receptor-Binding Domain of SARS-CoV Spike Protein Induces Long-Term Protective Immunity in an Animal Model. *Vaccine* **2007,** *25*, 2832–8.

Edridge, A. W. D.; Kaczorowska, J. M.; Hoste, A. C.; Bakker, M.; Klein, M.; Jebbink, M. F., et al. Human Coronavirus Reinfection Dynamics: Lessons for SARS-CoV-2. *Med Rxiv* **2020.**

Fehr, A. R.; Perlman, S. Methods I Coronaviruses: An Overview of Their Replication and Pathogenesis. Coronaviruses. In *Molecular Biology*, Vol. 1282; Maier H. J., Bickerton E., Britton P., Eds.; Springer, 2015; pp 1–23.

Giacomelli, A.; Pezzati, L.; Conti, F.; Bernacchia, D.; Siano, M., et al. Self-Reported of Factory and Tasted is Orders in Patients with Severe a Cute Respiratory Coronavirus 2 Infection: Across-Sectional Study. *Clin. Infect. Dis.* **2020,** *71*, 889–890.

Graham, R. L.; Donaldson, E. F.; Baric, R. S. A Decade After SARS: Strategies for Controlling Emerging Coronaviruses. *Nat. Rev. Microbiol.* **2013,** *11*, 836–48.

Guan, W. J.; Ni, Z. Y.; Hu, Y.; Liang, W. H.; Ou, C. Q., et al. Clinical Characteristics of Coronavirus Disease 2019 in China. *N. Engl. J. Med.* **2020,** *382*, 1708–20.

Gupta, A.; Madhavan, M. V.; Sehgal, K.; Nair, N.; Mahajan, S., et al. Extra Pulmonary Manifestations of COVID-19. *Nat. Med.* **2020,** *26*, 1017–1032.

Huang, C.; Wang, Y.; Li, X.; Ren, L.; Zhao, J.; Hu, Y., et al. Clinical Features of Patients Infected with 2019 Novel Coronavirus in Wuhan, China. *Lancet* **2020,** *395*, 497–506.

Jaurigue, J. A.; Seeberger, P. H. Parasite Carbohydrate Vaccines. *Front. Cell. Infect. Microbiol.* **2017,** *7*, 248.

Kimberlin, D.; Brady, M.; Jackson, M. Active and Passive Immunization. In *Report of the Committee on Infectious Diseases*, 31st ed; Red Book Ed., American Academy of Pediatrics: Itasca, IL, 2018; pp 13–64.

Kimbrell, D. A.; Beutler, B. The Evolution and Genetics of Innate Immunity. *Nature Rev. Genet.* **2001,** *2*, 256–267.

Kindler, E.; Thiel, V.; Weber, F. Interaction of SARS and MERS Coronaviruses with the Antiviral Interferon Response. *Adv. Virus Res.* **2016,** *96*, 219–43.

Lauer, S. A.; Grantz, K. H.; Bi, Q.; Jones, F. K.; Zheng, Q., et al. The Incubation Period of Coronavirus Disease 2019 (COVID-19) from Publicly Reported Confirmed Cases: Estimation and Application. *Ann. Intern. Med.* **2020,** 172, 577–582.

Lodoen, M. B.; Lanier, L. L. Natural Killer Cells as an Initial Defense Against Pathogens. *Curr. Opin. Immunol.* **2006,** *18*, 391–398.

Malonis, R. J.; Lai, J. R.; Vergnolle, O. Peptide-Based Vaccines: Current Progress and Future Challenges. *Chem. Rev.* **2020,** *120*, 3210–3229.

Maruggi, G.; Zhang, C.; Li, J.; Ulmer, J. B.; Yu, D. mRNA as a Transformative Technology for Vaccine Development to Control Infectious Diseases. *Mol. Ther.* **2019,** *27*, 757–772.

Medzhitov, R.; Janeway, C. A. 2000. Innate immunity. *N. Eng. J. Med.* **2000,** *343*, 338–344.

Pan, L.; Mu, M.; Yang, P.; Sun, Y.; Wang, R., et al. Clinical Characteristics of COVID-19 Patients with Digestive Symptoms in Hubei, China: A Descriptive, Cross-Sectional, Multicenter Study. *Am. J. Gastroenterol.* **2020,** *115*, 766–773.

Pardi, N.; Hogan, M. J.; Porter, F. W.; Weissman, D. mRNA Vaccines – A new Era in Vaccinology. *Nat. Rev. Drug. Discov*. **2018,** *17*, 261–279.

Park, K. S.; Sun, X.; Aikins, M. E.; Moon, J. J. Non-Viral COVID-19 Vaccine Delivery Systems. *Adv. Drug Deliv. Rev*. **2021,** *169*, 137–151.

PHG Foundation. RNA Vaccines: An Introduction. University of Cambridge. Retrieved 18 November 2020.

Plotkin, S. Vaccines, Vaccination, and Vaccinology. *J. Infect. Dis.* **2003,** *187*, 1349–1359.

Plotkin, S. A.; Farquhar, J. D.; Katz, M.; Buser, F. Attenuation of RA 27–3 Rubella Virus in WI-38 Human Diploid Cells. *Am. J. Dis. Child.* **1969,** *118*, 178–185.

Recalcati, S. Cutaneousmanife Stations in COVID-19: A First Perspective. *J. Eur. Acad. Dermatol. Venereol.* **2020,** *34*, e212–e213.

Roper, R. L.; Rehm, K. E. SARS Vaccines: Where are We? *Expert Rev. Vaccines* **2009,** *8*, 887–898.

Ruan, Q.; Yang, K.; Wang, W.; Jiang, L.; Song, J. Clinical Predictors of Mortality Due to COVID-19 Based on an Analysis of Data of 150 Patients from Wuhan, China. *Intensive Care Med.* **2020,** *46*, 846–848.

Schoeman, D.; Fielding, B. C. Coronavirus Envelope Protein: Current Knowledge. *Virol. J.* **2019,** 27, *16*(1), 69.

Siegrist C. *Vaccine Immunology*, 7th ed.; Plotkin, S., Orenstein, W., Offit, P., et al., Eds.; Elsevier, 2018; pp 16–34.

Song, Y.; Liu, P.; Shi, X. L.; Chu, Y. L.; Zhang, J.; Xia, J.; Gao, X. Z.; Qu, T.; Wang, M. Y. SARS-CoV-2 Induced Diarrhoeaasonset Symptom in Patient with COVID-19. *Gut* **2020,** *69*, 1143–1144.

Takahashi, M.; Okuno, Y.; Otsuka, T.; Osame, J.; Takamizawa, A. Development of a Live Attenuated Varicella Vaccine. *Biken J.* **1975,** *18*, 25–33.

Tang, N.; Li, D.; Wang, X.; Sun, Z. Abnormal Coagulation Parameters are Associated with Poor Prognosis in Patients with Novel Coronavirus Pneumonia. *J. Thromb. Haemost.* **2020,** *18*, 844–847.

Tseng, C. T.; Sbrana, E.; Iwata-Yoshikawa, N.; Newman, P. C.; Garron, T.; Atmar, R. L.; Peters, C. J.; Couch, R. B. Immunization with SARS Coronavirus Vaccines Leads to Pulmonary Immunopathology on Challenge with the SARS Virus. *PLoSONE* **2012,** 7e35421.

Ura, T.; Okuda, K.; Shimada, M. Developments in Viral Vector-Based Vaccines. *Vaccines* **2014,** *2*, 624–41.

Wang, D.; Hu, B.; Hu, C.; Zhu, F.; Liu, X., et al. Clinical characteristics of 138 Hospitalized Patients with 2019 Novel Coronavirus–Infected Pneumonia in Wuhan, China. *JAMA* **2020,** *323*, 1061–1069.

World Health Organization. Weekly Epidemiology Update, Edition 54, published 24 August 2021. Available online https://www.who.int/emergencies/diseases/novel-coronavirus-2019/situation-reports.

Zhao, J.; Zhao, J.; Legge, K.; Perlman, S. Age-Related Increases in PGD2 Expression Impair Respiratory DC Migration, Resulting in Diminished T Cell Responses Upon Respiratory Virus Infection in Mice. *J. Clin. Invest.* **2011,** *121*, 4921–4930.

Zhou, F.; Yu, T.; Du, R.; Fan, G.; Liu, Y., et al. Clinical Course and Risk Factors for Mortality of Adult Inpatients with COVID-19 in Wuhan, China: A Retrospective Cohort Study. *Lancet* **2020,** *395*, 1054–1062.

Zhou, P.; Yang, X. L.; Wang, X. G.; Hu, B.; Zhang, L., et al. A Pneumonia Outbreak Associated with a New Coronavirus of Probable Bat Origin. *Nature* **2020,** *579*, 270–273.

CHAPTER 6

Traditional System of Medicine and Lifestyle for the Management, Prevention, and Treatment of COVID-19

SHANTI BHUSHAN MISHRA[1], SHRADHANJALI SINGH[2], AMIT KUMAR SINGH[3], and ANIL KUMAR SINGH[3]

[1]*Department of Pharmacognosy, United Institute of Pharmacy, Prayagraj, Uttar Pradesh, India*

[2]*Department of Pharmaceutical Chemistry, United Institute of Pharmacy, Prayagraj, Uttar Pradesh, India*

[3]*Department of Pharmaceutics, United Institute of Pharmacy, Prayagraj, Uttar Pradesh, India*

ABSTRACT

All of humanity is affected by COVID-19 caused by a novel coronavirus (SARS-CoV-2) that is a viral pneumonia that was highly contagious and pathogenic. A few common symptoms of COVID-19 patients include fever, dry cough, loss of taste, loss of smell, and acute respiratory distress syndrome. Since the ancient period, herbal remedies have been conventionally used to treat flu and cold symptoms, as well as infections of the upper and lower respiratory system. Certain medicinal foods recipes could be used to inhibit the infection and as well strengthen immunity. Most of the population believes that consuming herbal medicines can prevent or even cure COVID-19 infection. Ayurveda and Yoga can certainly play an essential role to augment preventive measures for COVID-19. This chapter

COVID-19 and Immunomodulation with Special Emphasis on Nutraceutical and Herbal Formulation. Rajesh K. Kesharwani & Raj K. Keservani (Eds)

explicates about medicinal plants that are used traditionally to prevent or treat viral infections and some Yoga protocols to improve respiratory and cardiac efficiency and strengthen immunity.

6.1 INTRODUCTION

COVID-19 is a transmittable respiratory infection caused by a highly infectious and communicable type of novel coronavirus, SARS-CoV-2, noticed at the end of the year 2019. The pandemic has caused considerable damage to human lives and created unprecedented challenges for the public health system not only in India but also across the globe (Abebe, 2020). COVID-19 sick people showed various undefined symptoms, from slight to severe, namely, fever which is the most frequent manifestation followed by cough, weakness, mucus production, sore throat, nasal congestion, runny nose, and headache that is described by all the patients suffering from COVID-19. The old age people and those having previous medical conditions, such as asthma, cardiovascular disorders, diabetes, and cancer are more possible to create serious illnesses from SARS-CoV-2.2 (Lima, 2020).

Presently, there is no exact medication for COVID-19. Several vaccines are currently used as a preventive measure. According to an estimation of WHO, approximately 86 vaccines are under clinical trials around the world and 186 in preclinical stage. Vaccines like AstraZeneca/AZD1222 vaccines, Pfizer-BioNtech Comirnaty vaccine, Janssen/Ad26.COV 2.S, Covishield manufactured by Johnson & Johnson, and Sinopharm and Moderna COVID-19 vaccine (mRNA 1273) developed by Beijing Bio-Institute of Biological Products were listed by WHO in emergency use listing and the mass immunization program started in December 2020. Additionally, countless efforts have been committed to discovering effective prophylactics against COVID-19 (Sharma et al., 2020).

Furthermore, people in the scientific community and researchers are searching for the best approach to treat or prevent the disease, including the use of natural products and herbal medicine (Rane et al., 2020). Herbs offer a wide range of viral protein inhibitors for the curing of SARS. Generally, plants contain various types of secondary metabolites that can provide a preventive effect on the spread or proliferation of the virus (Jahan and Onay, 2020) In the current situation, a recent movement among the people is the consumption of herbal remedies containing certain phytoconstituents, which have anti-inflammatory, antimicrobial, immunostimulatory activities, and antiviral such as quinine, echinacea, curcumin, and ginseng. These herbal constituents are assumed to have the ability to adjust the immune response; consequently, they are supposed to have beneficial effects on preventing or curing COVID-19 as immunity of people plays an important role in COVID-19 infection (Nugraha et al., 2020). Since the immunogenic response of patients plays an central role in COVID-19 infection, a herbal remedy with immunomodulatory action may have therapeutic potential as a preventive measure for patients with COVID-19 infections. Several foods and herbs might be used as a supplementary therapy to prevent infection and enhance immunity (Nugraha et al., 2020). The long-lasting use of dietary therapy, life-style management, and herbal medicine could prevent and treat the diseases. This chapter provides strong evidence in confirmation of dietary therapy and herbs as preventive agents against COVID-19, as well as for enhancing immunity.

6.2 MEDICINAL PLANTS AS IMMUNITY BOOSTER AGAINST COVID-19

6.2.1 GILOY/GUDUCHI (TINOSPORA CORDIFOLIA)

Giloy herb has heart-shaped leaves and has been used and prescribed in the Indian system of medicine for centuries. In the pandemic, when immunity-boosting foods and healthy eating rapidly gained importance, Giloy became well-liked herb even among individuals who have not tried it before. Giloy is one such blessing of Mother Nature, which has helped people from breathing problems, cough, cold, and several other ailments (Chowdhury, 2020). These are also the main indications of the coronavirus infection. The plant has been used from a long time for its therapeutic actions. Ayurveda named it as *guduchi*, which means "protector from diseases," or as nectar or *amrita* which has the activity of immortalizing the user. In Ayurvedic literature, giloy is mentioned as a *patra shaka*, as a vegetable. This Ayurvedic herb is a source of antioxidants that scavenge-free radicals and prevent swelling (Borse et al., 2021). It augments the action of macrophages (the cells are sensible for fighting microorganisms or foreign bodies and thus help in rapid recovery). It cleans the blood, boosts immunity, cleans up toxins from the body, and helps diminish respiratory problems like frequent cough, cold, tonsils, and fights against virus and bacteria efficiently. The antiviral properties of Guduchi against H1N1 and Chikungunya virus have already been documented by a number of researchers (Saha and Ghosh, 2012). The immunomodulatory property of Giloy is well recognized due to the presence of compounds like *N*-methyl-2-pyrrolidone, tinocordiside, syringin, 11-hydroxymustakone, *N*-formylannonain, and cordifolioside (Sagar and Kumar, 2012). Kadha (tea), Giloy churna, gutika, and vati (tablets), and so on dosages form could be used for numerous skin complications as it eliminates various toxins from the body. It also shows pharmacological properties like immunomodulation, hypoglycemic, hepatoprotective, and anticancer (Sharma et al., 2012).

6.2.2 AMLA (PHYLLANTHUS EMBLICA)

Phyllanthus emblica L. (Indian gooseberry), belongs to the family Euphorbiaceae, is a medium-sized deciduous tree having great therapeutic importance. It helps in removing toxins from the whole organ system for good health and immune power. Amla fruits contain high amounts of vitamin C (ascorbic acid) and also rich in polyphenolics that are accepted to fight against the expansion of cancer cells. Amla is also useful in controlling metabolic disorders like diabetes and also reduces cholesterol levels. Amla possesses human immunodeficiency virus (HIV) reverse transcriptase activity and can also be analyzed against SARS-CoV-2 (Murugesan et al., 2021). It also contains numerous phytoconstituents, namely, a higher amount of polyphenols like ellagic acid, gallic acid, minerals, and vitamins, and different flavonoids like quercetin, rutin, tannins, amino acids, and fixed oils (Variya et al., 2016).

6.2.3 ASHWAGANDHA (WITHANIA SOMNIFERA)

Ashwagandha, a shrub with pale green flowers, red berries, and elliptic leaves is commonly known as winter cherry. Traditionally, the greatest benefits of ashwagandha come from the root and leaves. The roots can be taken in many forms but commonly as dried powdered as a supplement these days. The drug is well explored for miscellaneous pharmacological activities including immunomodulatory, antioxidant, antihypertensive, anti-inflammatory, antidiabetic, and anti-stress, along with organ-protective effects (Mishra et al., 2000). It also helps to increase strength, muscle, and improve brain function as well. Recently, an in-silico study explained that withaferin A showed antiviral activity against SARS-CoV-2 through inhibition of RNA polymerase with high binding energy than hydroxychloroquine and other drugs used in treatment of SARS-CoV-2. A new study on withanone also confirmed the inhibition of SARS-CoV-2 entry and subsequent infection by disrupting the electrostatic interaction between ACE2 and RBD (Balkrishna et al., 2020). Ashwagandha improves the body's immune system against ailments by improving cellular immunity. It also possesses antioxidant activities that help to protect against oxidative injury caused by free radicals species. It also revealed inhibitory activity against many cancers, (prostate, ovarian, breast, colon, colon, lung, and brain), accompanied by various pathways and mechanism of actions (Dutta et al., 2019).

6.2.4 NEEM (AZADIRACHTA INDICA)

Neem (*Azadirachta indica*) have a place in Meliaceae family and is often found in India and titled as "Free tree of India." "Nimba" is an alternative name of it which means "conferring good health." It is also known for "40 cures." In the Ayurvedic system of medicine, Neem is known as a healer of all ailments that is why known as Sarva Roga Nivarini. Neem is also useful in boosting immunity of body. It contains antifungal and antibacterial activities that help keep individuals' skin glowing, clean, and healthy. Neem also has blood-purifying nature, boosting both the cellular and lymphocytic immune systems (Gupta et al., 2017). Daily dose of Neem capsules can also prevent viral flu, malaria, high fever, dengue, and other infectious diseases. Neem extracts significantly constrain the HIV, poliovirus, HSV, influenza virus, and coxsackie B group virus by virus inactivation. About more than 70 numerous terpenoids have been identified in different parts of the Neem tree. A terpenoid obtained from Neem, beta-caryophyllene, is scientifically explored for anti-inflammatory, antioxidant, and pain-reducing benefits. Over 300 structurally different chemical constituents, including limonoids like azadirachtin, nimbolide, and gedunin, have been investigated as modulators of cell-signaling pathways. COVID-19 is responsible for serious cytokine-induced problems and coagulopathies. Neem also acts as an inhibitor of pro-inflammatory cytokines along with thrombolytic actions. Thus, Neem can be considered as a prominent herb due to its immunomodulator other than its broad-spectrum antiviral properties in slight, trivial, and severe cases of the COVID-19 virus (Baildya et al., 2021).

6.2.5 TULSI (OCIMUM SANCTUM)

According to ancient literature, different parts of Tulsi plant have been utilized for the treatment of different ailments. This herb contains abundant vitamin C and possesses antioxidants, antiseptic, and antiviral properties. Tulsi is useful to intensify the bronchial system due to its actions on the chemical alterations that occur in the body. Tulsi relieves physical, chemical, psychological, and metabolic stress through a distinct combination of healing actions (Ghoke et al., 2018). Several pure compounds isolated and recognized from Tulsi extracts like eugenol, carvacrol, 1,8-cineole, apigenin, quercetin, ursolic acid, methyl eugenol, linalool, luteoline, and oleanolic acid have exhibited activity against certain DNA and RNA viruses like DENV, CMV, HPAI (H5N1), NDV, HSV, EV71, HBV, HIV, CVB, and so on. Moreover, Tulsi extracts and volatile oils isolated from the leaves have shown promising antiviral activities against H9N2 virus. These chemical compounds are potential inhibitors of SARS-CoV-2 protease, which would suggest that Tulsi plants have anti-SARS-CoV-2 effect (Tshilandaa et al., 2020).

6.2.6 DRUMSTICK TREE (MORINGA OLEIFERA)

The most important nutrients which are needed for immunity are vitamin C, vitamin A, protein, and minerals (zinc, potassium, calcium, and magnesium), all of which are abundant in *Moringa*. This is a native Indian vegetable that has antiviral, antifungal, and anti-inflammatory properties (Stohs and Hartman, 2015). Drumsticks have more vitamin C as compared to oranges. Vitamin C is the primary nutrient that our body needs to build strong immunity, and during the COVID-19 pandemic, it should be a go-to herb for immunity strengthening. The investigators used computer-docking modeling to establish that phytoconstituents recognized from the drumstick plant could inhibit the SARS-CoV-2 virus and found that many phytochemicals unveil high binding affinity with the viruses and act as virus inhibitors. A report illustrates that the most active compound of *Moringa* is apigenin-7-O-rutinoside against the viruses and most of the phytochemicals have antioxidant properties that will ameliorate the secondary infection that arises after COVID (Sen et al., 2021).

6.2.7 WILD CARROT (DAUCUS MARITIMUS)

Daucus maritimus seed extracts were investigated for antiviral activities against a series of RNA-dependent RNA polymerases of dengue virus, HIV type 1, hepatitis C virus (HCV), and West Nile virus. A study showed that the extract of wild carrot showed trivial to potent inhibition against the four viral polymerases. The volatile oils from floral parts and roots of *Daucus carota* L. var. *maritimus* were obtained by distillation and studied by gas chromatography/mass spectrometry, and carbon-nuclear magnetic resonance. Their antibacterial effect resulted in the inhibition of a range of common human pathogenic bacteria, and some clinically and naturally isolated strains with significant MIC and MBC values (Jabrane et al., 2009).

6.2.8 PIPPALI (PIPER LONGUM)

In Indian medicine, *Piper longum* is used to treat respiratory disorders such as asthma, bronchitis, many stomach-related dysentery, pyrexia, and other sleep disorders called "insomnia." Bioactive compounds derived from plant sources have long been known as viral inhibitors. *P. longum* contains ribosomal inactivating proteins that protect against viral infection. The efficacy of *P. longum* against a number of viruses has been investigated. *P. longum* was found to be remarkable against hepatitis B virus, having double-stranded DNA, circular in shape, and belongs to Hepadna virus family. The virus causes acute and chronic infection of the hepatic region. Pippali is a main Rasayana in Ayurveda that exhibit inhibition of TNF-α-induced intercellular adhesion molecule-1 and vascular cell adhesion molecule-1 expression and also inhibits the TNF-α-induced expression of cell molecules by inhibiting nuclear factor-κB activation in endothelial cells (Subramaniam et al., 2021). *Ashtanga Sangraha* (Literature of the eighth century) illustrates decoction of Giloy and Pippali for the prevention of a disease (Vata, Kapha, and Sannipatik Jvara) that has manifestations similar to COVID-19. These two plants are very common in the clinical practice of Ayurveda and being used for various respiratory diseases (Choudhary et al., 2020). Hence, the combination is suggested for treatment of COVID-19 as an adjunct modality as well as for improving immunity and to arrest progression of COVID-19.

6.2.9 STINGING NETTLE (URTICA DIOICA)

Stinging nettle (*Urtica dioica*) has been used as a folklore medicine in various countries for years. It contains multiple phytochemicals and nutrients including vitamins B and C, magnesium, copper, iron, zinc, and potassium. It is caring to the lungs especially in the presence of excess mucous, to the kidneys, the joints, for malabsorption syndromes, and general inflammatory conditions. Stinging nettle has been noted to assist with chronic pain when given topically in the form of a wash (water extraction) or tincture as well. *Urtica* has been reported for its therapeutic effects on immunity, cardiovascular, digestive systems, and neuronal disorders (Dhouibi et al., 2020). Earlier reports recommend that the agglutinin lectin is derived from the rhizomes of the *U. dioica* (UDA) and NICTABA lectin of *Nicotiana tabacum* were able to show the very best inhibition tendency to ban the multiplication of the virus. Similarly, further studies also confirmed that the UDA have an impression on the inhibition of the SARS-CoV in vitro. Researches showed that lectins will affect the viral attachment, and lectins have the best effects once they are delivered at the first stage of the viral infection cycle. The study also demonstrated that the UDA prohibits the virus attachment by inhibition of SARS-CoV spike (S) glycoprotein. The recommendations from the previous research showed that UDA are often an appropriate compound for further research within the COVID-19 pandemic (Vander Meer et al., 2007). Stinging nettles are very safe plant that can be used by patients of any age.

6.2.10 GARLIC (ALLIUM SATIVUM)

Garlic is from the onion family Allium. It is a vital element of most foods around the world. Garlic is loaded with so many health benefits if consumed in the right way. It is a functional food documented for its antitumor, cardioprotective, germicide, antimutagenic, immunomodulatory, anti-inflammatory, anti-atherosclerotic, and antidiabetic features due to the presence of sulfur-containing phytochemicals. The most important compounds of garlic are alliin, allicin, vinyldithiins (2-vinyl-(4*H*)-1,3-dithiin, 3-vinyl-(4*H*)-1,2-dithiin), ajoenes (E- and Z-ajoene), diallyl (di and tri) sulfide, and some alliin-derived organosulfur compounds like *S*-allyl-cysteine, *S*-allyl-mercaptocysteine, and *N*-acetylcysteine. The anti-viral effect of garlic against numerous viruses like herpes simplex virus, influenza B, HIV (type 1), coxsackievirus species, vesicular stomatitis virus, and gamma-retrovirus was earlier demonstrated (Khubber et al., 2020). It is a wonderful source of minerals and vitamins such as vitamin B complex, phosphorus, folate, zinc, magnesium, sodium, iron, calcium, and manganese among others. Garlic is considered as a natural immunity booster due to the occurrence of allicin, which helps in fighting against several illnesses. Angiotensin-converting enzyme-2 is a fundamental membrane glycoprotein which is known for the highest expression in most of the tissues such as endothelium, kidneys, heart, and lungs (Donma and Donma, 2020). The ACE2 protein contains same functional host–cell receptor shared by SARS-CoV-2 and SARS. Therefore, apart from inhibiting SARS-CoV-2, the blockage of the ACE2 protein is certainly essential to reduce the activity of the host receptor of SARS-CoV-2. If the ACE2 protein is inhibited, it means that coronavirus is inhibited and treated. The volatile oil from garlic was found to be suitable for the prevention and cure of pneumonia caused by SARS-CoV-2 in definite and other viruses causing flu or pneumonia as it inhibits the ACE2 protein. Garlic is helpful in reverse of some signs and symptoms observed in COVID-infected persons, namely, to re-increase or regain the lost gustative sense, to expand the number of Treg cells, to increase cytotoxic, and helper T cells, to reduce the levels of leptin receptor, leptin, and PPAR-γ, to increase appetite, to prevent the inhibition of $CD4^+$ $CD25^+$ $FoxP3^+$, Treg cells, to decrease IL-6 concentrations, to suppress TNF-α and C-reactive protein, and to stimulate NK cells (Thuy et al., 2020).

6.2.11 KALMEGH (ANDROGRAPHIS PANICULATA)

Kalmegh also recognized as "King of bitters" belongs to the Acanthaceae family generally used to cure fever, diarrhea, and common cold. It has considerable extent of pharmacologically active compounds such as andrographolides and its derivatives that have been explored for anticancer, antimalarial, hepatoprotective, antioxidant activities, and reported to have potent antiviral activity against different group of viruses. It is also been involved in suppression of increased interleukin-1β molecules, caspase-1, and NOD-like receptor protein 3 which are significantly implicated in the pathogenesis of SARS-COV (Enmozhi et al., 2020). Andrographolide is also recognized for its broad-spectrum antiviral activity. Earlier studies showed andrographolide has been applicable against influenza A, Chikungunya virus, HCV, herpes simplex virus 1, HIV, hepatitis B virus, Epstein–Barr virus, and human papillomavirus. Kalmegh extract and its active constituent andrographolide had strong inhibitory effect against SARS-CoV-2 and this study opens an opportunity to develop its extract and andrographolide for COVID-19 treatment (Hiremath et al., 2021).

6.2.12 GINGER (ZINGIBER OFFICINALE)

Ginger (*Zingiber officinale*, family: Zingiberaceae) is a frequently consumed herbal supplement all over the world. Although used as spices, patients also use it as medicine for many conditions. Ginger has incredible antimicrobial activity and is effective in preventing several fungal, viral, and bacterial infections. Oleoresin from rhizome part includes several bioactive constituents such as 6-gingerol, the chief pungent element identified to perform a variety of remarkable pharmacological activities. 6-Gingerols are the main constituents of fresh ginger, while 6-shogaol is of dry ginger. Studies revealed isolation of various sesquiterpenes including beta-sesquiphellandrene that was very effective in inhibiting rhinovirus. The decoction of fresh and dried gingers has been found efficacious against human respiratory syncytial virus-induced plaque formation on epithelium by preventing viral attachment as it stimulates mucosal cells to secrete IFN-β that possibly contributed to counteracting viral infection (Chang et al., 2013). Ginger exerts anti-inflammatory properties by decreasing the levels of PGE2, nitrite, IL-8, and IL-6 via NF-κB inhibition that removes toxins from the respiratory tract. It contains several vitamins and minerals including magnesium, potassium, beta-carotene, and zinc. It acts as anti-oxidants to help support and boost the immune system. The use of ginger and its composition with other herbs such as bitter kola, turmeric, Giloy, garlic, and lime could be recommended for use in the prevention and cure of COVID-19 sign and symptoms or as a home remedy for prophylaxis against COVID (Singh et al., 2021).

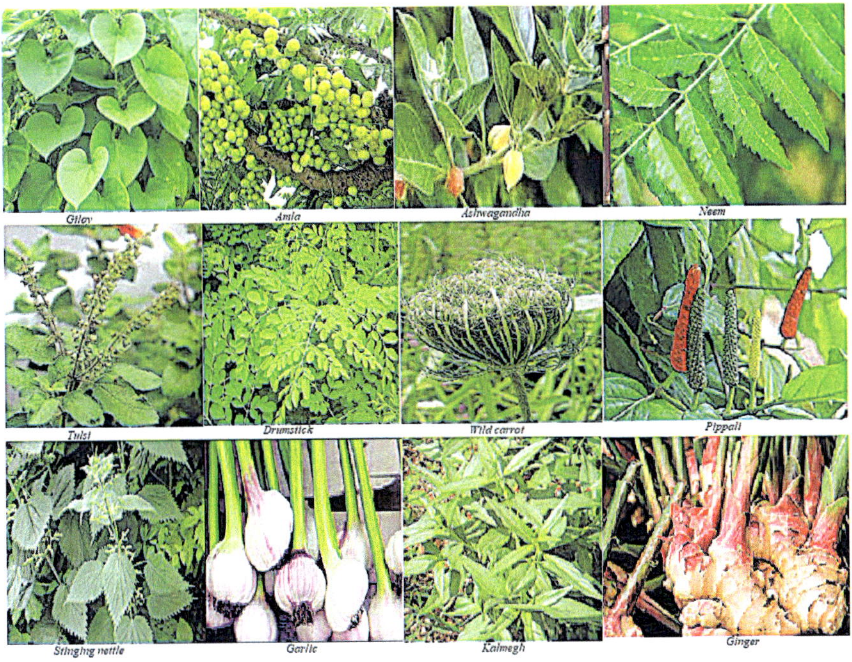

FIGURE 6.1 Plants used for prevention and mitigation of viral infections and COVID-19.

6.3 ROLE OF NATURAL PRODUCTS AS POTENTIAL CONTOUR IN TREATING COVID-19

To implement the use of antiviral drugs worldwide is challenging due to side effects of drugs and mutations of virus causing drug-resistant mutants. Natural products provide scientific literature, mechanism of action, and probable targets including entry of viral load, replication, assemblage, discharge, and virus–host-specific associations (Cheng et al., 2006; Lin et al., 2014). Table 6.1 shows the possible natural compounds with their possible mechanism of action against SARS-CoV infection.

6.4 YOGA PRACTICES, MEDITATION, AND MANAGEMENT OF CORONAVIRUS DISEASE

Most of the people know the benefits of Yoga and think of it as a form of exercise, but Yoga is more than that. It truly is a unique lifestyle; asanas are only one piece of it. Although Yoga has, usually, been a system of improving well-being on the physical, emotional, psychological, and spiritual levels,

TABLE 6.1 Possible Natural Compounds from Plants with Their Possible Mechanism of Action against SARS-CoV Infection.

S. No.	Name of the plant	Name of natural product	Mechanism of action compound	References
1	*Tinospora cordifolia*	Berberine and palmatine	Inhibition of viral replication	Singh et al. (2003), Wink (2007)
2	*Phyllanthus emblica*	Quercetin and rutin	Inhibits viral life cycle in the host, inhibition of viral entry in host cell	Kumar et al. (2017), Ghosh et al. (2020), da Silva et al. (2020), Nguyen et al. (2012)
3	*Azadirachta indica*	Quercetin	Inhibits viral life cycle in the host, inhibition of viral entry in host cell	Venmathi Maran et al. (2021), Nguyen et al. (2012), Ghosh et al. (2020)
4	*Moringa oleifera*	Rutin	Inhibits life cycle of virus in the host	Tshabalala et al. (2019), da Silva et al. (2020)
5	*Daucus maritimus*	Luteolin	Inhibition of viral entry in host cell	Al-Snafi (2017), Yi et al. (2004)
6	*Piper longum*	Demethoxycurcumin	Inhibition of viral entry in host cell	Liu et al. (2009), Yamamoto et al. (2016)
7	*Urtica dioica*	Quercetin, rutin	Inhibits viral life cycle in the host, inhibition of viral entry in host cell	Ji et al. (2007), Ghosh et al. (2020), da Silva et al. (2020), Nguyen et al. (2012)
8	*Zingiber officinale*	Citral	Inhibition of viral life cycle inside host	Shaghaghi (2020)

it is not generally regarded as a set of religious beliefs. Yoga can be practiced in a purely secular way and is practiced by persons of all religious traditions, alongwith agnostics and atheists. A healthy lifestyle, regular practice of Yoga/meditation, balanced nutrition, and good sleep are linked to a healthy immune system. Figure 6.3 shows different health benefits of Yoga. The comprehensive approach of Yoga includes a safe, simple, and easily implementable set of postures (asanas), regulated breathing practices (pranayam), and meditation (dhyan) to conquer the peak level of consciousness and achieve optimum physical and mental health. Such practices do not require any equipment, little space, and can be practiced at any time at home. Several physicians and specialists have recommended that those suffering from mild symptoms of COVID and those who have been directed to self-isolate at home may get benefited from Yoga asanas and breathing exercises with caution (Nagarathna et al., 2020). Yogic

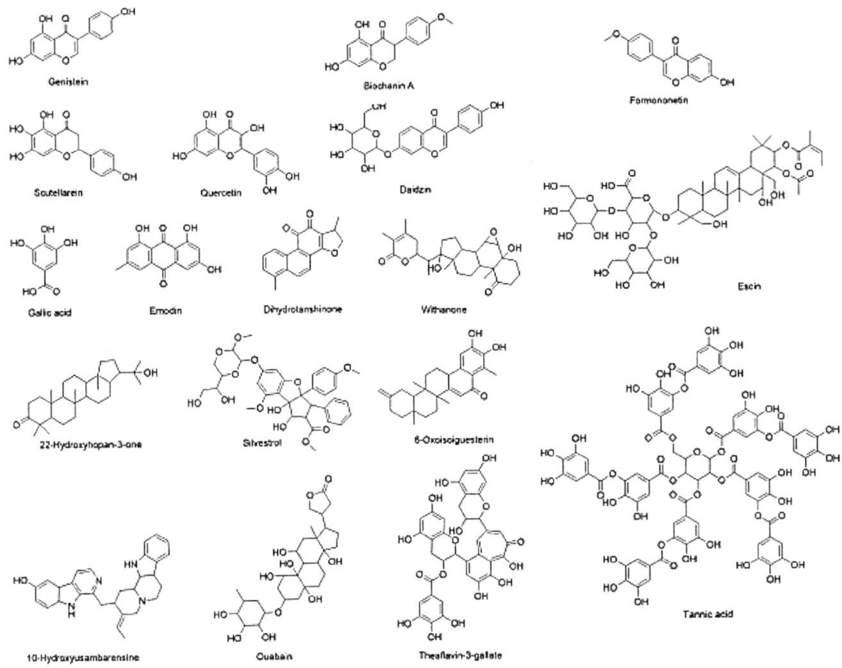

FIGURE 6.2 Lead compounds that exhibit potential in the prevention of COVID-19.

pranayam, training-level Yoga, meditation, and asanas bring harmony of mind, which is an important factor in the recovery for those who have had a stressful experience of contracting COVID-19. Apart from these, altered breathing practices and Yoga postures suggested by specialists can help to reduce exhaustion and gradually restore energy levels among COVID-19 patients, who are recovering (Patange and Sawarkar, 2020).

Yogic posture practices like a downward-facing dog (adho mukha svanasana), cobra pose (bhujangasana), seated vertebral twist Yoga pose (ardha matsyendrasana), eagle pose (garudasana), bridge pose (setu bandha sarvangasana), and legs up the wall pose (viparita karani) can help boost immunity to fight against COVID-19 infection as well as help to curb depression and anxiety. Yogic breathing practices like bhastrika, anulom vilom, nadi shodhna pranayama, and kapalbhati and meditation in savasana are simple techniques and now becoming progressively popular globally to treat several complex diseases like anxiety, depression, glaucoma, cardiovascular disorders, unexplained male factor infertility, and so on. All these complex lifestyle diseases have shared underlying mechanisms like psychological stress, oxidative stress, dysregulated immune system, shorter telomeres, and thus need an integrated approach which targets the mind and body (Deepak and Rao, 2021). There is a lot of supportive evidences that breathing exercises have beneficial effects on the respiratory system. Pranayama, a Yoga-based breathing exercise, is a simple and lucrative intervention that can be racially

TABLE 6.2 Common Protocol for Yoga (Asana).

Practices	Name of the asana	Time
Starting	Prayer	1 min
Loosening practices	Shoulder movement	2 min
	Neck bending	2 min
	Trunk movement	1 min
	Knee movement	1 min
Yoga practices		
Asanas performed in standing posture	Tadasana (the palm tree posture)	1 min
	Vrikshasana (the tree posture)	2 min
	ArdhaChakrasana (the half-wheel posture)	1 min
	Pada-hastasana (the hands to the feet posture)	1 min
	Trikonasana (the triangle posture)	2 min
Asanas performedin sitting posture	Vajrasana (the thunderbolt/diamond posture)	1 min
	Bhadrasana (the firm/auspicious posture)	1 min
	ArdhaUshtrasana (the half-camel posture)	1 min
	Sasakasana (the hare posture)	1 min
	Ushtrasana (the camel posture)	1 min
	Utthana Mandukasana (the stretched-up-frog posture)	1 min
	Vakrasana (the seated twist posture)	2 min
Asanas performed while lying on thestomach	Bhujangasana (the cobra posture)	1 min
	Makarasana (the crocodile posture)	1 min
	Shalabhasana (the locust posture)	1 min
Asanas performed while lying on theback	Setubandhasana (the bridge posture)	1 min
	ArdhaHalasana (the half-plough posture)	30 s
	Utthanapadasana (the raised leg posture)	30 s
	PawanaMuktasana (the wind-releasing posture)	2 min
	Kaphalabhati (the shining skull practice)	2 min
Kriya	Shavasana (the corpse posture)	2 min
Pranayama	AnulomaViloma Pranayama (the alternate nostril breathing)	2 min
	Bhramari Pranayama (the bee sound breathing) (5 rounds)	2 min
	Ujjayee Pranayama (the hissing breathing) (5 rounds)	2 min
Dhyana	The meditation	5 min
Closing	Sankalpa shanti patha	1 min

mixed into the daily routine and has been helpful in subjects of various age groups. Yoga exercise has been described to improve the strength of respiratory muscles. Many investigators stated positive effects of a 45-day course of pranayama on ventilatory lung functions. The authors reported enhanced ventilatory functions with respect to lowered respiratory rate and forced expiratory volume, prolongation of breath-holding time, increased forced vital capacity, peak expiratory flow rate, and maximum voluntary ventilation (Thangavel et al., 2013). Repeated practice of pranayama confirms that it enhances the cardiorespiratory connection and increases parasympathetic activity in healthy people. The breathing exercise, called Kapalabhati, involves powerful exhalation, followed by contraction of the abdominal muscles and diaphragm, followed by passive inhalation. Kapalbhati aids in proper exercise and toning of the diaphragm and abdominal muscles. It is also useful in the removal of secretions from the bronchial tree and cleans the respiratory tract and alveoli. Pattern of yogic breathing techniques improved pulmonary function in competitive swimmers (Bagade et al., 2018).

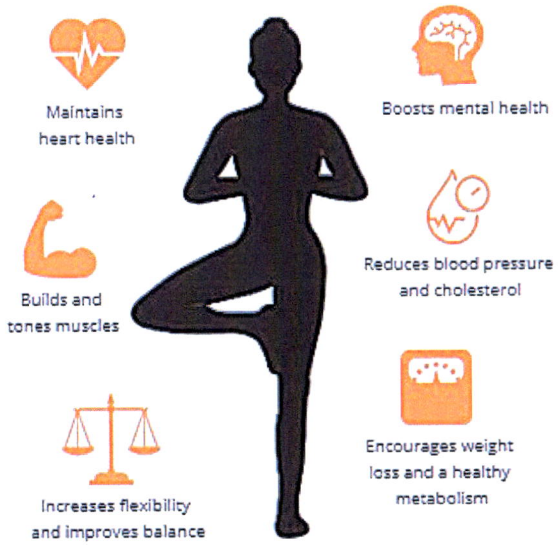
Maintains
heart health
Boosts mental health
Builds and
tones muscles
Reduces blood pressure
and cholesterol
Encourages weight
loss and a healthy
metabolism
Increases flexibility
and improves balance

FIGURE 6.3 Health benefits of Yoga.

Existing medical and health-care systems are being rigorously tested to ensure that COVID-19 is effectively managed. However, there are many gaps. We must remember the basic principle of medicine that "prevention is better than cure." Ayurveda, Yoga, and meditation have a promising role to connect the community in forming a more positive healthy environment. This narrative chapter has not been drafted according to the PRISMA guidelines due to lack of literature on the effect of Ayurveda and Yoga for COVID-19. The abovementioned suggestions were drawn to support the efficacy of Yoga practices and Ayurvedic drugs as preventive and curative measures. Collaborative multicenter studies are now needed to assess the safety, feasibility, and effectiveness of Ayurvedic and Yoga lifestyle interventions in the treatment of the various stages and severity of COVID-19 infection. This will permit the references of specific Ayurveda, Yoga, and meditation protocols for each stage of the illness. The inclusion of Yoga in your daily life can be a useful way to help fight coronavirus. It is necessary to understand that there is yet no cure for coronavirus, and this is only achieved through such effective measures and maintaining a holistic lifestyle in the direction of health and general safety that we will be ready to keep our bodies safe from coronavirus.

KEYWORDS

- **COVID-19**
- **functional food**
- **immunomodulator**
- **life style**
- **traditional medicines**
- **Yoga**

REFERENCES

Abebe, G. M. Emerging and Re-emerging Viral Diseases: The Case of Coronavirus Disease-19 (COVID-19). *Int. J. Virol. AIDS* **2020,** *7*, 067. doi:10.23937/2469-567X/1510067.

Al-Snafi, A. E. Nutritional and Therapeutic Importance of *Daucus carota*—A Review. *IOSR J. Pharm.* **2017,** 7, 72–88.

Bagade, A. H.; Bhonde, M. S.; Dhokane, N. B. Effect of Pranayama on Respiratory Endurance in Young Adults. *Natl. J. Physiol. Pharm. Pharmacol.* **2018,** 8, 1175–1178.

Baildya, N.; Khan, A. A.; Ghosh, N. N.; Dutta, T.; Chattopadhyay, A. P. Screening of Potential Drug from *Azadirachta indica* (Neem) Extracts for SARS-CoV-2: An Insight from Molecular Docking and MD-Simulation Studies. *J. Mol. Struct.* **2021,** *1227*, 129390. doi:10.1016/j.molstruc.2020.129390.

Balkrishna, A.; Pokhrel, S.; Singh, H.; Joshi, M.; Mulay, V. P.; Haldar, S.; Varshney, A. Withanone from *Withania somnifera* Attenuates SARS-CoV-2 RBD and Host ACE2 Interactions to Rescue Spike Protein Induced Pathologies in Humanized Zebrafish Model. *Drug Des. Dev. Ther.* **2021,** *15*, 1111–1133. doi:10.2147/DDDT.S292805.

Borse, S.; Joshi, M.; Saggam, A.; Bhat, V.; Walia, S.; Marathe, A.; Sagar, S.; Chavan-Gautam, P.; Girme, A.; Hingorani, L.; Tillu, G. Ayurveda Botanicals in COVID-19 Management: An In Silico Multi-target Approach. *PLoS One* **2021,** *16*, e0248479. doi:10.1371/journal.pone.0248479.

Chang, J. S.; Wang, K. C.; Yeh, C. F.; Shieh, D. E.; Chiang, L. C. Fresh Ginger (*Zingiber officinale*) Has Anti-viral Activity against Human Respiratory Syncytial Virus in Human Respiratory Tract Cell Lines. *J. Ethnopharmacol.* **2013,** *145*, 146–151. doi:10.1016/j.jep.2012.10.043.

Cheng, P. W.; Ng, L. T.; Chiang, L. C.; Lin, C. C. Antiviral Effects of Saikosaponins on Human Coronavirus 229E in Vitro. *Clin. Exp. Pharmacol. Physiol.* **2006,** *33*, 612–616. doi:10.1111/j.1440-1681.2006.04415.x.

Choudhary, P.; Chakdar, H.; Singh, D.; Selvaraj, C.; Singh, S. K.; Kumar, S.; Saxena, A. Computational Studies Reveal Piperine, the Predominant Oleoresin of Black Pepper (*Piper nigrum*) as a Potential Inhibitor of SARS-CoV-2 (COVID-19). *Curr. Sci.* **2020,** *119*, 1333–1342. doi:10.18520/cs/v119/i8/1333-1342.

Chowdhury, P. In Silico Investigation of Phytoconstituents from Indian Medicinal Herb "*Tinospora cordifolia* (giloy)" against SARS-CoV-2 (COVID-19) by Molecular Dynamics Approach. *J. Biomol. Struct. Dyn.* **2020,** *7*, 1–18. doi:10.1080/07391102.2020.1803968.

da Silva, F. M. A.; da Silva, K. P. A.; de Oliveira, L. P. M.; Costa, E. V.; Koolen, H. H.; Pinheiro, M. L. B.; de Souza, A. Q. L.; de Souza, A. D. L. Flavonoid Glycosides and Their Putative Human Metabolites as Potential Inhibitors of the SARS-CoV-2 Main Protease (Mpro) and RNA-Dependent RNA Polymerase (RdRp). *Mem. Inst. Oswaldo Cruz* **2020,** *115*, e200207. doi:10.1590/0074-02760200207.

Deepak, K. K.; Rao, M. R. Yoga and Meditation as an Adjunct Interventional Strategy for COVID-19 Management. *Ann. Natl. Acad. Med. Sci. (India)* **2021,** *57*, 65–67. doi:10.1055/s-0041-1731611.

Dhouibi, R.; Affes, H.; Ben Salem, M.; Hammami, S.; Sahnoun, Z.; Zeghal, K. M.; Ksouda, K. Screening of Pharmacological Uses of *Urtica dioica* and Others Benefits. *Prog. Biophys. Mol. Biol.* **2020,** *150*, 67–77.

Dinesh, T.; Gaur, G.; Sharma, V.; Madanmohan; Harichandra, K. T.; Grrishma, B. Effect of 6 Weeks of Kapalabhati Pranayama Training on Peak Expiratory Flow Rate in Young, Healthy, Volunteers. *Sch. Acad. J. Biosci.* **2013,** *1*, 111–114.

Donma, M. M.; Donma, O. The Effects of *Allium sativum* on Immunity within the Scope of COVID-19 Infection. *Med. Hypoth.* **2020,** *144*, 109934. doi:10.1016/j.mehy.2020.109934.

Dutta, R.; Khalil, R.; Green, R.; Mohapatra, S. S.; Mohapatra, S. *Withania somnifera* (Ashwagandha) and Withaferin A: Potential in Integrative Oncology. *Int. J. Mol. Sci.* **2019,** *20*, 5310. doi:10.3390/ijms20215310.

Enmozhi, S. K.; Raja, K.; Sebastine, I.; Joseph, J. Andrographolide as a Potential Inhibitor of SARS-CoV-2 Main Protease: An In Silico Approach. *J. Biomol. Struct. Dyn.* **2021,** *39*, 3092–3098. doi:10.1080/07391102.2020.1760136.

Ghoke, S. S.; Sood, R.; Kumar, N.; Pateriya, A. K.; Bhatia, S.; Mishra, A.; Dixit, R.; Singh, V. K.; Desai, D. N.; Kulkarni, D. D.; Dimri, U.; Singh, V. P. Evaluation of Antiviral Activity of *Ocimum sanctum* and *Acacia arabica* Leaves Extracts against H9N2 Virus Using Embryonated Chicken Egg Model. *BMC Complement. Altern. Med.* **2018,** *18*, 174. doi:10.1186/s12906-018-2238-1.

Ghosh, R.; Chakraborty, A.; Biswas, A.; Chowdhuri, S. Evaluation of Green Tea Polyphenols as Novel Corona Virus (SARS-CoV-2) Main Protease (Mpro) Inhibitors—An *In-Silico* Docking and Molecular Dynamics Simulation Study. *J. Biomol. Struct. Dyn.* **2020,** *39*, 4362–4374. doi:10.1080/07391102.2020.1779818.

Gupta, S. C.; Prasad, S.; Tyagi, A. K.; Kunnumakkara, A. B.; Aggarwal, B. B. Neem (*Azadirachta indica*): An Indian Traditional Panacea with Modern Molecular Basis. *Phytomedicine* **2017,** *34*, 14–20. doi:10.1016/j.phymed.2017.07.001.

Hiremath, S.; Kumar, H. D. V.; Nandan, M.; Mantesh, M.; Shankarappa, K. S.; Venkataravanappa, V.; Basha, C. R. J.; Reddy, C. N. L. In Silico Docking Analysis Revealed the Potential of Phytochemicals Present in *Phyllanthus amarus* and *Andrographis paniculata*, Used in Ayurveda Medicine in Inhibiting SARS-CoV-2. *3 Biotech* **2021,** *11*, 44. doi:10.1007/s13205-020-02578-7.

Jabrane, A.; Jannet, H. B.; Harzallah-Skhiri, F.; Mastouri, M.; Casanova, J.; Mighri, Z. Flower and Root Oils of the Tunisian *Daucus carota* L. Ssp. Maritimus (Apiaceae): Integrated Analyses by GC, GC/MS, and 13C-NMR Spectroscopy, and In Vitro Antibacterial Activity. *Chem. Biodivers.* **2009,** *6*, 881–889.

Jahan, I.; Onay, A. Potentials of Plant-Based Substance to Inhabit and Probable Cure for the COVID-19. *Turk. J. Biol.* **2020,** *44*, 228–241. doi:10.3906/biy-2005-114.

Ji, T.; Liu, C.; Wang, A.; Yang, J.; Su, Y.; Yuan, L.; Feng, X. Studies on the Chemical Constituents of *Urtica dioica* L. Grown in Tibet Autonomous Region. *J. Chin. Med. Mater.* **2007,** *30*, 662–664.

Khubber, S.; Hashemifesharaki, R.; Mohammadi, M.; Gharibzahedi, S. M. T. Garlic (*Allium sativum* L.): A Potential Unique Therapeutic Food Rich in Organosulfur and Flavonoid Compounds to Fight with COVID-19. *Nutr. J.* **2020,** *19*, 124. doi:10.1186/s12937-020-00643-8.

Kumar, S.; Singh, A.; Kumar, B. Identification and Characterization of Phenolics and Terpenoids from Ethanolic Extracts of *Phyllanthus* Species by HPLC-ESI-QTOF-MS/MS. *J. Pharm. Anal.* **2017,** *7*, 214–222. doi:10.1016/j.jpha.2017.01.005.

Lima, C. Information about the New Coronavirus Disease (COVID-19). *Radiol. Bras.* **2020,** *53*, V–VI. doi:10.1590/0100-3984.2020.53.2e1.

Lin, L. T.; Hsu, W. C.; Lin, C. C. Antiviral Natural Products and Herbal Medicines. *J. Tradit. Complement. Med.* **2014,** *4*, 24–35. doi:10.4103/2225-4110.124335.

Liu, W.; Jiang, Z.; Chen, J.; Zhang, X.; Ma, Y. Chemical Constituents from *Piper longum*. *Zhongguo Zhong Yao Za Zhi* **2009,** *34*, 2891–2894.

Mishra, L. C.; Singh, B. B.; Dagenais, S. Scientific Basis for the Therapeutic Use of *Withania somnifera* (ashwagandha): A Review. *Altern. Med. Rev.* **2000,** *5*, 334–346.

Murugesan, S.; Kottekad, S.; Crasta, I.; Sreevathsan, S.; Usharani, D.; Perumal, M. K.; Mudliar, S. N. Targeting COVID-19 (SARS-CoV-2) Main Protease through Active Phytocompounds of Ayurvedic Medicinal Plants—*Emblica officinalis* (Amla), *Phyllanthus niruri* Linn. (Bhumi Amla) and *Tinospora cordifolia* (Giloy)—A Molecular

Docking and Simulation Study. *Comput. Biol. Med.* **2021,** *136*, 104683. doi:10.1016/j.compbiomed.2021.104683.

Nagarathna, R.; Nagendra, H. R.; Majumdar, V. A Perspective on Yoga as a Preventive Strategy for Coronavirus Disease 2019. *Int. J. Yoga* **2020,** *13*, 89–98. doi:10.4103/ijoy.IJOY_22_20.

Nguyen, T. T.; Woo, H. J.; Kang, H. K.; Nguyen, V. D.; Kim, Y. M.; Kim, D. W.; Ahn, S. A.; Xia, Y.; Kim, D. Flavonoid-Mediated Inhibition of SARS Coronavirus 3C-Like Protease Expressed in *Pichia pastoris*. *Biotechnol. Lett.* **2012,** *34*, 831–838. doi:10.1007/s10529-011-0845-8.

Nugraha, R.; Ridwansyah, H.; Ghozali, M.; Khairani, A. F.; Atik, N. Traditional Herbal Medicine Candidates as Complementary Treatments for COVID-19: A Review of Their Mechanisms, Pros and Cons. *Evid. Based Complement. Alternat. Med.* **2020**. Article ID 2560645. doi:10.1155/2020/2560645.

Patange, A.; Sawarkar, P. Role of Yoga for the Prevention & Management of COVID-19—A Review. *Int. J. Res. Pharm. Sci.* **2020,** *11*, 1720–1724. doi:10.26452/ijrps.v11iSPL1.4472.

Rane, B. R.; Patil, A. S.; Keservani, R. K.; Jain, A. S. Novel Approaches in Herbal Formulation. In *Enhancing the Therapeutic Efficacy of Herbal Formulations through Novel Drug Delivery Systems*; Kesharwani, R. K., Keservani, R. K., Sharma, A. K., Eds.; IGI Global International Publisher, Pennsylvania, USA, 2020; Chapter 2, pp 43–68. ISBN13: 9781799844532.

Sagar, V.; HS Kumar, A. Efficacy of Natural Compounds from *Tinospora cordifolia* against SARS-CoV-2 Protease, Surface Glycoprotein and RNA Polymerase. *BEMS Rep.* **2020,** *6*, 06–08. doi:10.5530/bems.6.1.2.

Saha, S.; Ghosh, S. *Tinospora cordifolia*: One Plant, Many Roles. *Ancient Sci. Life* **2012,** *31*, 151–159.

Sen, D.; Bhaumik, S.; Debnath, P.; Debnath, S. Potentiality of *Moringa oleifera* against SARS-CoV-2: Identified by a Rational Computer Aided Drug Design Method. *J. Biomol. Struct. Dyn.* **2021,** *15*, 1–18. doi:10.1080/07391102.2021.1898475.

Shaghaghi, N. *Molecular Docking Study of Novel COVID-19 Protease with Low Risk Terpenoids Compounds of Plants*, 2020. https://chemrxiv.org/engage/chemrxiv/article-details/60c74898f96a001f292870ad (accessed Aug. 29, 2021).

Sharma, U.; Bala, M.; Kumar, N.; Singh, B.; Munshi, R. K.; Bhalerao, S. Immunomodulatory Active Compounds from *Tinospora cordifolia*. *J. Ethnopharmacol.* **2012,** *141*, 918–926. doi:10.1016/j.jep.2012.03.027.

Sharma, O.; Sultan, A. A.; Ding, H.; Triggle, C. R. A Review of the Progress and Challenges of Developing a Vaccine for COVID-19. *Front. Immunol.* **2020,** *11*, 585354. doi:10.3389/fimmu.2020.585354.

Singh, S. S.; Pandey, S. C.; Srivastava, S.; Gupta, V. S.; Patro, B.; Ghosh, A. C. Chemistry and Medicinal Properties of *Tinospora Cordifolia* (Guduchi). *Ind. J. Pharmacol.* **2003,** *35*, 83–91.

Stohs, S. J.; Hartman, M. J. Review of the Safety and Efficacy of *Moringa oleifera*. *Phytother. Res.* **2015,** *29*, 796–804. doi:10.1002/ptr.5325.

Singh, N. A.; Kumar, P.; Jyoti, Kumar, N. Spices and Herbs: Potential Antiviral Preventives and Immunity Boosters during COVID-19. *Phytother. Res.* **2021**. doi:10.1002/ptr.7019.

Subramaniam, K.; Subramanian, S. K.; Bhargav, S.; Parameswari, R.; Praveena, R.; Ravikumar, R.; Yuvaraj, E.; Manoj Kumar, V. Review on Potential Antiviral and Immunomodulatory Properties of *Piper longum*. *IOP Conf. Ser. Mater. Sci. Eng.* **2021,** *1145*, 012099.

Thuy, B. T. P.; My, T. T. A.; Hai, N. T. T.; Hieu, L. T.; Hoa, T. T.; Thi Phuong Loan, H.; Triet, N. T.; Anh, T. T. V.; Quy, P. T.; Tat, P. V.; Hue, N. V.; Quang, D. T.; Trung, N. T.; Tung, V. T.; Huynh, L. K.; Nhung, N. T. A. Investigation into SARS-CoV-2 Resistance of Compounds in Garlic Essential Oil. *ACS Omega* **2020,** *5*, 8312–8320. doi:10.1021/acsomega.0c00772.

Tshabalala, T.; Ncube, B.; Madala, N. E.; Nyakudya, T. T.; Moyo, H. P.; Sibanda, M.; Ndhlala, A. R. Scribbling the Cat: A Case of the "Miracle" Plant, *Moringa oleifera*. *Plants (Basel)* **2019,** *8*, 510. doi:10.3390/plants8110510.

Tshilandaa, D.; Ngoyi, E.; Kabengele, C.; Matondo, A.; Bongo, G. N.; Inkoto, C.; Mbadiko, M. C.; Gbolo, B. Z.; Lengbiye, E.; Kilembe, J.; Mwanangombo, D.; Kasiama, G.; Tshibangu, D.; Ngbolua, K. T. N.; Mpiana, P. T. *Ocimum* Species as Potential Bioresources against COVID-19: A Review of Their Phytochemistry and Antiviral Activity. *Int. J. Pathogen Res.* **2020,** *5*, 42–54.

Vander Meer, F. J. U. M.; Haan, C. A. M.; Schuurman, N. M. P.; Haijema, B. J.; Verheije, M. H.; Bosch, B. J.; Balzarini, J.; Egberink, H. F. The Carbohydrate-Binding Plant Lectins and the Nonpeptidic Antibiotic Pradimicin A Target the Glycans of the Coronavirus Envelope Glycoproteins. *J. Antimicrob. Chemother.* **2007,** *60*, 741–749.

Variya, B. C.; Bakrania, A. K.; Patel, S. S. *Emblica officinalis* (Amla): A Review for Its Phytochemistry, Ethnomedicinal Uses and Medicinal Potentials with Respect to Molecular Mechanisms. *Pharmacol. Res.* **2016,** *111*, 180–200. doi:10.1016/j.phrs.2016.06.013.

Venmathi Maran, B. A.; Josmeh, D.; Tan, J. K.; Yong, Y. S.; Shah, M. D. Efficacy of the Aqueous Extract of *Azadirachta indica* against the Marine Parasitic Leech and Its Phytochemical Profiling. *Molecules* **2021,** *26*, 1908. doi:10.3390/molecules26071908.

Wink, M. Molecular Modes of Action of Cytotoxic Alkaloids: From DNA Intercalation, Spindle Poisoning, Topoisomerase Inhibition to Apoptosis and Multiple Drug Resistance. *Alkaloids Chem. Biol.* **2007,** *64*, 1–47. doi:10.1016/s1099-4831(07)64001-2.

Yamamoto, M.; Matsuyama, S.; Li, X.; Takeda, M.; Kawaguchi, Y.; Inoue, J. I.; Matsuda, Z. Identification of Nafamostat as a Potent Inhibitor of Middle East Respiratory Syndrome Coronavirus S Protein-Mediated Membrane Fusion Using the Split-Protein-Based Cell–Cell Fusion Assay. *Antimicrob. Agents Chemother.* **2016,** *60*, 6532–6539. doi:10.1128/AAC.01043-16.

Yi, L.; Li, Z.; Yuan, K.; Qu, X.; Chen, J.; Wang, G.; Zhang, H.; Luo, H.; Zhu, L.; Jiang, P.; Chen, L.; Shen, Y.; Luo, M.; Zuo, G.; Hu, J.; Duan, D.; Nie, Y.; Shi, X.; Wang, W.; Han, Y.; Li, T.; Liu, Y.; Ding, M.; Deng, H.; Xu, X. Small Molecules Blocking the Entry of Severe Acute Respiratory Syndrome Coronavirus into Host Cells. *J. Virol.* **2004,** *78*, 11334–11339. doi:10.1128/JVI.78.20.11334-11339.2004.

CHAPTER 7

Role of Synthetic Medicines as Immunomodulators for the Cure of COVID-19

EKNATH D. AHIRE[1], KHEMCHAND R. SURANA[2], VIJAYRAJ N. SONAWANE[2], SWATI G. TALELE[3], SANJAY J. KSHIRSAGAR[1], UMESH D. LADDHA[1], and GOKUL S. TALELE[4]

[1]*Department of Pharmaceutics, MET's Institute of Pharmacy, Bhujbal Knowledge City, Affiliated to Savitribai Phule Pune University, Nashik, Maharashtra, India*

[2]*Department of Pharmaceutical Chemistry, SSS's, Divine College of Pharmacy, Satana, Maharashtra, India*

[3]*Department of Pharmaceutics, Sandip Institute of Pharmaceutical Sciences, Nashik, Maharashtra, India*

[4]*Department of Pharmaceutics, Matoshri College of Pharmacy, Nashik, Maharashtra, India*

ABSTRACT

Immunomodulation is a therapeutic approach in which we attempt to intervene in the defense system's autoregulating processes, and immunomodulators modulate immune system activity, which reduces the inflammatory response. Immunomodulators are most commonly used in organ transplantation to prevent organ rejection and in autoimmune diseases such as rheumatoid arthritis. To speed up the response during active flares

COVID-19 and Immunomodulation with Special Emphasis on Nutraceutical and Herbal Formulation.
Rajesh K. Kesharwani & Raj K. Keservani (Eds)

of disease, immunomodulators may be combined with corticosteroids. In this shell, lower steroid doses with fewer side effects are required. Corticosteroids can also be eliminated faster when combined with immunomodulators. As a result, immunomodulators are sometimes referred to as "steroid-sparing" medications. This chapter discusses the pharmacological effects of immunomodulators as well as specific immunomodulator agents such as immunostimulators and immunosuppressants, as well as cases of immunity and different immunomodulator agents.

7.1 BACKGROUND

Immunology is one of the quickly growing fields in the medical biotechnology research area and has great promise in the prevention and handling of extensive range of illnesses such as the inflammatory sicknesses of the skin, gut, respiratory tract, joints, and central organs. In addition, infectious illnesses are now chiefly measured by immunological disorders, although neoplastic diseases and organ transplantation and numerous autoimmune diseases are occupied in an immunosuppressive state. Immunomodulators are natural or manmade substances that help in controlling or regularizing the immune scheme. Immunomodulators are precise immune systems that are out of proportion. Natural immunomodulators are less authoritative than prescription immunomodulators and also less viable to have side effects.

The paybacks of immunomodulators stem from their strength to stimulate innate and adaptive safety mechanisms, along with cytokines, which allows the body to help itself. Immunostimulants are agents which are known to improve the body's resistance to infections; they improve the basal levels of immune response, and in individuals with deficiency of immune response, act as an immunotherapeutic agent. A number of disorders such as immunodeficiency state, autoimmune disease, malignant neoplastic diseases, and viral infections may be treated with immunostimulant drugs. Immunomodulators are proving to be a viable aid to recognize modalities' contribution, a novel methodology for the management of communicable diseases in the coming decades of the 21st century.

As a result, both immunostimulating and immunosuppressive agents have personal upright, and in the quest for better agents, applying these events is a revolving subject of primary interest all over the world. Natural adjuvant, artificial agents, and antibody reagents are used as immunosuppressive and immunostimulative agents. In that respect, major contributions of these agents to the worldwide purpose are factors such as extended hazard of infection and generalized effect throughout the resistant scheme. In recent years, an expansion in the clinical utilization of indigenous drugs is due to their being devoid of serious toxic effects and having better efficacy. Moreover, consistent growth within the antibiotic-resistant traces and numerous aspect outcomes brought through the synthetic drugs has led the scientists to search for herbal immunomodulators to deal with numerous infections. Herbal drugs are taken into consideration to elevate natural immunity of the body in opposition to infection, and their immunomodulatory activities have been defined by numerous plants (Rane et al., 2020). Indian medicinal plants and various "*Rasayanas*" have been declared to have immunomodulatory activities. Medicines of the *Rasayana* group are thought to boost health, immunity, and longevity. According to *Ayurveda*, they strengthen all the tissues of the body, prevent aging, promote intellect, and prevent diseases. Historically, herbal remedies have been the backbone of drug treatments and are currently getting attention as sources of synergistic combinations. In this chapter, recent developments in natural immune drug discovery are included.

7.2 INTRODUCTION

Immunomodulators are natural or manmade substances that help to regulate or normalize the immune scheme of human beings. Immunomodulators correct immune systems that are out of proportion. Immunomodulators correct weak immune systems and temper immune systems that are hyperactive, but they do not boost the immune system the way immunostimulants do. Immunomodulators are endorsed for patients with autoimmune illnesses and are broadly implemented in the treatment of persistent illness to repair immune system health in patients who have been on prolonged courses of antibiotics or antiviral therapies. Immunomodulators have become popular worldwide in the natural wellness industry as people have begun to understand the grandness of a healthy immune system for maintenance of health and prevention and recovery of diseases. It is thought to aid the immune system, allowing the torso to function more effectively. Nevertheless, on that point, a great deal of misinformation is going around about these natural compounds, much of it put out by companies attempting to sell their particular immunomodulators.

An immunomodulator is any core that serves to modulate the immune scheme. This "regulation" is a normalization process that facilitates immunomodulators to optimize immune response. Supplementation of an immunomodulator to an individual having low, healthful, and overactive immune system may also increase the immunity and may have partial impact and/or normalize the overactive immune system; immunomodulators now no longer promote immunity, but also normalize it. How immunomodulators work within the body continues to be usually a secret. Portion of their benefits seems to be their ability to naturally increase the body's production of messenger molecules, which includes cytokines, which mediate and modulate the immune scheme. Some of them, such as boron, can also lessen the production of inflammatory cytokines. The immune system is a remarkably versatile defense system that has evolved to protect animals from pathogenic microorganisms and cancer-related diseases. It is able to bring forth an enormous diversity of cells and molecules capable of specifically recognizing and getting rid of an apparently limitless variety of alien invaders. These cells and molecules are organized in a vigorous network whose difficulty matches that of the anxious organization.

Moreover, the immune system is capable of distinguishing subtle chemical alterations that discriminate one foreign pathogen from another. Additionally, the association is able to distinguish between foreign particles and the body's own cells and proteins. In such a case, when a foreign organism is recognized, the immune system recruits a diversity of cells and particles to mount a suitable reaction, known as an effector response, to eradicate or counteract the organism. In this manner, the association is capable of converting the initial acknowledgment event into a diversity of effector responses, each having exclusive response for a distinctive case of the pathogen. After revelation of the same foreign organism persuades a memory response, qualified by a more rapid and heightened immune reaction that helps in eliminating the pathogen and preventing diseases. The function and performance of the immune system can be determined through numerous exogenous and endogenous factors ensuing in both emancipation and immunostimulation. Several agents owning an activity to normalize or modulate pathophysiological strategies are known as immunomodulatory agents. Stress regularly results in oversecretion of glucocorticoids (GCs). Increase in the glucocorticoid level results in the suppression of immune characteristics in humans and animals. Environmental stress plays a significant part in the release of blood glucocorticoid level, which suppresses both innate as well as acquired immune functions and results in increased susceptibility to infections. Today, there may be a compelling proof that stress reactions will have clinically applicable immunosuppression and immune dysfunction. The term "immunity" implies resistance to injury, especially through poisons, overseas proteins, and invading pathogens. Also, immunostimulation and immunosuppression has to be undertaken in an effort to adjust to the normal.

7.3 CHEMICAL OR SYNTHETIC AGENTS AS IMMUNOMODULATORS

Certain chemical agents are capable of alkylate biological material, and in a while, it is observed that aliphatic nitrogen mustards have a particular impact on lymphoid tissue like spleen, bone marrow, thymus, and lymph nodes. Sellers of alkylate materials have boasted of various inaugural magnificence of chemical materials possessing immunosuppressive properties. Hektoen and Cooper confirmed that the formation of agglutinin and hemolysin for sheep red blood cells (SRBC) may be inhibited in rabbits and dogs after the management of sulfur mustard. Subsequently, it is identified that alkylating agents efficiently suppress the immune reaction and intervene with antibody formation in numerous animal species, while implemented on the very starting or 1–2 days earlier than the antigen stimulus. The most extensively used alkylating agent is cyclophosphamide, which provides an extensive spectrum of interest in animal and human malignancies. Arnold and Bourseaux first synthesized cyclophosphamide, which interferes with cell increase simply after activation of tissue. It is able to inhibit each humoral and cell-mediated immune reaction. In a few instances, the purine antagonists are the classical immunosuppressant drugs. Schwartz and Dameshek established that the antileukemic agent 6-marcaptopurine suppressed the immune reaction to human serum albumin in rabbits. Azathioprine is the drug of any other alternative in scientific immunosuppression, particularly for a kidney graft.

In addition, b,b-diethylcysteine, penicillamine,procarbazine, and other chemical agents are used for immunosuppression. Cinanserin is a potent serotonin antagonist, and it inhibits the formation of circulating antibodies, prolongs mouse-skin homograft, and actively exhibits in the EAE test in adjuvant-induced arthritis. In the last decades, some of the unrelated materials with immunopotentiating properties have come into awareness and greater interest is paid to using adjuvants, their nature, and the idea underlying immunostimulation. Adjuvants are materials that help in the improvement and manifestation of the immune system, while when injected with an antigen, they enhance the antigenic properties of a weak antigen or convert a nonantigenic substance to an effective antigen. They contribute to increasing antibody production and to bring on delayed hypersensitivity. For example, incorporation of an antigen into water, mineral, and oil emulsion leads to enhance and extend the period of antibody production. Certain salts of aluminum are useful adjuvants for immunization against diphtheria and tetanus. These aluminum salts preferentially enhance the humoral antibody response. Complementary copolymers that contain polyuridylic acid, polyadenylic acid, polyinosinic acid, and polycytidylic acid stimulate the formation of antibodies in mice immunized with SRBCs and seem to behave immediately on host cells in comparison with a unique complicated antigen. The absence of antigenicity of a few adjacent properties had been validated to have a modulatory effect on the immune response in experimental models and clinical trials. Cutting is an orally and parenterally active broad-spectrum antiviral substance and an effective interferon inducer. SRBC in mice is another synthetic agent that exhibits big promise to restore an impaired immune response.

Levamisole, an immunomodulator, has been employed efficaciously as an effective anthelmintic in human beings and animals in opposition to a wide variety of nematodal infections. In addition, isoprinosine is used to modulate immune responses, and it additionally stimulates the herbal process of thymic hormones. In improver, it works through a sense organ for an innocent-like compound on T-cell precursors.

7.3.1 ROLE OF VARIOUS DRUGS AS IMMUNOMODULATOR

Artificial immunomodulator medications such as azathioprine, 6-mercaptopurine, methotrexate, and mycophenolate mofetil work by overwhelming the immune system and reducing inflammation in the digestive tract in human beings with inflammatory bowel disease, ulcerative colitis, and Crohn's disease. Topical immunomodulators inclusive of tacrolimus and pimeocrolimus offer advantages in patients with eczema, vitiligo, and nickel allergy. Topical immunomodulators are well tolerated even in babies. However, herbal immunomodulators are widely used as immunosuppressive agents as they possess fewer side effects. Thus, there is scope to describe immunomodulator so that they are made in suitable courses to deal with pain relief. Side effects of prescription immunomodulator medications include nausea, emesis, diarrhea, stomach ulcers, rash, malaise, and liver inflammation. Natural immunomodulators are less powerful than prescription immunomodulators and also less probable to have side effects.

TABLE 7.1 Role of Different Synthetic Drugs as Immunomodulators.

Sr.No.	Name of drug	Mechanism of action	Uses
1.	Azathiopurine	Antagonizes purine metabolism	As adjust in prevention of kidney transplants
2.	Diphenyl cyclopemine	Inhibits maturation and activation of T cells	Immunosuppressive
3.	Cyclosporine A	Inhibits IL-2 activation	Prophylaxis of organ rejection in kidney and liver
4.	Beta-glucan	Stimulates cellular function	Analysis of sugar specificity
5.	Methotrexate	Inhibits metabolism of folic acid	Treatment of cancer autoimmune disease
6.	Mycophenolate mofetil	Inhibits T&B lymphocytes proliferation	Prophylaxis of organ rejection
7.	Licopid	Activation of phagocyte cells	As immunosuppressive agent
8.	Squaric acid dibutyl esters	Inhibits maturation and activation of T cells	As topical immunomodulator
9.	Sirolimus	Inhibits cell cycle (G1 to s phase)	Prophylaxis of organ rejection in kidney and liver

7.4 ROLE OF IMMUNOMODULATORS IN COVID-19

From the beginning of the outbreak of COVID-19 in China, the significance of immunomodulation within the scientific development of the contamination has been described. Passed at the rigor of the immunological image, a chain of etiopathogeneic mechanisms have been cautioned which can be tight to those worried within the different immunomediated disorders.

7.4.1 ANTIMALARIAL DRUGS

Old anti-infective drugs, such as chloroquine (CQ) and hydroxychloroquine (HCQ), firstly used as antimalarial drugs and later as immunomodulatory treatment for autoimmune and rheumatic diseases, mainly SLE and rheumatoid arthritis, have also shown a potential antiviral effect against SARS and avian influenza H5N1. Their consequences are connected to the extraction of cell membrane pH that is essential for viral fusion and the interference with glycosylation of viral proteins. Presently, at least 20 clinical trials have been filed to test the practicality of CQ and HCQ for the treatment of COVID-19. Recently, a completed Chinese clinical trial—ChiCTR2000029559—have validated the capacity of HCQ for the remedy of COVID-19. In vivo results, despite the fact that is hopeful, are confined to date. Therefore, seeing the antiviral and immunomodulatory nature of the antimalarial and the preclinical indication of efficiency and protection for a long-time clinical trial applied for other readings; clinical research on CQ/HCQ in patients with COVID-19 is necessary. As a result of the weak evidence available, behavior guidelines have previously combined the use of CQ/HCQ for treating COVID-19 patients. Accordingly, HCQ related with other drugs could perform a part in the treatment of SARS-2-CoV-19 infection.

7.4.2 IL-6 BLOCKADE [ANTI-IL-6]

Tocilizumab (TCZ) is an antihuman IL-6 receptor monoclonal antibody that prevents signal transduction by binding sIL-6R and mIL-6R. In 2017, the US Food and Drug Administration permitted TCZ for the treatment of cytokine-release syndrome consisting of a systemic inflammatory reaction triggered by the enormous release of proinflammatory cytokines in response to estrogenic or infective stimuli. In COVID-19 cases, IL-6 plasmatic levels were predominantly high in some serious cases. Histological analysis of lung tissue displayed longwinded alveolar impairment with cellular fibromyxoid exudates and interstitial mononuclear inflammatory penetrates signifying severe immune injury in a biopsy sample for a patient with severe COVID-19. A case series of 20 Chinese patients described that TCZ permitted the lung lesion opaqueness to be smeared out in 19 patients, oxygen consumption dropped in 15, and oxygen stopped in one illustration. Furthermore, raised C-reactive protein diminished suggestively in 84.2% of the patients and lymphocytes count regularized in 52.6% patients. In China, TCZ was permitted for patients affected by severe SARS-CoV-2 pulmonary difficulties. Beyond that, a randomized organized clinical test is continuing in China. Likewise, sarilumab is an antihuman IL-6 receptor monoclonal antibody launched for the management of rheumatoid arthritis. Presently, a phase II–III clinical trial has been initiated in the USA and five other European countries.

7.4.3 IL-1 BLOCKADE

Anakinra, an anti-IL-1, is an alternative therapeutic option for management of distress in patients with severe COVID-19. It is a recombinant and somewhat a different variation of the human IL-1 receptor antagonist protein. It is unsurprisingly unconfined by monocytes and tissue macrophages that selectively impasse to IL-R and modulate their activity. The inhibition of IL-1 leads to the destruction of inflammatory responses. In a phase III randomized controlled trial, the IL-1 blockade in sepsis has been seen as helpful in increased survival deprived of augmented adverse effects. Therefore, considering the similar "cytokine storm" between severe sepsis and severe COVID-19, anakinra may have played a part in the response of some severe or stubborn cases.

7.4.4 IL-2 INHIBITION

The cyclosporine–cyclophilin is a complex that prevents a calcium/calmodulin-dependent phosphatase, named calcineurin, with the exclusion of which is hypothetical to constrain organ denunciation by tentative construction of the proinflammatory molecules, TNF-α and IL-2. Due to these effects, cyclosporine has been established as beneficial in the management of autoimmune diseases. Cyclophilin is also predicted to be employed by the Gag polyprotein in HIV-1 virus infection and in managibg new virus particles responsible for HIV-1 infection. Observational studies revealed that cyclophilin inhibitors CyA have an inhibitory effect on SARS-CoV through the calcineurin pathway reserve, which also plays an important role in SARS-CoV virus replication. In addition, CyA and tacrolimus downmodulated the calcineurin/nuclear factor of activated T-cell inflammatory pathway triggered through SARS. In this way, pathogenic similarities in intense pulmonary COVID-19 and the anticancer differentiation-related gene 5-positive (anti-MDA-5) amyotrophic dermatomyositis-related unexpectedly modern interstitial lung disorder may be taken into account. MDA-5 cell sensor can be caused by viruses, which is fascinating. CyA or tacrolimus with or disadvantaged of intravenous immunoglobulins (IVIG) is a guide for pharmacologic control of the anti-MDA-5 syndrome. To conclude, instances of anti-MDA-5 syndrome complicated by a hemophagocytic syndrome had been designated. Accordingly, permitting antiviral and anti-inflammatory effects of calcineurin inhibitors, CyA and tacrolimus, could be potential operative drugs in treating severe forms of COVID-19.

7.4.5 OTHER CYTOKINE-TARGETED THERAPY

At the same time, other targets such as IL-37 and IL-38 could be beneficial options. IL-37 temporarily inhibits inflammation via the IL-18Ra receptor, mTOR, and the adenosine monophosphate kinase. IL-38 is likewise a suppressor cytokine that prevents IL-1b and other proinflammatory IL-family members. The behavior of WT mice with recombinant human IL-37 has been shown to be defensive in numerous models of inflammation and wound. These cytokines might signify novel therapeutic targets in patients with universal inflammatory syndromes.

7.4.6 INTRAVENOUS IVIG

Solicitations concerning immunoglobulin have been prolonged to include treatment for immunodeficiency ailments, immune thrombocytopenia, Kawasaki disease, neurologic disorders, SLE, and other undecorated or refractory autoimmune illnesses. Among the multiple effects on the innate and adaptive immune pathways related to IVIG, doses >0.5 g/kg weight/day can delay the symptoms of inflammatory cytokines formed by dissimilar stimuli. Although preliminary lessons have shown efficiency of IVIG in the management of patients with severe inflammatory grievances related to influenza and SARS-CoV infections, we require more clinical data of COVID-19 patients. Currently, a randomized clinical trial of IVIG in patients with severe SARS-CoV-2 infection is going on. TRALI is an immune-mediated procedure, and neutrophil-priming hypotheses have been predicted as conceivable treatments; thrombotic minutes related to IVIG treatment have a projected incidence of 1–16.9%. Interpreting to the doubtful practicality of IVIG treatment in patients with SARS-CoV and the risk of severe lung injury and thrombosis, we think that the IVIG option should be prudently analyzed before it is used in severe COVID-19 patients. In addition, the convalescent plasma (CP) and hyperimmune immunoglobulin neutralizing antibodies have been initiated for the treatment of severe acute respiratory syndrome of viral etiology, including MERS-CoV and SARS-CoV-2 infections. Despite preliminary evidence that CP/HIVIG can reduce mortality, particularly when administered early after symptoms appear, the true effectiveness is debatable, and this treatment should be evaluated within the context of well-designed clinical trials.

7.4.7 ANTICOAGULANTS

High levels of D-dimer are related to poor outcomes and high mortality rate. Even though D-dimer levels are elevated in maximum patients with blood clots, D-dimer levels also are significant in many other complaints counting infection. In any occasion, multiple pulmonary embolus has also been observed in these patients. Additionally, it has been observed that patients with severe COVID-19 may increase dispersed intravascular coagulation, PTE, and arterial thrombosis, in a similar way asfor SARS-CoV. Furthermore, distinct diagnostic tactics have been predicted in COVID-19 patients with medical history of PTE. Finally, autopsies of 50 COVID-19 patients revealed available microthrombosis and thrombus distressing big pulmonary arteries within the advanced vena cava and proper auricular veins. Interestingly, histologic evidence such as alveolar and interstitial irritation encompasses to the prudently contrasted pulmonary vasculature and the everyday circulatory fibrinogen stages and nearby fibrinolysis with raised D-dimer advent visible in preliminary COVID-19 pneumonia aren't systems of feature acute onset MAS/HPS. This hyperprovocative intrapulmonary inflammation strength inspire a tendency in severe local vascular dysfunction comprising microthrombosis and hemorrhage in lung-centric pulmonary intravascular coagulopathy performance rather than a DIC presentation.

7.4.8 GLUCOCORTICOIDS

GCs follow inhibitory property on a large variety of innate and adaptive immune responses. Since in their inhibitory consequences on severe kinds of immune cells, GCs are surprisingly powerful in dealing with the severity of extreme disorder appearances of inflammatory and autoimmune disorders. The anti-inflammatory and immunosuppressive effects of GCs rely on three main mechanisms that comprise (a)thorough effects on gene appearance by the binding of glucocorticoid receptors to glucocorticoid-responsive elements and (b) indirect effects on gene expression conclude the interactions of glucocorticoid receptors with other transcription factors. Effects of GCs have been proved for success of otherlife-threatening circumstances such as CID, sepsis, and acute distress respiratory syndrome. By its clinical comparison, GCs are presently empirically used in some hospitals in the management of severe COVID-19 patients, and different therapeutic local guidelines are made for them. Nonetheless, the current indication is unconvincing or does not support maintenance for GCs management of COVID- 19 patients to date. In selected cases, careful use with low-to-moderate doses and short courses of management could be recommended. According to Cochrane review, WHO recommendations, and professional agreement statement from Chinese Thoracic Society, some fundamental principles should be considered when administering corticosteroids to severe COVID-19 patients: Before using GCs, it is wise to weigh the benefits and risks. Additionally, GCs should be used with caution in patients with SARS-CoV-2 pneumonia who are disapprovingly ill. Additional corticosteroid use is also prudent for patients who frequently use corticosteroids for chronic diseases or who have hypoxemia due to fundamental diseases. Additionally, WHO and CDC recommend against routinely using corticosteroids in COVID-19 patients to treat viral pneumonia or ARDS unless indicated for a different reason. To sum up, doctors who decide to add corticosteroids to "goal standard" treatment for patients with dangerous septic COVID-19 should balance the potential small decrease in mortality with any long-term coronavirus shedding side effects.

7.5 CONCLUSION

These examples underline the significance of bioprospecting for more recent synergistic mixtures and pharmacological agents. Although many researchers have studied synergism and antagonism in botanicals, systematic medical investigations on pharmacodynamics, kinetics, dosing, and interactions are nonetheless required. Traditional expertise, specifically from the excellent traditions of, for example, *Ayurveda* and Chinese conventional medicines, can have a critical position in bioprospecting. *Rasayanas* are a particular branch of botanicals from *Ayurveda* with putative abilities to rejuvenate, build sturdiness, and refine health. In short, botanical immunotablets may offer a completely unique possibility to bioprospect numerous and synergistic chemical compounds moieties, which in mixture would possibly act on more than one goals and enhance the healing spectrum. Traditional expertise and practices carry experiential expertise to offer a more secure and extra cost-effective platform for more recent scaffolds and immunodrug discovery.

KEYWORDS

- **immunomodulator**
- **immunomodulation**
- **immune system**
- **immunity**
- **immunostimulators**
- **receptors**

REFERENCES

Adeboboye, C. F.; Oladejo, B. O.; Adebolu, T. T. Immunomodulation: A Broad Perspective for Patients' Survival of COVID-19 Infection. *Eur. J. Biol. Res.* **2020,** *10* (3), 217–224.

Ahire, E. D.; Sonawane, V. N.; Surana, K. R. Role of Drug Repurposing in Current Treatment Strategies against COVID-19: Systemic Review. *Pharm Reson.* **2020,** *1*, 24–29.

Alijotas-Reig, J.; Esteve-Valverde, E.; Belizna, C.; et al. Immunomodulatory Therapy for the Management of Severe COVID-19. Beyond the Anti-viral Therapy: A Comprehensive Review. *Autoimmun. Rev.* **2020,** *19*, 102569.

Bhargava, P.; Panda, P.; Ostwal, V.; Ramaswamy, A. Repurposing Valproate to Prevent Acute Respiratory Distress Syndrome/Acute Lung Injury in COVID-19: A Review of Immunomodulatory Action. *Cancer Res., Stat., Treat.* **2020,** *3* (5), 65.

Burrage, D. R.; Koushesh, S.; Sofat, N. Immunomodulatory Drugs in the Management of SARS-CoV-2. *Front. Immunol.* **2020,** *11*, 1844.

Courville, K.; Bustamante, N.; Pecchio, M. Cytokine Removal and Immunomodulation in COVID-19 Severe Pulmonary Respiratory Infection. *ScienceOpen Preprints* **2020.** doi:10.14293/S2199-1006.1.SOR-.PPWLC61.v1

Gasmi, A.; Tippairote, T.; Mujawdiya, P. K.; et al. Micronutrients as Immunomodulatory Tools for COVID-19 Management. *Clin. Immunol.* **2020,** *220*, 108545.

Jethwa H.; Sullivan, A.; Abraham, S. COVID-19 and Rheumatology Patients on Immunomodulatory Therapy—Can We Extrapolate Data from Previous Viral Pandemics? *J. Rheumatol.* 2020. doi:10.3899/jrheum.200527.

Kurya, A. U.; Toro, A. U.; Bello, U. R.; Sharma, D. C. A Review Study on Efficacy of Immunomodulatory Agents Used for the Treatment of COVID-19. *Asian J. Biol. Life Sci.* **2020,** *9* (2), 247.

Kwak-Kim, J.; Ota, K.; Sung, N.; et al. COVID-19 and Immunomodulation Treatment for Women with Reproductive Failures. *J. Reprod. Immunol.* **2020,** *141*, 103168.

Maldonado, V.; Alderete, J. C. Repositioning of Pentoxifylline as an Immunomodulator and Regulator of the Renin-Angiotensin System in the Treatment of COVID-19. *Med. Hypoth.* **2020,** *144*, 109988.

Nair, A.; Chattopadhyay, D.; Saha, B. Plant-Derived Immunomodulators. *New Look to Phytomedicine*; Elsevier: Amsterdam, 2019; pp 435–499.

Price, K. N.; Frew, J. W.; Hsiao, J. L.; Shi, V. Y. COVID-19 and Immunomodulator/Immunosuppressant Use in Dermatology. *J. Am. Acad. Dermatol.* **2020,** *82* (5), e173–e175.

Rane, B. R.; Patil, A. S.; Keservani, R. K.; Jain, A. S. Novel Approaches in Herbal Formulation, In *Enhancing the Therapeutic Efficacy of Herbal Formulations through Novel Drug Delivery Systems*; Kesharwani, R. K., Keservani, R. K., Sharma, A. K.; IGI Global International Publisher: Pennsylvania, USA, 2020, Chapter 2, pp 43–68. ISBN13: 9781799844532.

Ruscitti, P.; Berardicurti, O.; Di Benedetto, P.; et al. Severe COVID-19, Another Piece in the Puzzle of the Hyperferritinemic Syndrome. An Immunomodulatory Perspective to Alleviate the Storm. *Front. Immunol.* **2020,** *11*, 1130.

Smith, T.; Bushek, J.; LeClaire, A.; Prosser, T. *COVID-19 Drug Therapy*; Elsevier: Amsterdam, 2020.

Surana, K. R.; Ahire, E. D.; Sonawane, V. N.; Talele, S. G.; Talele, G. S. Informatics and Methods in Nutrition Design and Development. In *Natural Food Products and Waste Recovery*; Apple Academic Press: Cambridge, MA, 2021; pp 33–49.

Ye, Q.; Wang, B.; Mao, J. The Pathogenesis and Treatment of the "Cytokine Storm" in COVID-19. *J. Infect.* **2020,** *80*, 607–613.

Yessayan, L.; Szamosfalvi, B.; Napolitano, L.; et al. Treatment of Cytokine Storm in COVID-19 Patients with Immunomodulatory Therapy. *ASAIO J.* **2020,** *66*, 1079–1083.

CHAPTER 8

Immunomodulators as New Emerging Virus Infections (Zika Virus Infection, MERS, and COVID-19)

S. YASRI[1] and V. WIWANITKIT[2,3]

[1]*KMT Primary Care Center, Bangkok, Thailand*

[2]*Dr DY Patil University, Navi Mumbai, India*

[3]*Hainan Medical University, Haikou, China*

ABSTACT

Infectious disease is a common problem in clinical medicine. The infection results from the invasion of pathogen into the host and further cause inflammatory process that finalize into the clinical problem. The infectious disease is a challenge in medicine. There are many new emerging infectious diseases. Regarding the new disease, there is usually a limited knowledge on pathogenesis and this can result in difficulty in diagnosis and treatment. Within the past decade, many new emerging virus infections such as Zika virus infection, MERS, and Coronavirus disease 2019 (COVID-19) occurred. Those new emerging virus infections are usually problematic and become the global public health consideration. Those diseases can result in unwanted morbidity and mortality and it is the role of infectious medicine to control and manage those new emerging viral disease. The diagnosis and treatment become the two important processes in medicine regarding new emerging infections. An important knowledge is immunological mechanism related to that disease. Regarding an infection,

COVID-19 and Immunomodulation with Special Emphasis on Nutraceutical and Herbal Formulation.
Rajesh K. Kesharwani & Raj K. Keservani (Eds)

the triad, host, pathogen, and environment plays interrelationship at the same time and place that can result in final occurrence of infection. When a pathogen contacts with host, there will be a responsive interaction. Host usually has defensive mechanism against the pathogen. The specific response *via* immunological system is the important body defense to infection. This is also important in counteracting with new emerging virus infection. Since new emerging virus is a new disease, the knowledge on immunopathogenesis is limited. The clinical immunologist does usually not know the exact immunological pathway that host responded to the pathogenic agent. Many ongoing studies are on immunopathogenesis of the new diseases. The derived data will be useful for searching for new diagnostic and therapeutic techniques for the new diseases. The specific role of immunological system in the treatment of disease is very interesting since it is usually required a new effect method to contain the new emerging viral infection. Of several new therapeutic approaches, immunotherapy is a widely proposed therapeutic technique against the infection. For the new emerging viral infection, immunotherapy is also proposed as a new therapeutic alternative technique. There are many forms of immunotherapy such as passive immunity or immunoglobulin therapy, therapeutic vaccination, and immunomodulatory agent. The immunomodulator is a specific agent that has main pharmacobiomechanism in the modification of immunological reaction that will be useful in control and getting rid of the infectious pathogen. The immunomodulatory agent therapy for new emerging infection is a big challenge. In this chapter, the authors summarize and discussion on immunomolulator in the three important new emerging viral infections, Zika virus infection, MERS, and COVID-19. In the present new COVID-19 crisis, many classic immunomodulators are proposed for possible usefulness in disease management and there are many ongoing trials on those new immunomodulatory agents. Additionally, new studies aiming at searching for new effective and safe immunomodulatory agents for the treatment of the new are ongoing and it is the hope for the management of the COVID-19.

8.1 INTRODUCTION

The infectious disease is a common problem in clinical medicine. The infection results from the invasion of pathogen into the host and further cause inflammatory process that finalize into the clinical problem. The infectious disease is a challenge in medicine. There are many new emerging infectious diseases. Regarding the new disease, there is usually a limited knowledge on pathogenesis and this can result in difficulty in diagnosis and treatment. Within the past decade, many new emerging virus infections such as Zika virus infection, MERS, and Coronavirus disease 2019 (COVID-19) occurred. Those new emerging virus infections are usually problematic and become the global public health consideration. Those diseases can result in unwanted morbidity and mortality and it is the role of infectious medicine to control and manage those new emerging viral disease. The diagnosis and treatment become the two important processes in medicine regarding new emerging infections. An important knowledge is immunological mechanism related to that disease. Briefly, immune system is the specific body system that plays role in defense to an alien invader. The immunopathogensis can explain the pathobiological process that interrelates to the clinical feature of the disease.

Based on clinical epidemiological concept, the triad to fulfill the requirement for occurrence of an infection includes host, pathogen, and environment. The three things have to coexist at the same time and same place. When interrelationship occurs, infection might occur. When a pathogen enters into human body, there will be a reaction. The defensive mechanism will play roles in counteracting the invader (Furman and Davis, 2015). Immunological system is an important component of defense mechanism. Ideally, if immunological system of the host is strong enough, the pathogen will be successfully gotten rid of. This is a basic concept for cure of a disease. Therefore, it is no doubt that some infections might be self-limited without any treatment. However, many infections are serious and the immune mechanism might not able to get rid of the pathogen. In this case, the treatment is required. The treatment for infection might be by several ways. The use of antibiotic for treatment of bacterial infection is a good example.

For treatment, several therapeutic methods are available for therapy such as drug, vaccine, radio management, and surgical manipulation. However, an interesting approach is the immunotherapy. Immunotherapy is the treatment based on the immunological process. This is an approach that is widely used for the management of several diseases including to cancers and infections. Regarding infection, several forms of immunotherapy are available at present. The good examples are passive immunotherapy by sera or immunoglobulin, active immunotherapy by vaccine therapy or immunomodulatory therapy. To get a successful treatment outcome by immunotherapy, there must be these basic requirements: (1) effective immunotherapeutic agent, (2) safe immunotherapeutic agent, (3) sufficient immunotherapeutic agent, (4) good immunotherapeutic agent administration, and (5) good biotransportation biodistribution to the desired target (Tiligada et al., 2015). These issues are usually important focus in seeking for new effective and safe immunomodulatory agents.

TABLE 8.1 Examples of Some Important Immunotherapy Methods.

Techniques	Examples
Active immunotherapy	Immunoglobulin therapy
	Sera/plasma therapy
Passive immunotherapy	Therapeutic vaccine
Immunomodulatory therapy	Immunostimulant agent
	Immunosuppressive agent
	Immunomodification agent

Finally, there are many factors that are related to the success of treatment. The three main factors are host, pathogen, and drug. Regarding the host, the background underlying disease and strength of immune system are important determinants for responsiveness to immunomodulatory process. Some genetic backgrounds, genetic polymorphisms, are related to immune response. Regarding the pathogen, the invasiveness of the pathogen is an important factor determining severity of infection and it also implies the responsiveness to the therapy. Finally, different drugs have different pharmacomechanisms, which are related to treatment result. The dosage and time that drug is used are also important factors determining the treatment outcome. Hence, when one considered the outcome of therapy, this triad has to be recognized and assessed.

8.2 IMMUNOPHARMACOLOGY AND IMMUNOMODULATORY AGENT FOR MANAGEMENT OF INFECTION

Therapy is an important process in medicine. The aim of therapy is to cure or control of clinical disease. The therapy might be by different approaches such as medical and surgical. The specific treatment targeting immunological process is called immunotherapy. In fact, the medical application of immunotherapy is a really interesting present biomedical technology. The application can be either in single treatment or combined treatment with other therapeutic methods. The immunotherapy is an attempt to natural physiological response process in host to the foreign body. This is the way that uses the model of natural mechanism to get rid of illness. As already mentioned, the immunotherapy can be applied for the management of several medial diseases such as malignancies and infections. Effectiveness of immunotherapy leads the attention of medical society for application it in clinical purpose in the treatment of the patient. The immunopharmacology regarding the immunotherapy for treatment of infectious disease is interesting and should be mentioned.

Basically, immunopharmacology is based on the knowledge of immunopathogenesis. For any infection, the invasion of pathogen into human body will result in immunological response. This is a standard defense mechanism of human beings. The immunological reaction might be by cellular or humoral immune response. The result of immunological reaction might result in successful disease containment by human body. On the other hand, many infections can overcome immunological mechanism and cause pathology and finally results in diseases. In addition, the inappropriate immune reaction can also cause problem. Many diseases are the results from inappropriate immune response such as excessive immune reaction. Therefore, the pathology in many diseases might be an immunopathological process. On the other side of the coin, the too little immune response can also cause problem. The good example is the immunodeficiency status. If there is too low immune reactive, it is no doubt that the containment of pathogen will not be successful. Many diseases such as human immunodeficiency virus infection are due to immunodeficiency patholological process.

It is necessary to study and collect the knowledge on immunological reaction in any disease since such knowledge can be helpful for the proper therapeutic design. The specific immunopharmacological therapy for the management of infectious disease is the contemporary concept in modern medicine.

Conceptually, the immunotherapy follows a natural mechanism of disease containment. It should be safe if the immunotherapy is completely same as the defensive mechanism in human body. However, to achieve that ideal situation is usually difficult. Since the knowledge on immunopathogenesis is required for designing a good immunotherapy, the lack of data in many infections, especially for the new emerging infections, result in no complete data for the development of immunotherapy. In order to have a good immunotherapy, not only the knowledge on immunopathogenesis but also on immunopharmacology is necessary (van der Poll et al., 2017). In pharmacology, the details of drug mechanisms, biological process in host, effect on the pathogen and possible unwanted effect for usage are all requires data for any drug. This is also the same required knowledge in immunopharmacology. In immunopharmacology, the basic topics to be covered include (1) immunopharmaceutic, (2) immunopharmacostatic, and (3) immunopharmacodynamic (Tiligada et al., 2015).

At present, immunopharmacology in the management of infection is an important new therapeutic modality in clinical medicine. Many new immunological treatments are introduced and in use for the management of the infection. The specific researches on this area are interesting and should be promoted. Although there are already many data but more and more data are required from researching for continuous improvement of the immunotherapy. For the management on an infectious disease, there are two options of using immunopharmacotherapy. The first option is the use of classical known immunological agent and the second is the finding and use of the novel immunological agent. The two options are useful. In a routine situation, classical immunological agent with confirmed data on its efficacy and safety is routinely useful. However, the finding of the new immunological agent that can give a better effective and safer outcome is also useful and should be promoted. Nevertheless, the situation might be more complex in the case of new emerging infection. In that situation, there is no available drug and there is no knowledge on the pathogenesis of the disease. The use of classical drug in other similar infection might be done but it still requires a good control of usage. The clinical data from complete trial should be available from an actual implementation of the classical agent to the new disease management. Regarding the new therapeutic agent, it is still required a long time to get a new therapeutic agent and longer time to have complete data from standard trial to finally get a new agent for the management of new emerging infection. This might not be on time to correspond to the emerging crisis. The COVID-crisis is a good example that the use of either classical or new therapeutic agent is a challenge due to lack of data and rapid change of the outbreak crisis.

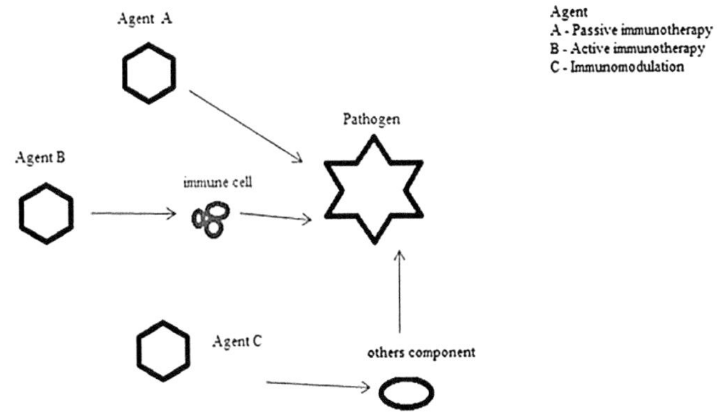

FIGURE 8.1 Different modes of immunotherapy against infectious pathogen.

8.3 IMMUNOPATHOGNESIS AND IMMUNOMODULATORY MANAGEMENT OF IMPORTANT NEW EMERGING INFECTIONS (ZIKA VIRUS INFECTION, MERS, AND COVID-19)

As already mentioned, immunotherapy is important medical therapy that directly relates to immunological principle. The application of immunotherapy in emerging infection is a big challenge. In clinical medicine, the use of immunotherapy to correspond the emerging and re-emerging infections is very interesting clinical issue. The data are little mentioned. The knowledge on immunopathology of a classic infection can be a good lesson learnt for the new disease. For example, knowledge from influenza can be a good data for the new emerging infectious disease. Newton et al. (2016) mentioned that "*The continuing threat posed by pandemic influenza as well as the emergence of novel respiratory viruses also capable of producing severe acute lung injury such as SARS-CoV, MERS-CoV, and enterovirus D68, highlights the need for an understanding of the immune mechanisms that contribute to virus elimination and immune-mediated injury.*" Here, the authors will discuss immunomodulator in the three important new emerging viral infections that emerged in the past decade. The three viral diseases are Zika virus infection, MERS, and COVID-19. The specific focus on the immunomodulatory agent in each emerging viral infection is hereby details.

8.3.1 ZIKA VIRUS INFECTION

There are many vector borne viral diseases in medicine. Some are common or endemic in the tropical region and it is called tropical arboviral diseases. The good examples of tropical arboviral diseases are dengue and Chikungunya virus infections. Many arboviral diseases become more important due to its rapid spreading worldwide. There are also some emerging arboviral diseases. Zika virus infection is a new emerging virus infection that becomes the global public health topic (Martins et al., 2020; Plourde and Bloch, 2016). Microbiologically, the Zika virus is in the virus family Flaviviridae. The virus has been known for many years but the large outbreak has just occurred for a few years. The big outbreak in America leads to many attempts to contain this infection.

This emerging viral infection has a multimodal transmission, including sexual contact transmission (Duarte et al., 2017). In general, the virus can cause a dengue-like illness. Asymptomatic infection is also common (Haby et al., 2017). The infection in pregnant women is a very interesting situation. Zika virus can spread from a pregnant woman to her child by transplacental transmission. The observation of offspring with neurological defect born to Zika virus infected mother lead to the worldwide concern on this new emerging virus infection (Chimelli and Avvad-Portari, 2018). Additionally, the virus can also cause neurological problem in adult. The Guillain–Barré syndrome is the possible serious neurological complication due to Zika virus infection (Nascimento and da Silva, 2017). Krauer et al. (2017) noted that available evidence from the outbreaks of Zika virus infection and Guillain–Barré syndrome showed that Zika virus infection is a trigger of Guillain–Barré syndrome. Piontkivska et al. (2018) noted that pathogenicity of congenital Zika disease and Guillain–Barré syndromes was also related to dysregulation of RNA editing.

The immunopathological process relating to Zika virus infection is an interesting issue in clinical pathophysiology. It is evidence that innate immunity might help restrict ZIKV infection and disease development (Xie et al., 2016). The Zika virus infection has a similar pathogenesis to dengue. The virus-specific immunity plays role in pathogenesis (Culshaw and Mongkolsapaya, 2017). Since Zika virus infection is a virus infection, the cellular immune response is the main human immunity system that corresponds to infection. Lima et al. (2017) noted that humoral immune response generated the primary correlate of protection from Zika disease but a more important role was corresponded by T-lymphocyte. Lima et al. (2017) also noted that pre-existing immunity to related flaviviruses could generate cross-reactive T cells. This fact is very important since the cross immunity might may affect immune responses upon any newly developed Zika virus vaccination (Lima et al., 2017). Priyamvada et al. (2017a) noted that humoral immune responses against Zika virus infection were significantly affected by pre-existing flavivirus immunity. The antibody-dependent enhancement is much affected from structural similarities between Zika virus and other flaviviruses, especially dengue virus (DENV). Indeed, the concurrent Zika virus infection and other arbovirus infection are the important clinical problem existing in the area that co-circulation of Zika virus and other arbovirus (Andrade et al., 2018). Priyamvada et al. (2017b) proposed that humoral cross-reactivity between Zika and dengue viruses plays role in both protection and pathology. Priyamvada et al. (2017a) concluded that the impact of pre-existing flavivirus immunity on Zika virus pathogenesis, in utero transmission of ZIKV infection and generation of protective responses were still the myth of Zika virus infection. Andrade and Harris (2018) found that investigating cross-neutralizing antibodies was very important for better understanding protection of Zika virus infection.

Pathophysiologically, the immunological response is mainly by T lymphocyte. Zika virus infection can induce the expression of CCR5, CX3CR1, and CXCR3 on CD4 and CD8 T cells (Badolato-Corrêa et al., 2018). The closed relationship between Zika virus and dengue can also affect the immunopathogenesis. Roth et al. (2018) noted that a pre-existing dengue immunity that could exacerbate Zika virus infection and disease, and given the lack of appropriate treatment for Zika virus infection. Several attempts are launched in order to understand the immunopathogenesis of Zika virus infection. The animal model is useful for the identification of Zika virus pathogenesis. The data from study on immunopathogenesis can help to finding the proper drug and vaccine. Also, the animal models are useful for evaluating new Zika virus vaccines and therapeutics as well as understanding disease pathogenesis (Lazear et al., 2016).

Immunotherapy for Zika virus infection is an interesting concept (Miner and Diamond, 2017). Antibody and vaccine are widely tested. Regarding immunomodulatory agent, a classical agent, methotrexate, is an example of agent proposed for usefulness in the management of Zika virus (Beck et al., 2019). Beck et al. (2019) found that methotrexate could cause the restriction of *de novo* synthesis of adenosine triphosphate (ATP) pools that can further result in the suppression of viral replication. Another drug that is proposed for the usefulness in immunotherapy for Zika virus infection is aminoglycoside (Gopinath et al., 2018). Topical mucosal application of aminoglycosides can prophylactically increase host resistance to Zika virus. After applying, aminoglycoside can promote interferon-stimulated genes by biopharmacological process *via* Toll-like receptor 3, and required Toll/interleukin-1-receptor-domain-containing adapter-inducing interferon-β signaling adaptor, and Interferon regulatory factors 3 and 7, and transcription factors (Gopinath et al., 2018; Xu et al., 2017). Additionally, interferon lambda is another agent that is proposed for usefulness in the management of Zika virus infection Caine et al. (2019). Interferon lambda is also proposed for its ability to reduce sexual transmission of Zika virus in female (Caine et al., 2019).

The immunosuppression by steroid is also proposed for the management of Zika virus infection. Li et al. (2020a) studied in animal model and found that 25-Hydroxycholesterol help protects animal against Zika virus infection and there is also a relationship with microcephaly. Xiao et al. (2020) proposed a new Zika virus therapy concept by targeting 7-dehydrocholesterol reductase. This approach can integrate cholesterol metabolism and activate IRF3 for eliminating the Zika virus infection (Chan et al., 2020). In real clinical practice, the steroid is reported for its usefulness in some patients with Zika virus infection. Burgueño-Montañés et al. (2018) reported using steroids and infliximab for clinical management non-para-neoplastic autoimmune retinopathy induced by Zika virus infection. Mancera-Páez et al. (2018) proposed that steroid therapy is useful for the management of patient with concurrent Guillain–Barré syndrome, transverse myelitis and encephalitis post-Zika. With steroid therapy and intensive care treatment, respiratory support, and intravenous immunoglobulin (IVIg), the outcome is favorable (Mancera-Páez et al., 2018). The Zika virus-infected patient did not die but still had residual flaccid paraparesis (Mancera-Páez et al., 2018). Nevertheless, the opposite finding is also observed in some reports. Chan et al. (2016) found that dexamethasone-immunosuppressed animal with Zika virus infection might demonstrate disseminated infection with multi-organ involvement.

Finally, there is also another interesting concept for the management of Zika virus infection, the immunometabolism therapy. Hooftman and O'Neill (2019) proposed for the Immunomodulatory potential of the metabolite itaconate. Hooftman and O'Neill (2019) performed a study in animal model of Zika virus infection and concluded that itaconate was the best example of such a moonlighting molecule that expressed multiple anti-inflammatory effects in macrophages. The main immunomodulative pharmacomechanism ofitaconate is *via* macrophage (O'Neill and Artyomov, 2019; Yu et al., 2019). Hooftman and O'Neill (2019) found that itaconate could be significantly upregulated under inflammatory conditions, and can promote an anti-inflammatory phenotype by reducing oxidative stress and blocking transcriptional responses to lipopolysaccharide in macrophages, which is beneficial in the treatment of Zika virus infection.

8.3.2 MERS

There are many viral respiratory infections in medicine. Some diseases are common and endemic such as common cold and influenza. An important group of respiratory viral infection is emerging viral respiratory syndrome. The Middle East Respiratory Syndrome (MERS) is a new emerging respiratory infection that occurred first in the Middle East (Chafekar and Fielding, 2018). The viral pathogen is MERS-CoV. This infection can result in severe respiratory problem and the patient might die of respiratory failure. The severity and transmissibility of MERS differ by outbreak region and patient characteristics (Park et al., 2018). The infection might be serious and severe pneumonia might occur (Yin and Wunderink, 2018). The specific treatment of this new disease is still not available and there is still no vaccine for MERS at present.

The immunopathological process relating to MERS is an interesting issue in clinical pathophysiology. Since MERS is a virus infection, the cellular immune response is the main human immunity system that corresponds to infection. The pathogenesis of MER is similar to a previously well-known coronavirus infection, SARS. Mubarak et al. (2014) noted that MERS-CoV has spike proteins as adhesive factors that are proinflammatory for host entry through a specific receptor called dipeptidyl peptidase-4 (DPP4). This cellular receptor is considered a key factor in signaling and activation of the acquired and innate immune responses to MERS (Mubarak et al., 2014). Focusing on immune response, lymphocyte plays important role. Mahallawi et al. (2018) found that MERS-CoV infection in humans is associated with a pro-inflammatory Th1 and Th17 cytokine profile. Rokni et al. (2020) proposed that a specific T-cell response against SARS-CoV-2 was very important for the recognition and getting rid of infected cells, particularly in the lungs of infected individuals. However, MERS can cause problem to lymphocyte. The lymphocytopenia is a common clinical presentation in MERS (Al-Tawfiq et al., 2017). MERS-CoV can induce IL-17 production in humans (Faure et al., 2014). Host recognition of viral dsRNA is an important determinant for the outcome of infection in the early stage of MERS (Faure et al., 2014). The host immune response in MERS can help to remove virus but it might also cause immunopathology (Newton et al., 2016). Generally, an effective immune response is important for viral pathogens elimination. Too much exaggerated or too long immune response can result in the respiratory tract damage (Newton et al., 2016). Immune-mediated pulmonary damage is possible and various degree of lung damage can occur (Newton et al., 2016). Chafekar and Fielding (2018) proposed that immunotherapy was a possible alternative therapeutic management for MERS.

Immunotherapy and antibody therapy are proposed as an effective therapeutic management for MERS (Arabi et al., 2016; Widjaja et al., 2019). The plasma therapy is a method that is widely studied (Arabi et al., 2016) and it is also the basic concept that is implemented for the later emerging COVID-19. Regarding immunomodulatory agent, alisporivir is an agent that is proposed for possible therapeutic role against MERS (de Wilde et al., 2017). In brief, alisporivir is a non-immunosuppressive cyclosporin A-analog that can inhibit the replication (de Wilde et al., 2017). The classic drug, hydroxychloroquine is also mentioned for managing MERS (Dyall et al, 2017). Statin is another classic drug that is proposed for usefulness in managing MERS. Regarding pharmacological mechanism, statin can inhibit MyD88 signaling and downstream NF-κB responses that can further result in improved disease outcomes in MERS (Totura and Baric, 2015).

The immunosuppression by steroid is also proposed for usefulness in MERS treatment (Alfaraj et al., 2019; Arabi et al., 2019). Arabi et al. (2018) noted that corticosteroid was helpful for managing MERS. Nevertheless, the adverse effects due to steroid therapy are a controversial issue. Alfaraj et al. (2019) noted that steroid therapy in MERS was associated with higher rate of mortality. Arabi et al. (2018) noted that steroid was not associated with a difference in mortality but it could result in delayed MERS coronavirus RNA clearance. Several therapeutic factors are also related to the outcome of steroid therapy in MERS. Extra Corporal Mechanical Oxygenation was reported to be useful in decreasing mortality in MERS patient treated with steroid (Alfaraj et al., 2019).

The role of steroids for the management of coronavirus infection is complex. Basically, steroids do not directly inhibit virus replication but it acts as anti-inflammatory and can suppress immune response (Montón et al., 1999; Yang et al., 2020) In the early stage of inflammation, steroid can reduce capillary dilation, inflammatory cell exudation, leukocyte infiltration, and phagocytosis whereas it can inhibit the excessive proliferation of capillaries and fibroblasts in the late stage (Yang et al., 2020). Steroid can also bind to specific receptor and further inhibits nuclear transcription factor-κB (NF-κB) signaling and further inhibit the transcription and translation of inflammatory factors (Yang et al., 2020). The mentioned biological process is useful for the management of viral infections including MERS.

8.3.3 COVID-19

Coronavirus disease 2019 (COVID-19) is another important emerging respiratory viral syndrome (Vieira et al., 2020). The viral pathogen is SARS-CoV2. This new viral respiratory infection is an important problem in medicine and public health. This new emerging respiratory infection firstly occurred in China then spread to Thailand and more than 200 countries around the world. More than nine millions of world population already got infection. COVID-19 can cause in severe respiratory problem and the patient might die of respiratory failure. The common serious lung disorder in COVID-19 is pneumonia (Hani et al., 2020). Similar to MERS, the specific treatment of this new disease is still not available and there is still no vaccine for COVID-19 at present. Nevertheless, COVID-19 might be asymptomatic and there are many possible atypical clinical presentations such as skin rashes.

The immunopathological process relating to COVID-19 is an interesting issue in clinical pathophysiology. Since COVID-19 is a new disease, still there is limited knowledge on its pathogenesis. Limited understanding of the immune effects caused by SARS-CoV-2, it is difficult to find therapeutic and preventive measurements against important complications of COVID-19, respiratory distress syndrome (ARDS) and pulmonary fibrosis

(PF) (Liang et al., 2020). Further research on this issue is recommended. Since COVID-19 is a coronavirus infection, its pathogenesis is believed to be similar to SARS and MERS. The lymphocyte plays important role in cellular immunity against COVID-19. But similar to MERS, COVID-19 can also induce the reduction in number of lymphocyte (Liang et al., 2020). Li et al. (2020b) noted that the immune response was essential for infection elimination. Jamilloux et al. (2020) noted that Cytokines are central to the pathophysiology of COVID-19. Some are beneficial (type-I interferon, interleukin-7), whereas the others, such as interleukin-1β, -6, and TNF-α, might induce unwanted problem (Jamilloux et al., 2020). Pathophysiologically, maladjusted, too longed or exaggerated immune responses may result in immunopathology. The immunopathology in COVID-19 is complex. The important immunological disturbance includes lymphopenia, exhausted lymphocytes, and a cytokine storm (Cao, 2020). García (2020) noted that the critical point where the progression of COVID-19 was related to center on loss of the immune regulation between protective and altered responses resulted from excessive inflammation process. An important emerging immunopathological problem in COVID-19 is cytokine storm (Chen et al., 2020; Vaninov, 2020). Cytokine storm is a pathological phenomenon result from an excessive immune response to external stimuli. Severe deterioration of COVID-19 patient has might be the result of cytokine storm (Ye et al., 2020). The cytokine storm can lead to severe clinical problem in COVID-19 (Ye et al., 2020). When there are immunologic complications like cytokine storm, a simple anti-viral treatment alone is not enough (Soy et al., 2020). Zhao (2020) noted that other immunomodulatory agents with effectiveness and safety profiles might be selected for use in combination with antiviral drugs for the treatment of severe COVID-19.

The immune response plays important role in the pathogenesis of COVID-19 (Yuki et al., 2020). Wang et al. (2020) found decreased total lymphocytes, CD4+ T cells, CD8+ T cells, B cells, and natural killer (NK) cells in COVID-19 patients. Wang et al. (2020) also noted that peripheral lymphocyte subset alteration played important role in the pathogenesis of COVID-19 and the alteration was associated with clinical characteristics and treatment efficacy of COVID-19. Liu et al. (2020a) found that neutrophil-to-lymphocyte ratio was related to COVID-19 outcome and concluded that this parameter was an independent risk factor for mortality in hospitalized patients with COVID-19. Liu et al. (2020b) noted that the degree of lymphopenia and proinflammatory cytokine storm is high in severe COVID-19 patients and this pathobiologial process was associated with the severity of COVID-19. The immunological-based therapy for COVID-19 is the contemporary issue in clinical medicine (Felsenstein et al., 2020). Many new treatment alternatives are proposed based on immunological process in COVID-19 (Barlow et al., 2020; Felsenstein et al., 2020).

Immunotherapy is an alternative treatment that is proposed as a possible useful therapeutic management for COVID-19. AminJafari and Ghasemi (2020) performed a meta-analysis on the use of immunotherapy in COVID-19 and noted that "*As a conclusion of these studies demonstrated that although no serious research has been done on this subject at the time of writing this article, similar studies on the related viruses showed notable results. So immunotherapy for this virus can also be a suitable option.*" Monoclonal antibody therapy is a good example of immunotherapy that might be useful for COVID-19 management (Shanmugaraj et al., 2020). Regarding immunomoulator, some medical scientists proposes ideas on some possible useful agents for the management of COVID-19 (Price et al., 2020). A good example is melatonin (Zhang et al., 2020). Conceptually, melatonin is an anti-inflammatory and anti-oxidative molecule (Zhang et al., 2020). It is proposed for advantage in respiratory distress syndrome in COVID-19 (Zhang et al., 2020). The exact efficacy of melatonin in COVID-19 management is an interesting research topic and there are many ongoing trials (García et al., 2020).

Another agent that is proposed for possible advantage in COVID-19 management is tocilizumab (Luo et al., 2020). In fact, tocilizumab is monoclonal antibody. But it is not an antibody against the virus but against interleukin-6 (IL-6). Since cytokine storm is an important immunopathogenesis in COVID-19, tocilizumab that focuses at IL-6 might be useful for the treatment of COVID19 (Luo et al., 2020). The action of tocilizumab is known as cytokine blockage. Anakinra, interleukin-1 receptor antagonist, is another agent that is based on this concept (Bilia et al., 2020; Wu et al., 2020). Dimopoulos et al. (2020) reported the use of anakinra in COVID-19 patient with secondary hemophagocytic lymphohistocytosis (sHLH) and noted that "*administration of Anakinra may be beneficial for treating severe COVID-19 patients with sHLH as determined by the Hscore.*" In another report by Aouba et al. (2020), a similar advantage is also observed.

Not only new immunomodulators, but some old drugs that have immunomodulatory property are also tested for the effectiveness in COVID-19 treatment. The good example is chloroquine (Zhso, 2020) and hydroxychloroquine (Zhou et al., 2020). Indeed, the patient who requires regular hydroxychloroquine is proposed for the low rate of COVID-19 infection (Joob and Wiwanitkit, 2020). Finally, attacking at cytokine storm is also an important immunopharmacotherapeutic concept in COVID-19. The exact efficacy of hydroxychloroquine in COVID-19 management is an interesting research topic and there are many ongoing trials. For example, Barnabas et al. (2020) studied on the efficacy of hydroxychloroquine for post-exposure prophylaxis to prevent SARS-CoV-2 infection among adults exposed to COVID-19. The results on this report would be good clinical evidences supporting or not supporting using hydroxychloroquine for managing severe COVID-19. Hydroxychloroquine also has potential for the management of cytokine storm problem in COVID-19 (Soy et al., 20200). However, there is still no conclusion on the exact usefulness of hydroxychloroquine for managing COVID-19. Some adverse effects of hydroxychloroquine such as induction of hemolysis in patient with underlying glucose-6-phosphase dehydrogenase deficiency is reported and there is a need to careful consider use hydroxychloroquine for managing patients with COVID-19 (Meyerowitz et al., 2020).

Regarding station that is proposed for the management of MERS, the similar proposal is raised for COVID-19 management (Castiglione et al., 2020; Dashti-Khavidaki and Khalili, 2020). Bifulco and Gazzerro (2020) noted that statin might be beneficial to manage COVID-19 *via* several pathways including modulating interleukin action. Statin can also counteract thrombohemostatic problem in COVID-19 by reducing thrombus plasminogen activator inhibitor-1 (PAI-1), tissue factor, neutrophils, and myeloperoxidase (Bifulco and Gazzerro, 2020). Nevertheless, its efficacy of statin for managing COVID-19 is presently not confirmed (Scicali et al., 2020).

The immunosuppression by steroid is also proposed for usefulness in COVID-19 treatment (Mehta, 2020). Mehta et al. (2020) noted that immunosuppression might be useful for the management of cytokine storm problem in COVID-19. Dai et al. (2020) reported two case studies of using corticosteroid treatment in severe COVID-19 pneumonia. Dai et al. (2020) mentioned that low-to-moderate doses of corticosteroids given to several severely ill COVID-19 patients were beneficial. Regarding standard clinical trial on steroid therapy in COVID-19, there are limited data. Abdolahi et al. (2020) presently registered a trial on dexamethasone for

COVID-19 treatment and the result is still pending. Selvaraj et al. (2020) reported on effective of short-term steroid therapy for managing COVID-19. Selvarj et al. (2020) found that the steroid therapy helped limit the severity of inflammation and prevented a severe hyperinflammatory phase in COVID-19. According to the study, turn reducing the length of hospitalization and ICU admissions is observed in case that steroid therapy is used (Selvarj et al., 2020). Selvarj et al. (2020) concluded that a short course of systemic corticosteroids, dexamethasone, among inpatients with SARS-CoV-2 with hypoxic respiratory failure was well tolerated, and most patients had improved outcomes. So et al. (2020) reported their experience on using high-dose, short-term corticosteroids for lung complication caused by COVID-19. So et al. (2020) concluded that short-term corticosteroid therapy early in COVID-19-related respiratory failure may provide a good prognosis of patients without any significant side effects of steroids. However, there is still no conclusive evidence of the effect of steroid therapy for managing COVID-19. The important consideration is on possible unwanted side effect induced by steroid in COVID-19 patient. Nasim et al. (2020) noted that the use of corticosteroid might cause possible unwanted problem and it was a double-edged sword. There are both reports supporting and against using steroid therapy for COVID-19 patient. Both usefulness and possible hazard of steroids are mentioned. Also, some repots mention for null effect of steroid on COVID-19. For example, Halpin et al. (2020) reported that there was no evidence on benefits or harms of inhaled steroids in COVID-19. It is essential that collective data from epidemiological studies of COVID-19 and clinical trials on steroid therapy should be summarized and analyzed for final conclusion on recommendations on using or not using steroid therapy for managing COVID-19.

Another interesting new therapy for the management of COVID-19 is immunomodulation by stem cell therapy. The mesenchymal stem cells-based immunomodulation treatment is proposed as a possible effective therapeutic approach (Golchin et al., 2020). Expanded umbilical cord mesenchymal stem cells are proposed stem cell technology as a new therapeutic strategy in managing COVID-19 patients (Atluri et al., 2020). Liu et al. (2020) proposed that mesenchymal stem cells could balance the inflammatory response. Liu et al. (2020c) mentioned that this new approach was effective for managing lung complications in COVID-19. Nevertheless, this approach is still only a new concept and there is still no approved mesenchymal stem cell-based approach for the treatment of COVID-19 (Colchin et al., 2020). Data from trials are required for final approval of this new concept (Colchin et al., 2020).

Finally, there is also a new concept based on immunonutrition principle (Caccialanza et al., 2020). Vitamin D is proposed as a nutrition supplementation that might help to promote immunity against COVID-19. The possible pharmacological mechanism include cathelicidins and defensins induction that resulting lowering of viral replication rates and reducing concentrations of pro-inflammatory cytokines which is the cause of the inflammation that injures the lining of the lungs, leading to pneumonia, as well as increasing concentrations of anti-inflammatory cytokines which is related to cytokine storm (Ebadi and Montano-Loza, 2020; Grant et al., 2020; Jakovac, 2020; Panarese and Shahini, 2020).

TABLE 8.2 Examples of Immunomodulatory Agents for New Emerging Viral Infections.

Diseases	Examples
Zika virus infection	Metrotrexate
MERS	Alisporivir
COVID-19	Tocilizumab, chloroquine, anakinra, steroid

8.4 FUTURE PROSPECTS

The immunotherapy will become more widely used around the world in the near future. The new immopharmacological advents will play important role in therapy of medical disorders including to infectious disease. There will be many new pharmaceutical manufacturers that will apply immunopharmacological principles for production of the new therapeutic agents. Based on the continuous improvement of immunopharmacological technology, many new immunological agents, including immunomodulatory agents, are expected to be available in the near future. Lessons learnt from studies on immunomodulatory agents in the three well-known emerging infections, Zika virus infection, MERS, and COVID-19 will be useful for the new emerging problematic situations. The new immunomodulatory agents will useful for medical therapy of several disorders including to new emerging viral infections.

It is no doubt that there will be new emerging infection in the future. The returned loop of lack of knowledge will occurs, when a new infectious disease emerges. The studies on immunopathogenesis of the new disease will be required. It will also be the attempts to find classical immunomodulatory drug that might be effective and safe in management of the new infection. The new reaching for searching on new immunomodulatory agents that will be effective in management of the new disease will also be widely performed. There will be new available treatments based on the new immunomodulatory concepts. The newly registered and proven immunomodulatory agents will be new hopes for management of the difficult-to-manage new emerging infection.

With the possible new immunomodulatory technology for management of new disease, the better outcome of treatment will be achieved. Nevertheless, there will be also new considerations on the possible unknown adverse effects of the newly developed immunomodulatory agent. With the rapid growth of the new technology, the closed monitoring of the unwanted adverse side effects of any newly available immunomodulatory agent will be required. There will also be the new standards and legal control of the production of the new immunomodulator or reuse of classic immunomodulation with the new indication in the management of new emerging infectious disease.

8.5 CONCLUSION

Immunological response plays important role in physiological homeostasis of human being. To correspond to an infectious disease, immunological system is the main defense against invasive pathogen. The knowledge on immunopathology is very important in clinical medicine. Within the past decade, there are many new emerging infections. The good examples are Zika virus infection, MERS, and COVID-19. Those new emerging virus infections become important global public health threatens. The immunological responses to those new diseases are important in pathogeneses of those new infections. The immunological response in different emerging viral infection is different and is the explanation for the clinical presentation of each disease. The host response might be different based on the genetic underlying factor and the environmental factor is also important determinant for clinical appearance of the infection. Additional, the knowledge on immunological mechanism in each disease is also important data for finding and development of new drug and vaccine search. The immunotherapy is the new concept that is usually proposed as an alternative new treatment for the new emerging infection. The immunotherapy is proposed in several forms such as immunoglobulin, vaccine, and immunomodulatory agent. The immunomodulatory is a specific group of substance that can affect the immune system in host and the alteration of immunological system is the biological process that is further useful for the management of the new disease. Many new immunomodulators are introduced and tested on clinical trials for the management of the new diseases, Zika virus infection, MERs, and COVID-19. For the newest COVID-19, many classic immunomodulators are presently proposed as useful therapeutic agents for treatment of the patient. There are many ongoing researches to find new immunomodulatory agent and produce in a large scale for disease containment. There are many concerns on the cost-effectiveness, safety, and adverse effects of those new alternative immunomodulators. There is still no proof for the role of alternative immunomodulatory for the management of COVID-19. The assessment on effectiveness and safety of the new alternative immunomodulatory agent is warranted.

KEYWORDS

- **COVID-19**
- **emerging**
- **immunomodulator**
- **MERS**
- **Zika**

REFERENCES

Abdolahi, N.; Kaheh, E.; Golsha, R.; Khodabakhshi, B.; Norouzi, A.; Khandashpoor, M.; Besharat, S.; Tavassoli, S.; Livani, S.; Azimi, S. A.; Gharib, M. H.; Peivandi, B.; Fazel, A.; Shirzad-Aski, H.; Roshandel, G. Letter to the Editor: Efficacy of Different Methods of Combination Regimen Administrations Including Dexamethasone, Intravenous Immunoglobulin, and Interferon-Beta to Treat Critically Ill COVID-19 Patients: A Structured Summary of a Study Protocol for a Randomized Controlled Trial. Version 2. *Trials* **2020,** *21*(1), 549. DOI: 10.1186/s13063-020-04499-5.

Alfaraj, S. H.; Al-Tawfiq, J. A.; Assiri, A. Y.; Alzahrani, N. A.; Alanazi, A. A.; Memish, Z. A. Clinical Predictors of Mortality of Middle East Respiratory Syndrome Coronavirus (mers-cov) Infection: A Cohort Study. *Travel Med. Infect. Dis.* **2019,** 29, 48–50.

Al-Tawfiq, J. A.; Hinedi, K.; Abbasi, S.; Babiker, M.; Sunji, A.; Eltigani, M. Hematologic, Hepatic, and Renal Function Changes in Hospitalized Patients with Middle East Respiratory Syndrome Coronavirus. *Int. J. Lab. Hematol.* **2017,** *39* (3), 272–278.

AminJafari, A.; Ghasemi, S. The Possible of Immunotherapy for COVID-19: A Systematic Review. *Int. Immunopharmacol.* **2020,** *83*, 106455.

Andrade, D. V.; Harris, E. Recent Advances in Understanding the Adaptive Immune Response to Zika Virus and the Effect of Previous Flavivirus Exposure. *Virus Res.* **2018,** *254*, 27–33.

Aouba, A.; Baldolli, A.; Geffray, L.; Verdon, R.; Bergot, E.; Martin-Silva, N.; Justet, A. Targeting the Inflammatory Cascade with Anakinra in Moderate to Severe COVID-19 Pneumonia: Case Series. *Ann. Rheum. Dis.* **2020,** DOI: 10.1136/annrheumdis-2020-217706. Online ahead of print.

Arabi, Y. M.; Hajeer, A. H.; Luke, T.; Raviprakash, K.; Balkhy, H.; Johani, S.; Al-Dawood, A.; Al-Qahtani, S.; Al-Omari, A.; Al-Hameed, F.; Hayden, F. G.; Fowler, R.; Bouchama, A.; Shindo, N.; Al-Khairy, K.; Carson, G.; Taha, Y.; Sadat, M.; Alahmadi, M. Feasibility of Using Convalescent Plasma Immunotherapy for MERS-CoV Infection, Saudi Arabia. *Emerg. Infect. Dis.* **2016,** *22* (9), 1554–1561.

Arabi, Y. M.; Mandourah, Y.; Al-Hameed, F.; Sindi, A. A.; Almekhlafi, G. A.; Hussein, M. A. Corticosteroid Therapy for Critically Ill Patients with Middle East Respiratory Syndrome. *Am. J. Respir. Crit. Care Med.* **2018,** *197* (6), 757–767.

Atluri, S.; Manchikanti, L.; Hirsch, J. A. Expanded Umbilical Cord Mesenchymal Stem Cells (UC-MSCs) as A Therapeutic Strategy in Managing Critically Ill COVID-19 Patients: The Case for Compassionate Use. *Pain Physician.* **2020,** *23* (2), E71–E83.

Badolato-Corrêa, J.; Sánchez-Arcila, J. C.; Alves de Souza, T. M.; Santos Barbosa, L.; Conrado Guerra Nunes, P.; da Rocha Queiroz Lima, M.; Gandini, M.; Bispo de Filippis, A. M.; Venâncio da Cunha, R.; Leal de Azeredo, E.; de-Oliveira-Pinto, L. M. Human T Cell Responses to Dengue and Zika Virus Infection Compared to Dengue/Zika Coinfection. *Immun. Inflamm. Dis.* **2018,** *6* (2), 194–206.

Barnabas, R. V.; Brown, E.; Bershteyn, A.; Miller, R. S.; Wener, M.; Celum, C.; Wald, A.; Chu, H.; Wesche, D.; Baeten, J. M. Hydroxychloroquine COVID-19 PEP Study Team. Efficacy of Hydroxychloroquine for Post-Exposure Prophylaxis to Prevent Severe Acute Respiratory Syndrome Coronavirus 2 (SARS-CoV-2) Infection Among Adults Exposed to Coronavirus Disease (COVID-19): A Structured Summary of a Study Protocol for a Randomised Controlled Trial. Version 2. *Trials* **2020,** *21* (1), 475.

Barlow, A.; Landolf, K. M.; Barlow, B.; Yeung, S. Y. A.; Heavner, J. J.; Claassen, C. W.; Heavner, M.S. Review of Emerging Pharmacotherapy for the Treatment of Coronavirus Disease 2019. *Pharmacotherapy* **2020,** *40* (5), 416–437.

Beck, S.; Zhu, Z.; Oliveira, M. F.; Smith, D. M.; Rich, J. N.; Bernatchez, J. A.; Siqueira-Neto, J. L. Mechanism of Action of Methotrexate Against Zika Virus. *Viruses* **2019,** *11* (4), 338.

Bifulco, M.; Gazzerro, P. Statin Therapy in COVID-19 Infection: Much more than a Single Pathway. *Eur. Heart J. Cardiovasc. Pharmacother.* **2020,** pvaa055.

Bilia, S.; Giannini, D.; Rizzelli, G. M. L.; Tavoni, A. Anakinra in COVID-19 Therapy: what have we Learned from Adult-Onset Still's Disease? *Clin. Exp. Rheumatol.* **2020,** *38* (3), 579.

Burgueño-Montañés, C.; Álvarez-Coronado, M.; Colunga-Cueva, M. Autoimmune Neuroretinopathy Secondary to Zika Virus Infection. *Arch. Soc. Esp. Oftalmol.* **2018,** *93* (7), 336–341.

Caccialanza, R.; Laviano, A.; Lobascio, F.; Montagna, E.; Bruno, R.; Ludovisi, S.; Corsico, A. G.; Di Sabatino, A.; Belliato, M.; Calvi, M.; Iacona, I.; Grugnetti, G.; Bonadeo, E.; Muzzi, A.; Cereda, E. Early Nutritional Supplementation in Non-critically Ill Patients Hospitalized for the 2019 Novel Coronavirus Disease (COVID-19): Rationale and Feasibility of a Shared Pragmatic Protocol. *Nutrition* **2020,** *74*, 110835.

Caine, E. A.; Scheaffer, S. M.; Arora, N.; Zaitsev, K.; Artyomov, M. N.; Coyne, C. B.; Moley, K. H.; Diamond, M. S. Interferon Lambda Protects the Female Reproductive Tract Against Zika Virus Infection. *Nat. Commun.* **2019,** *10* (1), 280.

Cao, X. COVID-19: Immunopathology and its Implications for Therapy. *Nat. Rev. Immunol.* **2020,** *20* (5), 269–270.

Castiglione, V.; Chiriacò, M.; Emdin, M.; Taddei, S.; Vergaro, G. Statin Therapy in COVID-19 Infection. *Eur. Heart J. Cardiovasc. Pharmacother.* **2020,** *6* (4), 258–259.

Chafekar, A.; Fielding, B. C. MERS-CoV: Understanding the Latest Human Coronavirus Threat. *Viruses* **2018,** *10* (2), 93.

Chan, J. F.; Zhang, A. J.; Chan, C. C.; Yip, C. C.; Mak, W. W.; Zhu, H.; Poon, V. K.; Tee, K. M.; Zhu, Z.; Cai, J. P.; Tsang, J. O.; Chik, K. K.; Yin, F.; Chan, K. H.; Kok, K. H.; Jin, D. Y.; Au-Yeung, R. K.; Yuen, K. Y. Zika Virus Infection in Dexamethasone-immunosuppressed Mice Demonstrating Disseminated Infection with Multi-organ Involvement Including Orchitis Effectively Treated by Recombinant Type I Interferons. *EBioMedicine* **2016,** *14*, 112–122.

Chen, C.; Zhang, X. R.; Ju, Z. Y.; He, W. F. Advances in the Research of Mechanism and Related Immunotherapy on the Cytokine Storm Induced by Coronavirus Disease 2019. *Zhonghua Shao Shang Za Zhi* **2020,** *36* (6), 471–475.

Chimelli, L.; Avvad-Portari, E. Congenital Zika Virus Infection: A Neuropathological Review. *Childs Nerv. Syst.* **2018,** *34* (1), 95–99.

Culshaw, A.; Mongkolsapaya, J; Screaton, G. R. The Immunopathology of Dengue and Zika Virus Infections. *Curr. Opin. Immunol.* **2017,** *48*, 1–6.

Dai, J.; Xiong, Y.; Li, H.; Qian, Y.; Xu, Y.; Xu, Q.; Yan, X.; Tang, J. Corticosteroid Treatment in Severe COVID-19 Pneumonia: Two Cases and Literature Review. *Clin. Rheumatol.* **2020,**
39 (7), 2031–2037.

Dashti-Khavidaki, S.; Khalili, H. Considerations for Statin Therapy in Patients with COVID-19. *Pharmacotherapy* **2020,** *40* (5), 484–486.

de Wilde, A. H.; Falzarano, D.; Zevenhoven-Dobbe, J. C.; Beugeling, C.; Fett, C.; Martellaro, C.; Posthuma, C. C.; Feldmann, H.; Perlman, S.; Snijder EAlisporivir Inhibits MERS- and SARS-Coronavirus Replication in Cell Culture, but not SARS-Coronavirus Infection in a Mouse Model. *J. Virus Res.* **2017,** *228*, 7–13.

Dimopoulos, G.; de Mast, Q.; Markou, N.; Theodorakopoulou, M.; Komnos, A.; Mouktaroudi, M.; Netea, M. G.; Spyridopoulos, T.; Verheggen, R. J.; Hoogerwerf, J.; Lachana, A.; van de Veerdonk, F. L.;, Giamarellos-Bourboulis, E. J. Favorable

Anakinra Responses in Severe COVID-19 Patients with Secondary Hemophagocytic Lymphohistiocytosis. *Cell Host Microbe.* **2020**. DOI: 10.1016/j.chom.2020.05.007. Online ahead of print.

Duarte, G.; Moron, A. F.; Timerman, A.; Fernandes, C. E.; Mariani Neto, C.; Almeida Filho, G. L.; Werner, Junior H.; Espírito Santo, H. F. B. D.; Steibel, J. A. P.; Bortoletti Filho, J.; Andrade, J. B. B.; Burlá, M.; Silva de Sá, M. F.; Busso, N. E.; Giraldo, P. C.; Moreira de Sá, R. A.; Passini, Junior R.; Mattar, R.; Francisco, R. P. V. Zika Virus Infection in Pregnant Women and Microcephaly. *Rev. Bras. Ginecol. Obstet.* **2017,** *39* (5), 235–248.

Dyall, J.; Gross, R.; Kindrachuk, J.; Johnson, R. F.; Olinger, G. G. Jr.; Hensley, L. E.; Frieman, M. B.; Jahrling, P. B. Middle East Respiratory Syndrome and Severe Acute Respiratory Syndrome: Current Therapeutic Options and Potential Targets for Novel TherapiesDrugs **2017,** *77* (18), 1935–1966.

Ebadi, M.; Montano-Loza, A. J. Perspective: Improving Vitamin D Status in the Management of COVID-19. *Eur. J. Clin. Nutr.* **2020,** *74* (6), 856–859.

Faure, E.; Poissy, J.; Goffard, A.; Fournier, C.; Kipnis, E.; Titecat, M.; Bortolotti, P.; Martinez, L.; Dubucquoi, S.; Dessein, R.; Gosset, P.; Mathieu, D.; Guery, B. Distinct Immune Response in Two MERS-CoV-Infected Patients: Can we go from Bench to Bedside? *PLoS One* **2014,** *9* (2), e88716.

Felsenstein, S.; Herbert, J. A.; McNamara, P. S.; Hedrich, C. M. COVID-19: Immunology and Treatment Options. *Clin. Immunol.* **2020,** *215,* 108448.

Furman, D.; Davis, M. M. New Approaches to Understanding the Immune Response to Vaccination and Infection. *Vaccine* **2015,** *33* (40), 5271–5281.

García, L. F. Immune Response, Inflammation, and the Clinical Spectrum of COVID-19. *Front Immunol.* **2020,** *11,* 1441.

García, I. G.; Rodriguez-Rubio, M.; Mariblanca, A. R.; de Soto, L. M.; García, L. D.; Villatoro, J. M.; Parada, J. Q.; Meseguer, E. S.; Rosales, M. J.; González, J.; Arribas, J. R.; Carcas, A. J.; de la Oliva, P.; Borobia, A. M. A Randomized Multicenter Clinical Trial to Evaluate the Efficacy of Melatonin in the Prophylaxis of SARS-CoV-2 Infection in High-Risk Contacts (MeCOVID Trial): A Structured Summary of a Study Protocol for a Randomised Controlled Trial. Version 2. *Trials* **2020,** *21* (1), 466.

Golchin, A.; Seyedjafari, E.; Ardeshirylajimi, A. Mesenchymal Stem Cell Therapy for COVID-19: Present or Future. *Stem Cell Rev. Rep.* **2020,** *16* (3), 427–433.

Gopinath, S.; Kim, M. V.; Rakib, T.; Wong, P. W.; van Zandt, M.; Barry, N. A.; Kaisho, T.; Goodman, A. L.; Iwasaki, A. Topical Application of Aminoglycoside Antibiotics Enhances Host Resistance to Viral Infections in a Microbiota-Independent Manner. *Nat. Microbiol.* **2018,** *3* (5), 611–621.

Grant, W. B.; Lahore, H.; McDonnell, S. L.; Baggerly, C. A.; French, C. B.; Aliano, J. L.; Bhattoa, H. P. Evidence that Vitamin D Supplementation Could Reduce Risk of Influenza and COVID-19 Infections and Deaths. *Nutrients* **2020,** *12* (4), 988.

Haby, M. M.; Pinart, M.; Elias, V.; Reveiz, L. Prevalence of Asymptomatic Zika Virus Infection: A Systematic Review. *Bull. World Health Organ* **2018,** *96* (6), 402–413D.

Halpin, D. M. G.; Singh, D.; Hadfield, R. M. Inhaled Corticosteroids and COVID-19: A Systematic Review and Clinical Perspective. *Eur. Respir. J.* **2020,** *55* (5), 2001009.

Hani, C.; Trieu, N. H.; Saab, I.; Dangeard, S.; Bennani, S.; Chassagnon, G.; Revel, M. P. COVID-19 Pneumonia: A Review of Typical CT Findings and Differential Diagnosis. *Diagn. Interv. Imag.* **2020,** *101* (5), 263–268.

Hooftman, A.; O'Neill, L. A. J. The Immunomodulatory Potential of the Metabolite Itaconate. *Trends Immunol.* **2019,** *40* (8), 687–698.

Jakovac, H. COVID-19 and Vitamin D-Is There a Link and an Opportunity for Intervention? *Am. J. Physiol. Endocrinol. Metab.* **2020,** *318* (5), E589.

Jamilloux, Y.; Henry, T.; Belot, A.; Viel, S.; Fauter, M.; El Jammal, T.; Walzer, T.; François, B.; Sève, P. Should we Stimulate or Suppress Immune Responses in COVID-19? Cytokine and Anti-Cytokine Interventions. *Autoimmun. Rev.* **2020,** *19* (7), 102567.

Joob, B.; Wiwanitkit, V. SLE, Hydroxychloroquine and no SLE Patients with COVID-19: A Comment. *Ann. Rheum. Dis.* **2020,** *79* (6), e61.

Krauer, F.; Riesen, M.; Reveiz, L.; Oladapo, O. T.; Martínez-Vega, R.; Porgo, T. V.; Haefliger, A.; Broutet, N. J.; Low, N. WHO Zika Causality Working Group. Zika Virus Infection as a Cause of Congenital Brain Abnormalities and Guillain-Barré Syndrome: Systematic Review. *PLoS Med.* **2017,** *14* (1), e1002203.

Lazear, H. M.; Govero, J.; Smith, A. M.; Platt, D. J.; Fernandez, E.; Miner, J. J.; Diamond, M. S. A Mouse Model of Zika Virus Pathogenesis. *Cell Host Microbe.* **2016,** *19* (5), 720–730.

Li, C.; Deng, Y. Q.; Wang, S.; Ma, F.; Aliyari, R.; Huang, X. Y.; Zhang, N. N.; Watanabe, M.; Dong, H. L.;

Li, G.; Fan, Y.; Lai, Y.; Han, T.; Li, Z.; Zhou, P.; Pan, P.; Wang, W.; Hu, D.; Liu, X.; Zhang, Q.; Wu, J. Coronavirus Infections and Immune Responses. *J. Med. Virol.* **2020b,** *92* (4), 424–432.

Liang, Y.; Wang, M. L.; Chien, C. S.; Yarmishyn, A. A.; Yang, Y. P.; Lai, W. Y.; Luo, Y. H.; Lin, Y. T.; Chen, Y. J.; Chang, P. C.; Chiou, S. H.; Liang, Y.; et al. Highlight of Immune Pathogenic Response and Hematopathologic Effect in SARS-CoV, MERS-CoV, and SARS-Cov-2 Infection. *Front Immunol.* **2020,** *11*,1022.

Lima, N. S.; Rolland, M.; Modjarrad, K.; Trautmann, L. T Cell Immunity and Zika Virus Vaccine Development. *Trends Immunol.* **2017,** *38* (8), 594–605.

Liu, P.; Li. X. F.; Ye, Q.; Tian, M.; Hong, S.; Fan, J.; Zhao, H.; Li, L.; Vishlaghi, N.; Buth, J. E.; Au, C.; Liu, Y.; Lu, N.; Du, P.; Qin, F. X.; Zhang, B.; Gong, D.; Dai, X.; Sun, R.; Novitch, B. G.; Xu, Z.; Qin, C. F.; Cheng, G. 25-Hydroxycholesterol Protects Host Against Zika Virus Infection and Its Associated Microcephaly in a Mouse Model. *Immunity* **2017a,** *46* (3), 446–456.

Liu, Y.; Du, X.; Chen, J.; Jin, Y.; Peng, L.; Wang, H. H. X.; Luo, M.; Chen, L.; Zhao, Y. Neutrophil-to-lymphocyte Ratio as an Independent Risk Factor for Mortality in Hospitalized Patients with COVID-19. *J. Infect.* **2020a,** *81* (1), e6–e12.

Liu, J.; Li, S.; Liu, J.; Liang, B.; Wang, X.; Wang, H.; Li, W.; Tong, Q.; Yi, J.; Zhao, L.; Xiong, L.; Guo, C.; Tian, J.; Luo, J.; Yao, J.; Pang, R.; Shen, H.; Peng, C.; Liu, T.; Zhang, Q.; Wu, J.; Xu, L.; Lu, S.; Wang, B.; Weng, Z.; Han, C.; Zhu, H.; Zhou, R.; Zhou, H.; Chen, X.; Ye, P.; Zhu, B.; Wang, L.; Zhou, W.; He, S.; He, Y.; Jie, S.; Wei, P.; Zhang, J.; Lu, Y.; Wang, W.; Zhang, L.; Li, L.; Zhou, F.; Wang, J.; Dittmer, U.; Lu, M.; Hu, Y.; Yang, D.; Zheng, X. Longitudinal Characteristics of Lymphocyte Responses and Cytokine Profiles in the Peripheral Blood of SARS-CoV-2 Infected Patients. Version 2. *EBioMedicine* **2020b,** *55*, 102763.

Liu, S.; Peng, D.; Qiu, H.; Yang, K.; Fu, Z.; Zou, L. Mesenchymal Stem Cells as a Potential Therapy for COVID-19. Version 2. *Stem Cell Res Ther.* **2020c,** *11* (1), 169.

Luo, P.; Liu, Y.; Qiu, L.; Liu, X.; Liu, D.; Li, J. Tocilizumab Treatment in COVID-19: A Single Center Experience. *J. Med. Virol.* **2020,** *92* (7), 814–818.

Mahallawi, W. H.; Khabour, O. F.; Zhang, Q.; Makhdoum, H. M.; Suliman, B. A. MERS-CoV Infection in Humans is Associated with a Pro-Inflammatory Th1 and Th17 Cytokine Profile. *Cytokine* **2018,** *104*, 8–13.

Mancera-Páez, O.; Román, G. C.; Pardo-Turriago, R.; Rodríguez, Y.; Anaya, J. M. Concurrent Guillain-Barré Syndrome, Transverse Myelitis and Encephalitis Post-Zika: A Case Report and Review of the Pathogenic Role of Multiple Arboviral Immunity. *J. Neurol. Sci.* **2018,** *395*, 47–53.

Martins, M. M.; Medronho, R. A.; Cunha, A. J. L. A. D. Zika Virus in Brazil and Worldwide: A Narrative Review. *Paediatr. Int. Child Health* **2020,** 1–8. DOI: 10.1080/20469047.2020.1776044. Online ahead of print.

Mehta, P.; McAuley, D. F.; Brown, M.; Sanchez, E.; Tattersall, R. S.; Manson, J. J.; HLH Across Speciality Collaboration, UK. COVID-19: Consider Cytokine Storm Syndromes and Immunosuppression. *Lancet* **2020,** *395* (10229), 1033–1034.

Meyerowitz, E. A.; Vannier, A. G. L.; Friesen, M. G. N.; Schoenfeld, S.; Gelfand, J. A.; Callahan, M. V.; Kim, A. Y.; Reeves, P. M.; Poznansky, M. C. Rethinking the Role of Hydroxychloroquine in the Treatment of COVID-19. *FASEB J.* **2020,** *34* (5), 6027–6037.

Miner, J. J.; Diamond, M. S. Zika Virus Pathogenesis and Tissue Tropism. *Cell Host Microbe.* **2017,** *21* (2), 134–142.

Montón, C.; Ewig, S.; Torres, A.; El-Ebiary, M.; Filella, X.; Rañó, A. Role of Glucocorticoids on Inflammatory Response in Nonimmunosuppressed Patients with Pneumonia: A Pilot Study. *Eur. Respir. J.* **1999,** 14 (1), 218–220.

Mubarak, A.; Alturaiki, W.; Hemida, M. G. Middle East Respiratory Syndrome Coronavirus (MERS-CoV): Infection, Immunological Response, and Vaccine Development. *J. Immunol. Res.* **2019,** *2019*, 6491738.

Nascimento, O. J. M.; da Silva, I. R. F. Guillain-Barré Syndrome and Zika Virus Outbreaks. *Curr. Opin. Neurol.* **2017,** *30* (5), 500–507.

Nasim, S.; Kumar, S.; Azim, D.; Ashraf, Z.; Azeem, Q. Corticosteroid use for 2019-nCoV Infection: A Double-Edged Sword. *Infect. Control Hosp. Epidemiol.* **2020,** 1–2.

Newton, A. H.; Cardani, A.; Braciale, T. J. The Host Immune Response in Respiratory Virus Infection: Balancing Virus Clearance and Immunopathology. Version 2. *Semin. Immunopathol.* **2016,** *38* (4), 471–482.

O'Neill, L. A. J.; Artyomov, M. N. Itaconate: The Poster Child of Metabolic Reprogramming in Macrophage Function. *Nat. Rev. Immunol.* **2019,** *19* (5), 273–281.

Panarese, A.; Shahini, E. Letter: COVID-19, and vitamin D. *Aliment. Pharmacol. Ther.* **2020,** *51* (10), 993–995.

Park, J. E.; Jung, S.; Kim, A.; Park, J. E. MERS Transmission and Risk Factors: A Systematic Review. *BMC Public Health* **2018,** *18* (1), 574.

Piontkivska, H.; Plonski, N. M.; Miyamoto, M. M.; Wayne, M. L. Explaining Pathogenicity of Congenital Zika and Guillain-Barré Syndromes: Does Dysregulation of RNA Editing Play a Role? Bioessays **2019,** *41* (6), e1800239.

Plourde, A. R.; Bloch, E. M. A Literature Review of Zika Virus. *Emerg. Infect. Dis.* **2016,** *22* (7), 1185–1192.

Price, K. N.; Frew, J. W.; Hsiao, J. L.; Shi, V. Y. COVID-19 and Immunomodulator/ Immunosuppressant use in Dermatology. *J. Am. Acad. Dermatol.* **2020,** *82* (5), e173–e175.

Priyamvada, L.; Hudson, W.; Ahmed, R.; Wrammert, J. Humoral Cross-Reactivity Between Zika and Dengue Viruses: Implications for Protection and Pathology. *Emerg. Microbes Infect.* **2017a,** *6* (5), e33.

Priyamvada, L.; Suthar, M. S.; Ahmed, R.; Wrammert, J. Humoral Immune Responses Against Zika Virus Infection and the Importance of Preexisting Flavivirus Immunity. *J. Infect. Dis.* **2017b,** *216* (suppl_10), S906–S911.

Rokni, M.; Ghasemi, V.; Tavakoli, Z. Immune Responses and Pathogenesis of SARS-CoV-2 During an Outbreak in Iran: Comparison with SARS and MERS. *Rev. Med. Virol.* **2020,** *30* (3), e2107.

Roth, C.; Delgado, F. G.; Simon-Lorière, E.; Sakuntabhai, A. Immune Responses to Dengue and Zika Viruses-Guidance for T Cell Vaccine Development. *Int. J. Environ. Res. Public Health* **2018,** *15* (2), 385.

Scicali, R.; Di Pino, A.; Piro, S.; Rabuazzo, A. M.; Purrello, F. May Statins and PCSK9 Inhibitors be Protective from COVID-19 in Familial Hypercholesterolemia Subjects? *Nutr. Metab. Cardiovasc. Dis.* **2020,** *30* (7), 1068–1069.

Selvaraj, V.; Dapaah-Afriyie, K.; Finn, A.; Flanigan, T. P. Short-Term Dexamethasone in Sars-CoV-2 Patients. R I Med. J. (2013) **2020,** *103* (6), 39–43.

Shanmugaraj, B.; Siriwattananon, K.; Wangkanont, K.; Phoolcharoen, W. Perspectives on Monoclonal Antibody Therapy as Potential Therapeutic Intervention for Coronavirus Disease-19 (COVID-19). *Asian Pac. J. Allergy Immunol.* **2020,** *38* (1), 10–18.

So, S.; Ro, S.; Murakami, M.; Imai, R.; Jinta, T. High-Dose, Short-Term Corticosteroids for ARDS Caused by COVID-19: A Case Series. *Respirol. Case Rep.* **2020,** *8* (6), e00596.

Soy, M.; Keser, G.; Atagündüz, P.; Tabak, F.; Atagündüz, I.; Kayhan, S. Cytokine Storm in COVID-19: Pathogenesis and Overview of Anti-Inflammatory Agents used in Treatment. *Clin. Rheumatol.* **2020,** *39* (7), 2085–2094.

Tiligada, E.; Ishii M.; Riccardi, C.; Spedding, M.; Simon, H. U.; Teixeira, M. M.; Cuervo, M. L.; Holgate, S. T.; Levi-Schaffer, F. The Expanding Role of Immunopharmacology: IUPHAR Review 16. *Br. J. Pharmacol.* **2015,** *172* (17), 4217–4227.

Totura, A. L.; Whitmore, A.; Agnihothram, S.; Schäfer, A.; Katze, M. G.; Heise, M. T.; Baric, R. S. Toll-Like Receptor 3 Signaling via TRIF Contributes to a Protective Innate Immune Response to Severe Acute Respiratory Syndrome Coronavirus Infection. mBio **2015,** *6* (3), e00638–15.

Toturaa, A. L.; Baric, R. S. Reply to "Statins may Decrease the Fatality Rate of MERS Infection". mBio **2015,** *6* (5), e01303–15.

Ulrich, H.; Pillat, M. M. CD147 as a Target for COVID-19 Treatment: Suggested Effects of Azithromycin and Stem Cell Engagement. *Stem Cell Rev. Rep.* **2020,** *16* (3), 434–440.

Vaninov, N. In the eye of the COVID-19 Cytokine Storm. *Nat. Rev. Immunol.* **2020,** *20* (5), 277.

van der Poll, T.; van de Veerdonk, F. L.; Scicluna, B. P.; Netea, M. G. The Immunopathology of Sepsis and Potential Therapeutic Targets. *Nat. Rev. Immunol.* **2017,** *17* (7), 407–420.

Vieira, J. M.; Ricardo, O. M. P.; Hannas, C. M.; Kanadani, T. C. M.; Prata, T. D. S.; Kanadani, F. N. What do we know About COVID-19? A Review Article. *Rev. Assoc. Med. Bras.* (1992) **2020,** *66* (4), 534–540.

Wang, F.; Nie, J.; Wang, H.; Zhao, Q.; Xiong, Y.; Deng, L.; Song, S.; Ma, Z.; Mo, P.; Zhang, Y. Characteristics of Peripheral Lymphocyte Subset Alteration in COVID-19 Pneumonia. *J. Infect. Dis.* **2020,** *221* (11), 1762–1769.

Widjaja, I.; Wang, C.; van Haperen, R.; Gutiérrez-Álvarez, J.; van Dieren, B.; Okba, N. M. A.; Raj, V. S.; Li, W.; Fernandez-Delgado, R.; Grosveld, F.; van Kuppeveld, F. J. M.; Haagmans, B. L.; Enjuanes, L.; Drabek, D.; Bosch, B. J. Towards a Solution to MERS: Protective Human Monoclonal Antibodies Targeting Different Domains and Functions of the MERS-Coronavirus Spike Glycoprotein. *Emerg. Microbes Infect.* **2019,** *8* (1), 516–530.

Wu, R.; Wang, L.; Kuo, H. D.; Shannar, A.; Peter, R.; Chou, P. J.; Li, S.; Hudlikar, R.; Liu, X.; Liu. Z.; Poiani, G. J.; Amorosa, L.; Brunetti, L.; Kong, A. N. An Update on Current Therapeutic Drugs Treating COVID-19. *Curr. Pharmacol. Rep.* **2020,** 1—15.

Xiao, J.; Li, W.; Zheng, X.; Qi, L.; Wang, H.; Zhang, C.; Wan, X.; Zheng, Y.; Zhong, R.; Zhou, X.; Lu, Y.; Li, Z.; Qiu, Y.; Liu, C.; Zhang, F.; Zhang, Y.; Xu, X.; Yang, Z.; Chen, H.; Zhai, Q.; Wei, B.; Wang, H. Targeting 7-Dehydrocholesterol Reductase Integrates Cholesterol Metabolism and IRF3 Activation to Eliminate Infection. *Immunity* **2020,** *52* (1), 109.e6–122.e6.

Xie, X.; Shan, C.; Shi, P. Y. Restriction of Zika Virus by Host Innate Immunity. *Cell Host Microbe.* **2016,** *19* (5), 566–567.

Xu, Z.; Xu, X.; Qi, D.; Yang, L.; Li, B.; Li, L.; Li, X.; Chen, D. Effect of Aminoglycosides on the Pathogenic Characteristics of Microbiology. *Microb. Pathog.* **2017,** *113*, 357–364.

Yang, Z.; Liu, J.; Zhou, Y.; Zhao, X.; Zhao, Q.; Jing, J. The Effect of Corticosteroid Treatment on Patients with Coronavirus Infection: A Systematic Review and Meta-Analysis. *J. Infect.* **2020.** DOI: 10.1016/j.jinf.2020.03.062 [Epub ahead of print]

Ye, Q.; Wang, B.; Mao, J. The Pathogenesis and Treatment of the `Cytokine Storm' in COVID-19. *J. Infect.* **2020,** *80* (6), 607–613.

Yin, Y.; Wunderink, R. G. MERS, SARS and Other Coronaviruses as Causes of Pneumonia. *Respirology* **2018,** *23* (2), 130–137.

Yu, X. H.; Zhang, D. W.; Zheng, X. L.; Tang, C. K. Itaconate: An Emerging Determinant of Inflammation in Activated Macrophages. *Immunol. Cell Biol.* **2019,** *97* (2), 134–141.

Yuki, K.; Fujiogi, M.; Koutsogiannaki, S. COVID-19 Pathophysiology: A Review. *Clin. Immunol.* **2020,** *215*, 108427.

Zhang, R.; Wang, X.; Ni, L.; Di, X.; Ma, B.; Niu, S.; Liu, C.; Reiter, R. J. COVID-19: Melatonin as a Potential Adjuvant Treatment. *Life Sci.* **2020,** *250*, 117583.

Zhao, M. Cytokine Storm and Immunomodulatory Therapy in COVID-19: Role of Chloroquine and Anti-IL-6 Monoclonal Antibodies. *Int. J. Antimicrob. Agents* **2020,** *55* (6), 105982.

Zhou, D.; Dai, S. M.; Tong, Q. COVID-19: A Recommendation to Examine the Effect of Hydroxychloroquine in Preventing Infection and Progression. *J. Antimicrob. Chemother.* **2020,** *75* (7), 1667–1670. doi: 10.1093/jac/dkaa114.

CHAPTER 9

COVID-19 Infection and Recent Investigations and Future Prospects

BHUSHAN R. RANE[1], MOUNIKA BHARAT[1], and RAJ K.KESERVANI[2]

[1]*Department of Pharmaceutics, Shri D. D. Vispute College of Pharmacy & Research Center, Panvel, District Raigad, Maharashtra, India*

[2]*Faculty of B. Pharmacy, CSM Group of Institutions, Prayagraj, Uttar Pradesh, India*

ABSTRACT

The world is in a state of disarray today due to a coronavirus infection. In late 2019, December, the first reported case was reported in the Wuhan of China. The first patient with corona was first treated with pneumonia. The WHO has declared the coronavirus as an epidemic since the official platform in February 2020. Recent research has found the novel coronavirus (nCoV) to be found as a new species that has never been seen in human being and is a virus that causes illness from common colds such as Middle Ages East Respiratory Syndrome (MERS-CoV) and Severe Acute Respiratory Syndrome (SARS-CoV). More research is still being done to determine the exact cause but the virus is thought to have a zoonotic origin and is closely related to bat coronaviruses, pangolin coronaviruses, and SARS-CoV. Although there are no specific vaccines or drugs for COVID-19, scientists from around the world are struggling to find a solution. Various studies are underway to find appropriate treatment by trial method. The results of the study also revealed that strengthening the lungs and the practice of yoga is a step toward preventing coronavirus. The

COVID-19 and Immunomodulation with Special Emphasis on Nutraceutical and Herbal Formulation.
Rajesh K. Kesharwani & Raj K. Keservani (Eds)

current revised article will discuss the nature of the coronavirus and how it has caused a rapid epidemic and how the world is coping with its extinction. In February and March 2020, many countries began to close their mouths as a WHO suggestion to end the chain of social unrest. The review also aims to emphasize more ongoing research on methods and the role of different approaches. Research is still underway with plasma treatment, allopathic treatment (e.g., hydroxychloroquine, dexamethasone), herbal/Ayurvedic, and Unani as a traditional treatment for coronavirus.

9.1 INTRODUCTION

In early 2020, China reported a new type of respiratory disturbance of an unknown cause in the WHO Country workplace originated in the Chinese city of Wuhan—the provincial capital of Hubei in the month of December 2019 from bats in China. It was predicted in early March 2019 (Fan et al., 2019), no international preventive action has been taken. Finally, when more cases of respiratory disorders and related etiologies were discovered in late 2019, the Chinese National Health Commission released more information about the epidemic in early 2020 (Wang et al., 2020). It is thought that the country's food market in the Chinese city is the source of the epidemic. Although it was originally thought that COVID-19 patients in China may have used infected animals as food, or visited a food market; one study revealed that some patients did not visit the food market. The virus was spread from person to person through coughing, sneezing, and the spread of droplets while sneezing or aerosols are accepted. In addition, many continents around the world have reported the airborne aerosol-induced infections of the lungs (Rio and Althaus, 2020; Parry, 2019). This was followed by a rapid growth within cases worldwide. Coronaviruses (CoV) cause ill health starting from the respiratory disorder to a lot of severe diseases, such as Middle East Respiratory Syndrome (also known as MERS-CoV) and Severe Acute respiratory Syndrome (also known as SARS-CoV), and the viruses belong to a large family of viruses. A novel coronavirus (nCoV) is a unique virus and the new strain that has not been reported in human beings; and is a new single-stranded RNA virus, belonging to the β-Coronavirus genus (subfamily Orthoronavirinae, family Coronaviridae, taxonomic group Cornidovirineae, order Nidovirales) (Fan et al., 2019) (WHO). Officially declared as a world pandemic by the world Health Organization (WHO) on March 11, 2020, the COVID-19 pandemic has changed at an extraordinary rate. After its emergence in the city, Hubei, in December 2019, the total count of confirmed Covid cases universally has previously exceeded more than 11 million, and the death count was reported to be more than 5 lakhs as of June 5, 2020 (WHO), with real numbers supposed to be high. The main causative living creature, that is, virus to be responsible for the COVID-19 pandemic, at first was named as 2019 novel coronavirus or "2019-nCoV," which was later named to be severe acute respiratory syndrome coronavirus 2, that is, "SARS-CoV-2," it has its resemblance to the earlier SARS-CoV (Guo et al., 2020). There is no approved treatment available yet, so, the most effective resolution for controlling the pandemic is the use of prevention measures, sensitive diagnostic approaches, and exploitation of currently available medication, while still developing novel treatments (Mohamed et al., 2020; Momtazmanesh et al., 2020; Hanaei and Rezaei, 2020)

9.2 HUMAN CORONAVIRUS TYPES

Coronaviruses are named after it is revealed to have crown-like spikes on their surface when observed on the microscope. There are four basic sub-groupings of coronaviruses, which are categorized as alpha (α), beta (β), gamma (γ), and delta (δ). Human coronaviruses were first discovered somewhere in the mid-1960s. There are many coronaviruses known to be present in the environment, but only seven of them are known to affect people, and out of which, four human coronaviruses only cause very mild symptoms like cold or flu-like symptoms, while the other three coronaviruses cause more serious risks.

9.2.1 COMMON HUMAN CORONAVIRUSES

Common human coronaviruses are typically known to cause illness with mild or moderate symptoms. Most people around the world will develop a minimum of one or more of these viral infections in their lifespan. Those who contract these viruses are able to enhance their personal performance on occasion.

1. 229E (alpha-coronavirus)
2. NL63 (alpha-coronavirus)
3. OC43 (beta-coronavirus)
4. HKU1 (beta-coronavirus)

9.2.2 *OTHER HUMAN CORONAVIRUSES*

1. MERS-CoV (the beta-coronavirus that causes Middle East Respiratory Syndrome, or MERS)
2. SARS-CoV (the beta-coronavirus that causes severe acute respiratory syndrome, or SARS)
3. SARS-CoV-2 (the novel coronavirus that causes coronavirus disease 2019, or COVID-19)

Source: obtained online from (https://www.cdc.gov/coronavirus/types.html andhttps://www.healthline.com/health/coronavirus-types#types)

9.3 ORIGIN AND TRANSMISSION

Coronaviruses belong to the family Coronaviridae within the order of Nidovirales. Corona represents crown-shaped spikes on the outside of the virus; therefore, it is called coronavirus. Coronaviruses are much smaller than the nano-sized particles in size and contain single-stranded RNA as nucleic material (Shereen, 2020).

Coronaviruses (CoVs) are divided into four categories, including α– / β– / γ– / δ-CoV. A-, and β-CoV. They have the ability to infect mammals, while γ- and δ-CoVs tend to infect birds. The known coronavirus types are α-CoVs, HCoV-229E, and HCoV-NL63, as well as β-CoVs HCoV-HKU1, and HCoV-OC43 often causes low pathogenicity, causing mild respiratory symptoms almost like the flu normal, respectively. Two opposing β-CoVs, that is, SARS-CoV, and MERS-CoV cause serious and dangerous deadly diseases (Yin and Wunderink, 2018). It has been found that the SARS-CoV-2 gene is the CoV RaTG13 genus. According to this, the origin of virus is believed to be from bats, and SARS-CoV-2 can be transmitted from bats through unknown mammals, subsequently infecting people. It is now clear that SARS-CoV-2 could use ACE2 (angiotensin-converting enzyme 2), the same receptor as SARS-CoV (Zhou, 2020) to infect a person.

9.4 SARS-COV-2 CHARACTERISTICS

SARS-CoV-2 is an envelope, direct concept, and RNA beta-coronavirus whose nuclear material is a single-stranded RNA of 29.9 kb (Zhou et al., 2020; Wu et al., 2020). The SARS-CoV-2 genome study revealed that it had 88% similarity with bat-SL-CoVZC45 and bat-SL-CoVZXC21, and was 96.2% similar to other batCoV RaTG13. However, recent research has suggested that pangolin smuggled from Malaysia to China, with some potential intermediates, such as tortoises or snakes may be the source of the virus instead of bats (Lam et al., 2020). In addition, the SARS-CoV-2 protein-coding genes account for 79.5% and 51%, respectively for SARS-CoV and MERS-CoV. The SARS-CoV-2 virus utilizes the angiotensin-converting enzyme 2 (ACE2) receptor in cell signaling, such as SARS-CoV (Guo et al., 2020; Paraskevis et al., 2020). Therefore, previous treatments used to control SARS-CoV and MERS-CoV outbreaks may also apply to SARS-CoV-2.

9.5 SIGNS AND SYMPTOMS

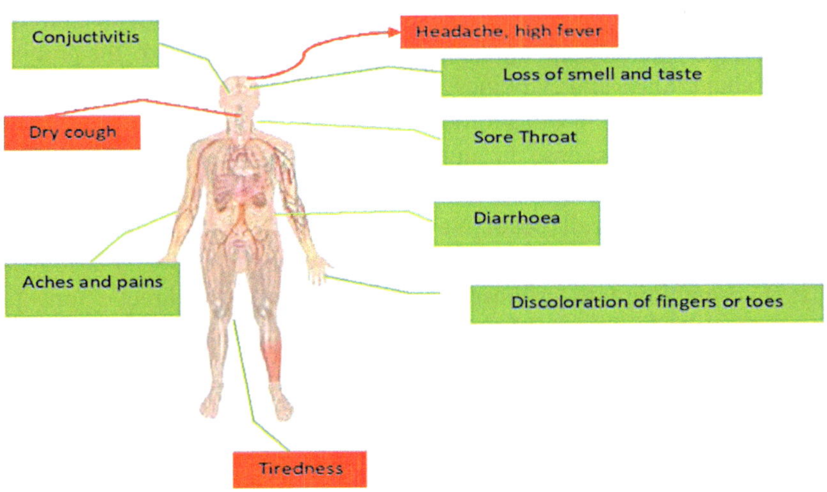

FIGURE 9.1 Signs and symptoms.

9.6 PATHOGENESIS

SARS-CoV-2 reaches the human cell via a clathrin-mediated endocytosis initiated by binding to the SARS-COV-2 Spike S protein and ACE 2 receptor (Hoffmann et al., 2020). ACE 2 enzyme is present in multiple human organs, such as lungs, intestines, heart, and kidneys. The role of ACE2 is in converting angiotensin II into angiotensin (Fan et al., 2020; Zimmerman and Curtis, 2020; Aderson et al., 2004; Hoffmann et al., 2020; Yan et al., 2020; Xudong et al., 2006), thus regulating renin homeostasis and lowers the expression of ACE2 aging (Xudong et al., 2006). Examination of genomics, epigenomics, and transcriptomics information included by Chen et al. (2020) showed a reduction in ACE2 expression suggesting that greater exposure to ACE2 in adolescents may play a protective role in COVID-19 pathogenesis (Chen et al., 2020; Newton et al., 2016; Prompetchara et al., 2020).

The interaction between SARS-CoV-2 and the management system may appear to play an important role in the pathogenesis of the disease, which explains in part the severity of the disease in children. Like other respiratory RNA viruses, the immune response begins as soon as SARS-CoV-2 is detected by the system. In such early stages, the type of Interferons (IFN-IFN-a and IFN-b) appears to play a single role not only in their internal antiviral activity but also in their ability to reactivate immune cells (monocytes-macrophages, natural killer cells); therefore, the production of chemokines and cytokines, such as tumor necrosis factor-a (TNF-a) and interleukin-6 (IL-6). In addition, type IFNs play a role in the onset of a dynamic immune response through dendritic cell activation, and therefore, stimulation of antigen presentation in CD4 T cells, as well as antagonist expression in CD8 T cells occur (Newton et al., 2016). Previous research and the first discovery of SARS-CoV, MERS-CoV, and SARS-CoV-2 suggest that abnormal immune responses occur in contrast to the direct cytopathic virus effect that appears to be responsible for pathogenesis, especially in severe cases of infection. In particular, it appears that the delayed response of IFN-I jeopardizes early viral control leading to a series of inflammatory processes mediated by excessive production of cytokines by neutrophils and monocytes-macrophages leading to "cytokine storm" (Prompetchara et al., 2020). In severe cases of COVID-19, the most common findings are lymphopenia and the creation of main pro-inflammatory cytokines, such as interleukin (IL) -2, IL-7, granulocyte colony-stimulating factor

(G-CSF), interferon-c-inducible protein 10 (IP-10), monocyte chemoattractant protein 1 (MCP-1), macrophage inflammatory protein 1-a (MIP-1a), and TNF-a. This cytokine storm results in hyperinflammatory syndrome almost which is identical to that of the inflammatory conditions of hemophagocytic lymphohistiocytosis (HLH). This appears to cause lung damage and extrapulmonary immune-mediated symptom, which leads to acute respiratory distress syndrome (ARDS) and failure of the lungs within the context of multiple organ failure, ultimately leading to shock and death (Sun et al., 2020; WHO).

9.7 CURRENT COVID-19 DIAGNOSIS

Collection of swabs or sputum samples from oropharyngeal and nasopharyngeal regions to detect viral RNA in the most widely used RT-qPCR (Reverse Transcription Quantitative Polymerase Chain Reaction) is a central method of identifying COVID-19. In addition, chest X-ray may be the only available diagnostic method for diagnosing pneumonia in two countries, showing multilobar ground glass opacities with asymmetric, peripheral, and posterior distribution.

9.7.1 SALIVARY DIAGNOSTICS

Saliva now has a broad base as a storehouse of biological indicators ranging from the conversion of nucleic acids, proteins, and biochemical chemicals to microorganism. As a diagnostic fluid, saliva is much stronger and more concentrated than other biological fluids, because the saliva sample method does not involve aggressive or aggressive disturbances, and is cheaper and more effective in regulating the system's health. In the foreseeable future, the creation of accurate and responsive saliva diagnostic tools and the use of well-known guidelines after detailed testing will allow the use of saliva diagnostics as a test for the adaptation of various diseases. The benefits of a salivary gland test are as follows:

1. Economical
2. Noninvasive
3. Results will be obtained in a short time
4. Healthier to apply than serum sampling

5. Specialized healthcare workers are not needed
6. A lot of samples can be obtained
7. Collecting and monitoring of samples are possible at home
8. Cross-infection is not observed,
9. No issue in the transportation of sampling,
10. During diagnosis, less agitation,
11. Assays are available commercially for screening.

Thus, salivary diagnostic testing offers a convenient and cost-effective mechanism for early diagnosis of COVID-19 (Santosh et al., 2020). The documented three methods to capture saliva are shown in Figure 9.2.

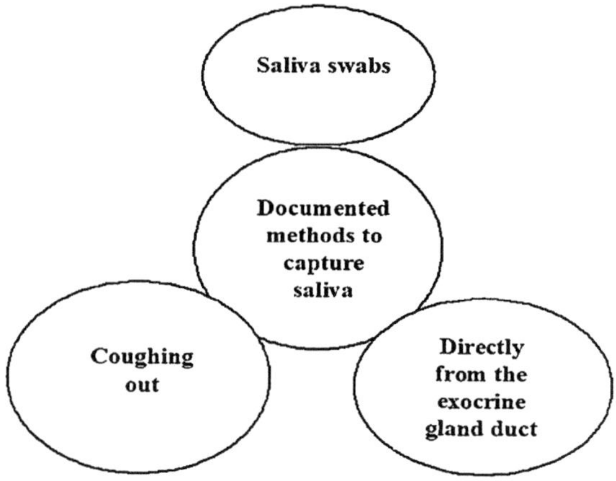

FIGURE 9.2 Methods to capture saliva.

Saliva from the deep throat can be collected as it provides the largest amount of COVID-19 initial detection and treatment programs that require a strict viral load. Saliva extracted from the salivary glands in conjunction with the harmful COVID-19 may be a reliable and noninvasive test in critically ill patients (Xu et al., 2011). Many diagnostic procedures are available that will be performed before starting dental treatment at the appropriate dental clinics.

- LAMP (loop-mediated isothermal amplification) tests.
- Testing of antibody.

- RT-PCR microfluidic devices (Sabino-Silva et al., 2020; Sharma et al., 2020).

9.7.2 MICROBIOLOGICAL ANALYSIS

In children and adults, SARS-CoV-2 tests were performed on biological samples obtained from the nasopharyngeal swab, tracheal aspirate, or bronchoalveolar lavage, corresponding to the clinical status of patients. Trials of polymerase polymerase chain reaction (RT-PCR) identify and amplify the unique genetic sequence of viral RNA (N, E, and RdRP) (Corman et al., 2020)). The effects of RT-PCR are restored in about 4 h. The specification is close to 100% (Strunk et al., 2014). Sensitivity range is wide: 32–93%, associated with a variety of clinical examples, appears to be higher with bronchoalveolar discharge, followed by sputum, nasal swabs, pharyngeal swabs, feces, and blood (Wang et al., 2020). The use of a rapid nasopharyngeal swab test has been instantly permitted officially by the FDA. The tests will help to identify the target genes ORF1ab and S. Results usually return within an hour, with significant results between the individual patient management (USFDA).

9.7.3 SEROLOGICAL ASSAY (ELISA)

Investigate the presence of specific Immunoglobulin M and/or IgG antibodies against the SARS-COV-2 Rp3 nucleocapsid protein. Previous studies conducted on SARS-CoV have shown that IgM antibodies can be detected after 3–6 days from the onset of symptoms while IgG antibodies are detected after 8 days. Further research is to confirm testing and to determine when the immune response is needed (Li et al., 2020).

9.7.4 IMAGING

Thinking techniques, such as the chest radiograph, lung ultrasound, and high-resolution computed tomography (HRCT) of the chest have been used in patients with COVID-19. The penetration of bronchovascular bundles, the reduction of clarity, and the thickening of the leaflets are common features found on the chest radiograph. The stiffness and instability of the pleural line, subpleural fusion, turning the B-line into the image of the white lung in the most severe cases, where the disappearance of the A-line is often shown in ultrasound of the lungs (Peng et al., 2020). Low glass opacities, intersecting areas (multilobar and sub-pleural), local or combined two-dimensional and reticular patterns with interstitial intensity, insignificant compression, and rare nodules are exposed in Chest HRCT (Li et al., 2020; Guan et al., 2020).

9.8 PREVENTIVE MEASURES

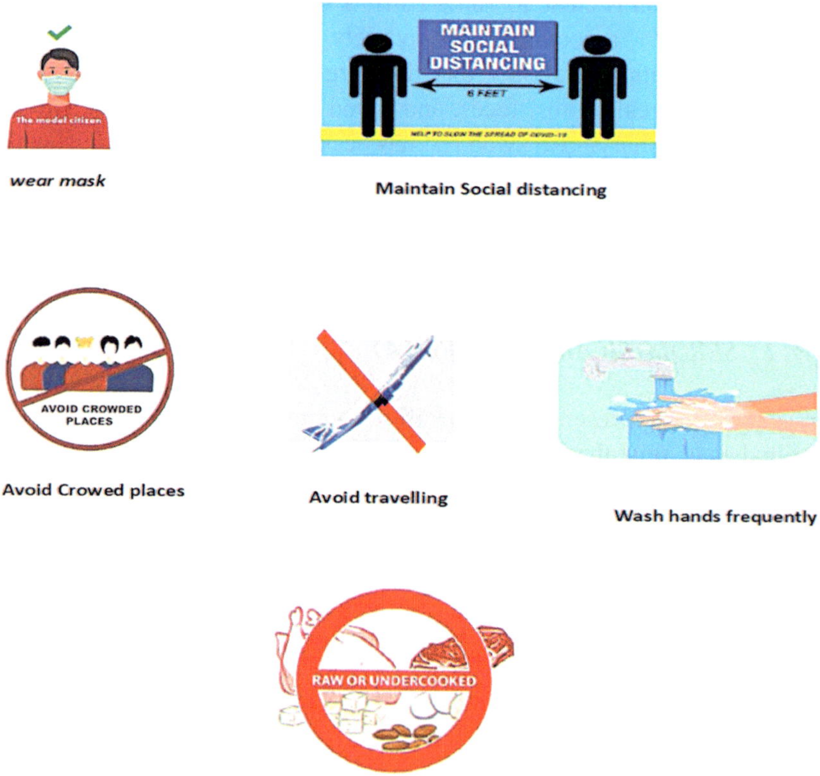
The model citizen
wear mask
MAINTAIN SOCIAL DISTANCING
6 FEET
Maintain Social distancing
AVOID CROWDED PLACES
Avoid Crowed places
Avoid travelling
Wash hands frequently
RAW OR UNDERCOOKED

FIGURE 9.3 Preventive measures.

9.9 APPROACHES AVAILABLE FOR TREATMENT OF COVID-19

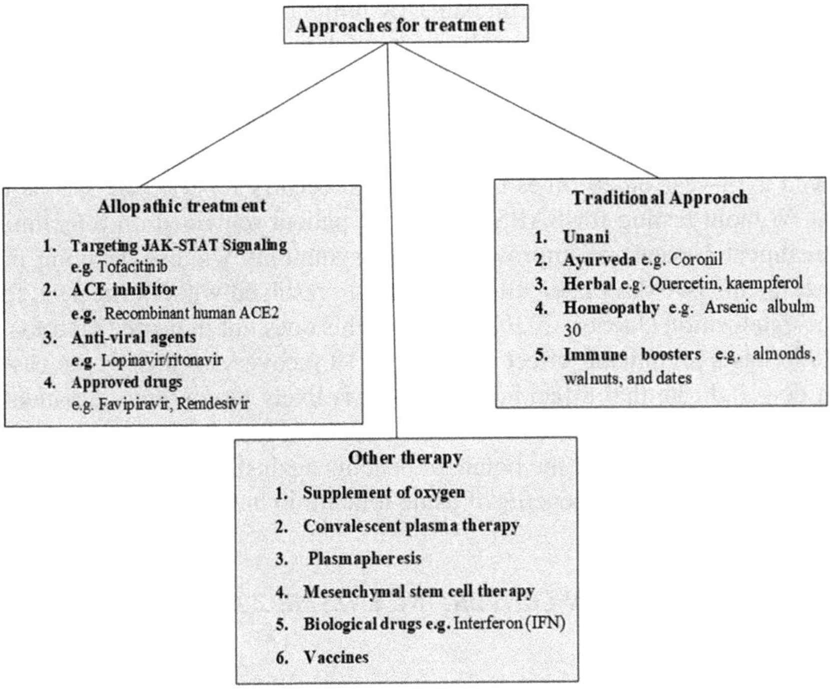

FIGURE 9.4 Different approaches available for treatment of COVID-19.

9.9.1 TARGETING JAK-STAT SIGNALING

It has earlier been investigated in patients with SARS that COVID-19 causes a cytokine storm similar to the second hemophagocytic lymphohistiocytosis (sHLH) (Nicholas et al., 2003). Often caused by severe viral infections, sHLH may be a life-threatening complication of the hyperinflammatory syndrome (La Rosee et al., 2019), and has been described by CRS, cytopenias, and organ dysfunction (Hutchinson et al., 2019). In addition to elevated serum cytokines, improperly activated macrophages are also an indicator of sHLH and are affected due to increased ferritin sources. Therefore, sHLH is also called macrophage activation syndrome (MAS). Cao et al. (2020) recently confirmed the efficiency of the drug ruxolitinib in patients with high-risk COVID-19, as quicker improvement clinically and improved protection compared with the control group (Cao et al., 2020) were observed.

Tofacitinib is a useful oral pan-JAK inhibitor that is permitted for use in RA, autoimmune, and illness, where cytokines take part in pathogenesis of the disease (Feldmann, 2002). It can effectively block Interlukin (IL)-2, 4, 6, and 7 as a potent JAK3 and TYK2 inhibitor (EC50 but less than 5 nM) (Roskoski, 2016). A case of SARS-CoV-2 infection in a female patient with a 13-year olden times of colitis was recently reported by Jacobs et al. Without testing for SARS-CoV-2, the patient remained on tofacitinib treatment because of improved clinical symptoms without delaying the treatment. Two days later, all symptoms are resolved without the need for hospitalization (Jacobs, 2020). Although this does not indicate that tofacitinib has a significant effect on COVID-19 recovery in this whole case, it does indicate that tofacitinib treatment is likely to continue in patients infected with SARS-CoV-2. A variety of clinical trials are presented for research to understand the potential benefits against the disease, but very few studies show the benefits of using tofacitinib in COVID-19.

9.9.2 ANGIOTENSIN-CONVERTING ENZYME-2 AS THERAPEUTIC TARGET

The interaction between SARS-CoV-2 virus and ACE2 is suspected to be a factor in their infection (Kuba et al., 2005). Another possible way to deal with ACE2-mediated SARS-CoV-2 virus is that it can deplete ACE2 (but not ACE) proteins by binding spike proteins and leading to increased lung damage (For et al., 2005). As the ACE2/angiotensin 1–7 axis is often effective in lung protection in developing acute breathing distress syndrome (ARDS) as a major coronavirus problem, recently, human ACE2 recombinant (rhACE2; APN01, GSK2586881) has acquired a lot of attention (Zhang and Baker, 2017; Guo et al., 2020). According to the literature found in previous studies, purification of ACE2 potentially invasive viral cells, that is, rhACE2 when used have the ability to decrease plasma angiotensin II and to enhance plasma angiotensin 1–7 and thus demonstrate the ability to stop angiotensin II, which induces angiotensin II, diastolic dysfunction, as well as myocardial infarction, fibrosis (Colafella et al., 2018).

In general, it was thought that excessive ACE2, especially the soluble form of ACE2, could delay the entry and spread of the virus. Making the virus dangerous and releasing ACE2 cell phones and improving its function can prevent the lung from being damaged. RhACE2 can reduce severe lung damage in mice deficient in ACE2 mice demonstrated in numerous animal experimental studies (Gu et al., 2016; Zou et al., 2014). Also, rhACE2 is safe and has no side or special effects in patients with ARDS and healthy human volunteers as revealed in human studies (Haschke et al., 2013; Khan et al., 2017; Zhang and Baker, 2017). Reduction of interleukin-6 (IL-6) concentration in patients with ARDS with rhACE2 supplementation was observed when the results of experimental studies were revealed (Khan et al., 2017). Recent studies have confirmed an elevated level of IL-6 in human beings with COVID-19 pneumonia, and it has been shown that the IL-6 level indicates a direct correlation with disease severity (Wu et al., 2020; Wan et al., 2020). Considering the importance of mutant cytokines in patients with COVID-19, rhACE2 may also be considered a promising treatment option.

9.9.3 INHIBITION OF THE INTERACTION BETWEEN SARS-COV-2 VIRUS AND ACE2–THE ENTRY INHIBITORS OF THE ACE2

Recently, in the management of this outbreak, ACE2 receptor entry inhibitors were considered. Other compounds, such as morphine and codeine that have a direct binding to highly affluent ACE2 receptors are often suggested in competition (Yan et al., 2020). Since ancient times, morphine has been used to control acute pain and anesthesia. Morphine as a painkiller and natural opioid mediates its effects through three receptors called m, d, and k opioid receptors (Alimian et al., 2014; Borner et al., 2012). The administration of morphine sulfate can regulate respiration in lethal COVID-19 human beings in their end days of life based on primary care and a public respiratory package to be used during COVID-19 provided under the National Health Service (NHS) health authority in England (Eng). In addition, Swedish researchers suspect that morphine may be one of the main therapies for controlling asthma, coughing, and pain in patients with COVID-19 (Ekstrom and Dahalnder, 2020).

9.9.4 TRANSFUSION-RELATED TREATMENTS USED IN PATIENTS WITH COVID-19

The pathogenesis of SARS-CoV-2 is complex, and a more detailed treatment approach should be used to address the various pathogenic mechanisms. Once patients have been infected with SARS-CoV-2, they receive certain humoral and cellular responses over a period of time, and patients show severe infection after recovery. Because the epidemic continues, little information is available about the status of the system after the 2019-nCoV infection. Immune levels are found in the serum of some patients in the final stage of SARS-CoV-2 infection, and serum levels IL-2, IL-7, IL-10, G-CSF, MCP-1, MIP1A, and TNF-α are higher in patients in most serious cases than in patients with mild issues. SARS-CoV-2 is isolated from a single patient with severe COVID-19 and is usually administered by serum from several other patients with COVID-19. The current technology related to the transfusion of COVID-19 is discussed below:

9.9.4.1 CONVALESCENT PLASMA THERAPY

There is currently no specific vaccine available against COVID-19 that is safe and approved. Some drugs that are believed to have antiretroviral effects are currently being tested in clinical trials. Convalescent plasma in patients recovered from COVID-19 contains specific antibodies that will successfully treat SARS-CoV-2 infections. The basis of convalescent plasma therapy is that it is best for patients with a high viral titer, so it is ideal for patients with a rapidly growing disease or who are very sick or critically ill. Convalescent plasma may increase or worsen lung damage in patients suffering from multiple sclerosis, and they may experience adverse reactions to transfusions, so in such cases, they should not be included. COVID-19 is not the primary viral infection to be treated with convalescent plasma previously SARS-CoV, MERS-CoV, Ebola virus, and H1N1 infections are all treated with convalescent plasma (Chen et al., 2005; Zhou et al., 2007; Mair Jenkins et al., 2015; Marano et al., 2016).

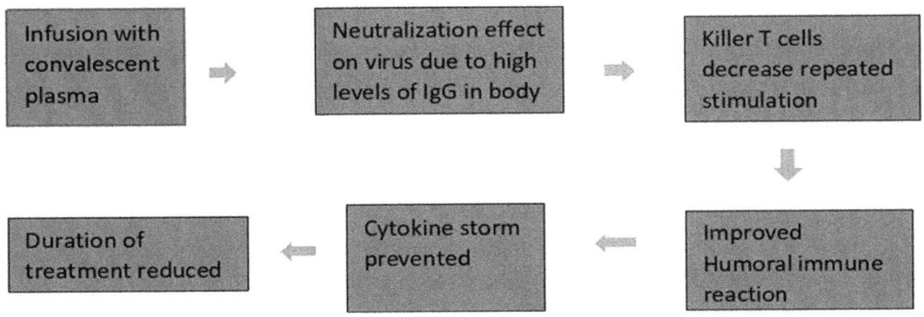

FIGURE 9.5 Mechanism of plasma therapy.

Special attention is required on plasma donor values, duration, and evaluation of convalescent plasma treatment of COVID-19. The prerequisites for following a convalescent plasma donation are:

(1) The donor must be fully recovered and free of SARS-CoV-2; pharyngeal swabs, sputum, alveolar cleansing fluid, blood, and feces sample should all be negative by macromolecule testing; (2) Donors produce high-dose antibodies, namely, SARS-CoV-2-specific IgG antibodies. Convalescent plasma with antibody titer ≥1: 160 or ≥1: 320, if possible, has a very simple effect. The presence of IgM antibodies indicates a recent viral infection or recurrence of a virus, or residual virus; so, convalescent plasma that strongly binds or has high titers of IgM antibodies should not be used to give it to a clinician.

(3) Donor eligibility must meet basic blood donation standards and testing for hepatitis B surface antigens, hepatitis C antibodies, AIDS antibodies, and *Treponema pallidum* antigens must be negative.

(4) Donors must give a clear signal that they are willing to donate plasma. After being stimulated by the antigens of the virus, the body triggers an initial immune response, lasting about 10 days, and then produces IgM and IgG antibodies that are slightly compatible.

The closest IgG antibodies are produced as soon as the immune system is repeated. Theoretically, the easiest time to treat patients with convalescent plasma is within the first stage of the disease, when IgG antibodies are not yet produced, macromolecule testing is very good, so the viral load is high. The best time to evaluate the effectiveness of plasma therapy is 24–48 h after convalescent plasma implantation. Indications that need to be evaluated for efficacy include clinical signs, laboratory indicators, lung imaging, and macromolecule detection.

9.9.4.2 PLASMAPHERESIS

Plasmapheresis involves the use of a blood fraction to separate plasma from a patient's blood. The pathogenic substances present in the plasma are discarded, and other parts of the blood are returned to the patient, supplemented with a flexible fluid, such as a fresh frozen plasma or human blood albumin. SARS and MERS have been treated with plasmapheresis therapy (Tsang and Zhong, 2003; Koch et al., 2018; Arabi et al., 2016). By removing excess cytokines, it prevents the cytokine storm and thus minimizes damage to the body. In addition, plasmapheresis plays an important role in preventing and minimizing severe damage. Plasmapheresis may be the most common procedure performed by transfusion recipients (Li et al., 2010; Luo et al., 2017; Sivakumaran et al., 2009); therefore, transfusion departments have technological advantages in treating patients with COVID-19.

9.9.4.3 MESENCHYMAL STEM CELL THERAPY

Mesenchymal stem cells have immunomodulatory effects where they inhibit the uncontrolled production of cytokines or inflammatory substances, inhibit immune responses, and reduce tissue damage to tissues and organs. Mesenchymal stem cells not only play a role in suppressing immune damage through immunomodulation, but also restore and repair damaged tissue and prevent lung fibrosis. Good results were achieved with mesenchymal stem cell treatment (Leng et al., 2020). Somatic cell therapy can suppress systemic overuse, promote endogenous regeneration by improving the microenvironment, slow down the progression of acute lung inflammation, and relieve symptoms of respiratory depression. Preliminary reports indicate that this is usually a safe and effective treatment for patients with COVID-19.

9.9.5 *ALLOPATHIC TREATMENT*

9.9.5.1 *CHLOROQUINE PHOSPHATE*

It is mainly used in patients with confirmed malaria and as an anti-inflammatory agent in the treatment of rheumatic diseases (Bijker et al., 2013). Previous studies have also found that it shows broader antiviral effect (Delvecchio et al., 2016; Mizui et al., 2010). Chloroquine can bind to the protein and reduce the helix of DNA, making it posh and preventing the DNA replication or RNA transcription. In addition, chloroquine can cause changes in the pH of endosomes and is an effective inhibitor of autophagy, which disrupts viral infections and reproduces by affecting autophagy (Schultz and Gilman, 1997). In addition to the antiviral activity, chloroquine 1 has antibacterial properties, which can improve its viral immunity in vivo. With the exception of chloroquine phosphate, hydroxychloroquine 1 is in addition to the antimalarial agent used in the clinical setting, having a structure and mechanism similar to that of chloroquine but less toxic (Ben-Zvi et al., 2012). Azithromycin alongside hydroxychloroquine successfully lowered the viral load to D6 implants and resulted in lower moderate administration compared with controls. The potential effect of hydroxychloroquine against COVID-19 may also be enhanced by azithromycin (Gautret et al., 2020).

9.9.5.2 *ARBIDOL*

Abidol may be a non-nucleoside antiviral developed by the research center of the former Soviet Union Pharmaceutical Chemistry, which demonstrates antibacterial activity against multiple viruses (Kadam and Wilson, 2017; Pécheur et al., 2007), a major indicator of abidol that disease caused by flu viruses A and B. Abidolexpressly prevents contact, adhesion, and adhesion of the viral lipid envelope as well as the host cell wall, and prevents viral genes from entering the nucleus, preventing the formation of viral DNA or RNA by activating 2-oligoadenylate synthetase (an anti-protein and viruses) in vivo. Abidolhas is not approved by Western countries but first approved in Russia in 1993 and is now widely used in Russia and China but an effective solution for preventing SARS-CoV-2 in vitro infection with EC50 at 4.11 (3.55–4.73) μM indicated by Abidol (Wang et al., 2020b). It was predicted in structural and molecular dynamics studies that arbidol may target SARS-CoV-2 spike glycoprotein and prevent the formation of spike glycoprotein, which may be important for cell adhesion and motor hijacking (Vankadari, 2020). A recent cohort study found that a combination of arbidol and lopinavir/ritonavir treatment showed a positive clinical response to the treatment of COVID-19 (Deng et al., 2020).

9.9.5.3 FAVIPIRAVIR (AVIGAN®)

RdRp inhibitor with anti-flu activity (Furuta et al., 2013) was developed by the Toyama industry and licensed in Japan in 2014. Favipiravir may inhibit the selectivity of RNA polymerase that is associated with viral replication. and may be phosphoribosylated by the host cell enzyme to provide the bioactive favipiravir furylribo-5-triphosphate-inositol (favipiravir RTP). Repetitive disturbances of viral RNA sequences are detected when Virus RNA polymerase does not detect favipiravir RTP, resulting in favipiravir RTP activation in the RNA viral chain or binding to the viral domain of RNA polymerase, that is, (Furuta et al.). Due to the specific mechanism, favipiravir has a detrimental effect on the Ebola virus, the yellow jacket virus, norovirus, and so on (Furuta et al., 2009; Oestereich et al., 2014; Rocha-Pereira et al., 2012). Nowadays, favipiravir has been used in antiretroviral therapy A and B. Favipiravir has shown significant inhibitory effect on SARS-CoV-2 in vitro (EC50 = 61.88 μM). On February 16, favipiravir was approved by the NMPA for the treatment of recent or recurrent fevers in adults. Four trials of favipiravir for COVID-19 are still ongoing in China (Khambholja and Asudani, 2020). Preliminary clinical study results (ChiCTR2000029600) have shown that favipiravir may release COVID-19 progression by accelerating viral load. Other open-label control studies showed that favipiravir showed better treatment effects in disease progression and viral clearance, with a better rate of 91.43% compared with 62.22% (P = 0.004) compared with lopinavir/ritonavir.

9.9.5.4 LOPINAVIR/RITONAVIR (ALUVIA®/KALETRA®)

Lopinavir/ritonavir (Aluvia®/Kaletra®) developed by Alberta, may be used in the treatment of human immunodeficiency virus (HIV) PI, which may enhance the antiretroviral activity by inhibiting cytochrome P450 (Cvetkovic et al., 2003). Lopinavir/ritonavir was approved to treat HIV infection among us in 2000 and became available in China in 2008. During the SARS epidemic, it was found that patients with SARS were treated with a combination of lopinavir/ritonavir and rizvirin during the threat of ARDS or death compared with those treated with rizvirin alone (Chuet al., 2004), within DTPNCP (trial version 2) released on January 22, it has been announced that no drug is available against COVID-19 yet, and lopinavir/ritonavir may be tried in as little as 14 days during a study involving 47 patients with COVID-19, combination therapy of lopinavir/ritonavir with pneumonia-related drugs showed significant therapeutic effect in lowering blood pressure and restoring normal nontoxic pathways and side effects related to adjuvant drug treatment only (Wang et al., 2020c). There were no benefits to the treatment by lopinavir/ritiomnavir (Cao et al., 2020), which were achieved and trials within small cases of COVID-19 also showed similar results when Bin Cao et al. performed a randomized controlled trial (Cheng et al., 2020). In addition, lopinavir/ritonavir was found to be associated with abnormal liver function that occurs after ingestion.

9.9.6 *BIOLOGICAL DRUGS*

9.9.6.1 *INTERFERON (IFN)*

IFN may be a secreted cytokine by mammals during viral resistance, which may interfere with viral replication and improve cell antiviral capacity (C E 2001). It is known that IFN is usually classified into three types: type I, type II, and type III (Chen et al., 2020). Type I IFN (IFN-α, IFN-β) is also called "viral IFN." Both RNA and DNA viruses inhibited by IFN-α but it does not directly kill them (C E 2001). IFN-α can inhibit viral gene and protein synthesis by activating signaling pathways, thereby activating immune cell proliferation and improving the immune system. IFN-β is activated by blocking the advertising of certain viruses, promoting phagocytosis of natural killer cells, and mononuclear macrophages to viruses. It has been used in combination with other antiretroviral drugs (such as rivatirin) to treat patients with SARS-CoV and MERS-CoV IFN-α as it can effectively prevent the recurrence of MERS-CoV and SARS-CoV in vitro or in animal models (Omrani et al., 2014). A clinical trial with an open, randomized, phase II clinical trial concluded that triple antiviral therapy with IFN β-1b, lopinavir/ritonavir, and r flirting was safer and higher than lopinavir/ritonavir only in reducing viral load, as well as reducing COV symptoms in patients. -19. It has also been suggested that inhaled IFN-α is commonly used as a therapeutic effort against COVID-19.

9.9.6.2 TOCILIZUMAB

Analysis of adjacent blood samples in severe patients with COVID-19 showed that significant lung damage induced by SARS-CoV-2 was associated with inflammatory cytokine responses. Pathogenic T cells quickly activate viruses and produce cytokines, such as granulocyte-macrophage colony-stimulating factor (GM-CSF) and interleukin 6 (IL-6), two important inflammatory factors. The continuous increase in IL-6 is considered to be a warning sign of clinical degeneration (Alzghari and Acuna, 2020; Fu et al., 2020). Tocilizumab may be a recombinant humanized anti-IL-6 receptor (IL-6R) antibody, and it reduces inflammation and block COVID-19-induced cytokine storm by binding directly to soluble receptors 1 and membrane-bound IL-6 and inhibits signal transmission mediated by IL-6 (Scheinecker et al., 2009). Tocilizumab was first used in a study of 21 Chinese patients with severe COVID-19. Based on its stimulant therapeutic effect, multicenter clinical trials (ChiCTR2000029765) were resumed, and approximately 500 critically ill or critically ill patients were included within DTPNCP (Trial Version 7). Tocilizumab was recommended in the treatment of patients with multiple lung ulcers or laboratory tests of elevated IL-6 levels (Antinori et al., 2020). Italy and 20 other countries monitor the use of tocilizumab. Tocilizumab was combined with other drugs and used in trials (Toniati et al., 2020).

9.9.7 APPROVED DRUGS

9.9.7.1 REMDESIVIR

Like the Gilead-developed nucleotide analogue prodrug, remdesivir can also block RdRp in a similar way to the action of favipiravir (Tchesnokov et al., 2019). A double-stranded RNA template is embedded in the central RdRp channel where remdesivir is integrated into the primer strand into a double-nucleotide nucleus, thus breaking the chain extension of the RdRp-Remdesivir complex structure. When placed in position i, the inhibitor causes the binding of RNA synthesis in the area +3 (Gordon et al., 2020). in addition, the importance of balance between input and nucleoside analogue output structures between RdRp and exonuclease has also received growing attention. In general, remdesivir may be an effective antiretroviral drug (Agostini et al., 2018). On January 31, the clinical symptoms of a SARS-CoV-2-infected patient within us improved significantly after treatment with remdesivir, so oxygen saturation returned to 94–96% (Holshue et al., 2020). Four days later, remdesivir was reported to have the strongest in vitro inhibitory effect on SARS-CoV-2 among the six drugs that were tested against the virus (EC50 = 0.77 μM). Phase III 8, a randomized, double-blind, 85-day placebo-controlled clinical trial and comprising 237 cases with mild-to-moderate SARS-CoV-2 infection (NCT04257656) was conducted in China. Results showed that the use of remdesivir was not related to time difference in clinical development, however, patients receiving remdesivir experienced rapid clinical improvement with symptoms lasting 10 days or less, so adverse events were reported in 66%, compared with 64% of the placebo group. In addition, the results of a Gilead III trial study suggested that remdesivir had a very positive effect on the 10-day group. Remdesivir has also been found to have a synergy effect with emetine, and remdesivir at 6.25 μM and emetine at 0.195 μM may achieve a 64.9% inhibition on viral harvesting (Choy et al., 2020). In support of these clinical findings, the USFDA has made remdesivir available under the official use of emergency treatment for adults and adolescents with severe COVID-19 (Hendaus, 2020). Although remdesivir was considered a promising option for COVID-19, its safety and impact on humans still require further evidence from additional clinical trials.

9.9.8 THE HUMAN ANTIBODY C5 MONOCLONAL 1

Numerous studies on major lung injuries caused by viruses that cause many diseases, such as the flu pandemic and coronavirus have found that concomitant overdose (especially C5a) can also be a major issue there. In the treatment of severe lung damage caused by the C5a virus, it is very important as an effective anti-inflammatory agent. BDB-001 may be an antibody directed to human C5a developed in China; it can regulate the further development of inflammation without inhibiting the function of the immune system (Barratt-Due et al., 2013). It is expected to halt the spread of pneumonia in a coronavirus infection and it also reduces the incidence of severe pneumonia and acute respiratory infections.

9.9.9 VACCINE DEVELOPMENT

Vaccines encourage the individual's immune system to fight off future pathogen attacks. this is usually done by exposing the person in advance to kill or weaken the germs, or the number of parts of the pathogen structure, which leads the body to trigger an immune response, and this exact approach is considered by the Serum Institute of India and Sanofi Pasteur vaccine preparation. Another strategy is to get antibodies against the virus's spike proteins, followed by Moderna Inc., MA, USA. In addition, German Enterprise, CureVac, seeks to develop a RNA-based vaccine. In this manner, the RNA encoding a few proteins from viruses is administered into the body. This RNA normally produces viral proteins, in which the body is unable to synthesize antibodies, thus preparing for the invasion of the virus.

Some of the most promising vaccines are listed in Table 9.1. Among all modern vaccines, Oxford vaccines are the most promising vaccines, with commercial use predicted by the end of 2020. These vaccines may be available soon, but in the future. It will take this as market success depending on the positive results from all the three phases of clinical trials (Obtained online from https://indiabioscience.org/columns/general-science/COVID-19-vaccine-development-and-therapeutic-strategies).

9.9.10 BACILLUS CALMETTE–GUÉRIN (BCG)

To decrease the COVID-19 morbidity and mortality rates Bacillus Calmette–Guérin (BCG) vaccination is being considered in clinical trials to test its efficacy (Caly et al., 2020).

9.9.11 TRADITIONAL AND AYURVEDIC MEDICINE

Naturally manufactured products and their derived products have possible utility within the treatment of bacterial infections (Denaro et al., 2020). To

TABLE 9.1 Various Vaccines Clinical Trial.

Sr no.	Vaccine name	Company name	Status	Strategy used	Result
1.	mRNA-1273	Moderna Therapeutics	Phase 1 and 2 completed Phase 3 ongoing	mRNA-based vaccine	Participants showed good immune response to COVID-19 and recovered soon
2.	ChAdOx1	Astrazeneca and Oxford	Phase 1 and 2 completed Phase 3 ongoing	Weakened version of adenovirus	Two vaccine doses induce a significantly greater antibody response, with a significant rise in neutralizing antibodies that bind to the virus and block infection
3.	Ad5-nCoV	CanSino Biologics	Phase 1 ongoing	Recombinant novel coronavirus vaccine	Moral responses against SARS-CoV-2 sharp at day 28 after vaccination in healthy human beings, the vaccine is tolerable and immunogenic at day 28 after vaccine. Moreover, specific T-cell responses were observed from day 14 post-vaccination
4.	BBV152 Covaxin	Bharat biotech	Phase 1 and 2 ongoing	Inactive version of the SARS-COV-2 virus	-
5.	BNT162	BioNTech	In preclinical trial	mRNA-based vaccine	These preliminary data suggest that BNT162b1 targets the RBD SARS-CoV-2 and is capable of generating antibody reaction in patients at or above the levels observed in convalescent sera – and that it does so at relatively low dose levels
6.	SCB-2019	GlaxoSmithkline & Clover Biopharmaceuticals	In preclinical trial	Engineering adjuvants with proteins	The primary study revealed the positive results of GSKs SCB-2019 vaccine contender, with high neutralizing antibody levels obtained in various animals

TABLE 9.1 *(Continued)*

Sr no.	Vaccine name	Company name	Status	Strategy used	Result
7.	INO-4800	Inovio Pharmaceuticals	In preclinical trial	DNA-based coronavirus vaccine	In Initial clinical data, INO-4800 has been shown to protect mice in SARS-CoV-2 viral challenge studies, where vaccination with INO-4800 prevented viral replication in the lungs of animals challenged with SARS-CoV-2
8.	Ad26	Johnson & Johnson	In preclinical trial	Deactivated virus	–
9.	ZyCov-D	Zydus Cadila	Phase 1 ongoing	DNA-based coronavirus vaccine	The vaccine was responsible for good immune response' in various species, like rats, mice, guinea pigs, and rabbits. The antibodies produced were found to totally neutralize the virus when tested during assay

date, dozens of herbal remedies have been shown to be effective antiviral. However, there are not enough studies in the event that anti-COVID-19 agents are dispensed with herbal remedies (Clinical trial govt). Such herbal ingredients are essential to stopping and combating COVID-19. In general, Chinese Medicine (CM) has favored good clinical experience, effective, and effective herbal formulas for the prevention and treatment of respiratory diseases (Cui et al. 2020). Chinese Traditional Medicine (CTM) suggests that Chinese herbal remedies support the symptoms of patients in line with Chinese diagnostic patterns. CTM may be another strategy to prevent COVID-19 in high-risk individuals (Zumla et al., 2020). The results showed that the duration of clinical symptoms disappeared, the patient's stay in the hospital decreased, alone or with western medicines such as antimicrobials or type of antimicrobials. China has used traditional medicines, and it was reported that these traditional medicines are found good in treating patients with COVID-19, and Chinese researchers have indicated that more than 90% of patients in Hubei province and nationwide are treated with traditional medicine. Studies have shown that certain formulas are generally effective in treating this condition.

Repetition of the virus and inhibition of viral replication is suggested as a possible alternative to Chinese medicine (Tong et al., 2004). Reduction of bacterial infections has been observed with the use of western herbal remedies. On January 24, 2020, the first patient with symptoms of COVID-19 pneumonia recovered from the hospital after being treated with traditional Chinese medicine (Li et al., 2014). Indian herbs with medicinal advantages are a promising platform for the treatment of a number of ailments (Vellingiri et al., 2020). Therefore, Indian medicinal plants are often regarded as a new option for this role in beating viral transmission (Balachandar et al., 2020).

9.9.11.1 COLCHICINE

Colchicine has an immunomodulatory effect and is often used to treat gout. Because of its antibody effects, it may be helpful in reducing the clinical manifestations of COVID-19 (Kaplan, 1997), due to the wide variety of treatment options, such as single-drug or combination-based therapies, it is difficult for clinical trials to be complete. That is why WHO conducted the Solidarity clinical trial; as of April 21, 2020, more than 100 countries have joined the clinical trial to win SARS-CoV-2 (WHO clinical trial of solidarity).

Some of the SARS-COV-2 operations are listed below in Table 9.2, but a thorough analysis must be done before use.

TABLE 9.2 Different Species Showing Anti-COVID-19 Activity.

Sr no.	Species name	Expected mechanism	Reference
1.	Quercetin, kaempferol	Interferes with SARS-CoV 2 3CL protease	(Zhang et al., 2020)
2.	*Gymnema sylvestre*	Anti-mouse coronavirus activity	(Vimalanathan et al., 2009)
3.	*Sphaeranthus indicus*	Known to decrease the provocative cytokine level using the NF-kB pathway, an vital pathway in respiratory distress in SARS-CoV	(Tiwari et al., 2009)
4.	*Allium sativum, Glycyrrhiza glabra*	Have negative result on SARS-CoV replication	(Keyaerts et al., 2004)
5.	*Ocimum sanctum, Solanum nigrum*	Have negative effect on reverse transcriptase of HIV and can be investigated for SARS-CoV-2	(Yu, 2004)
6.	*Citrus aurantium L, Allium sativum L*	Study revealed to have ACE inhibitory effects	(Ziai et al., 2005)
7.	*Rheum officinale, Polygonum multiflorum*	Hamper the bindings of SARS-CoV (S) spike protein to ACE2	(Ho et al., 2007)
8.	*Lycoris radiata, Artemisia annua,*	Have anti-SARS-COV-2 activity	(Li et al., 2005)
9.	*Canavalia ensiformis*	Combine to glycosylated membrane proteins and avoid the target cell recognition and virus entry	(Greig and Bouillant, 1977)
10.	*Clitoria ternatea*	Known to inhibit ADAM17 metalloproteinase which is concerned in ACR destruction	(Keyaerts et al., 2004)

9.9.12 PATANJALI'S CORONIL

Patanjali has developed an Ayurvedic drug called "coronil" which is ready to treat coronavirus patients within 5–14 days. Coronil is made from a mixture of current substances that promote the immune system, such as Mulethi (liquorice), Giloy (moonseed), Tulsi (basil), and Ashwagandha (Indian ginseng). Their goal was to find active agents and perform clinical trials and identify a combination that could fight the virus and stop its spread in the body, and then clinical case studies were performed on most positive patients and received 100% positive results. COVID patients reportedly recovered within 5–14 days and were found to be free after taking the drug.

However, the ayush department recommends the coronil tablet as an immune booster instead of a specific remedy. Available from (https://www.timesnownews.com/health/article/COVID-19-drug-patanjali-to-launch-ayurvedic-medicine-coronil-to-treat-coronavirus-infection-today/610441).

9.9.13 UNANI MEDICINES

Generally, Unani remedy (medicines obtained from plant) is nontoxic and has no side effects. Unani and Ayurvedic remedies are based on herbal remedies. Various components of various plants have been documented for a long time against infection (Li et al., 2005; Lin et al., 2014; Kim et al., 2010). The main vital plants are licorice, onion, garlic, *Ocimum sanctum, Ocimum tenuiflorum, pepper, Cinnamomumverum, Daucus maritimus*, turmeric, etc. The aqueous extract of herbs and honey was reported to be more useful in cold condition and traditional cold sores. The ingredients included in this recipe have antiviral properties. The licorice plant is known to report antiviral activities including SARS-related coronavirus, HIV-1, and sycytial-like respiratory infections and similar research was conducted by Fiore et al. (2008).

9.9.14 HOMEOPATHY

In homeopathy, arsenic in low concentrations is considered beneficial for a number of diseases including bacterial infections. Recently, the Directorate of AYUSH head quarter situated in New Delhi, India issued an order on January 30, 2020, requiring prophylactic treatment to prevent coronavirus infection. A dosage of 4 tablets of the Arsenic Album-30 drug once a day on empty stomach for 3 days is recommended by the directors. Arsenic Album-30 is a highly purified arsenic and acts as a homeopathic prophylaxis. It is significant to make a note that there is no scientific evidence available for Arsenic Album-30 drug as an effective drug. A piece of writing is published in Taiwan Medical News on February 18, 2020 (https://www.thailandmedical.news/news/india-slammed-forproposing-usage-of-homeopathy-to-prevent-coronavirus)

9.9.15 IMMUNE SYSTEM BOOSTERS

It is noteworthy that premature death was in the elderly, probably due to immunosuppression, which promotes the rapid development of COVID (Li et al., 2020; Wang et al., 2020). It is advised to add important spices in our food to boost our system. It is suggested that people should use other supplements also to make stronger their immune system. Healthy people should eat plenty of citrus fruits that contain a variety of vitamins. Some dried fruits (nuts and dates) are also helpful in improving the system. However, adults are therefore more likely to take vitamins and zinc supplements in consultation with a physician. Essential vitamins A, C, D, and E needed to boost the immune system and fight Covid situation. It is also good that you need zinc and iodine intake.

9.10 RECENT DEVELOPMENTS IN COVID-19

(Available from https://www.medicalnewstoday.com/coronavirus)

9.10.1 POSSIBILITY OF TRANSMISSION OF COVID-19 BY AIR

The World Health Organization (WHO) recently acknowledged that coronavirus may be spread through the air under certain conditions. The air transfer differs from droplet transfer which can be defined as the presence of bacteria in the nuclei of droplets, usually considered particles less than 5 μm in diameter.

9.10.2 THE ANTIBODY MIXTURE SHOWS PROMISE IN THE FIGHT AGAINST THE NOVEL CORONAVIRUS

It has recently been studied that the blood of a SARS-CoV patient has shown a good immune response. It was found to have weakened the virus in the study area and protected the animals from certain effects of infection. Combining the two antibodies may prevent the virus from becoming resistant to the virus, as other studies suggest. In general, it can take years to isolate and build up the immune system as a treatment, but recent technological advances have made it possible to speed up the process. Researchers have previously reported that Monoclonal antibodies are produced by a unique set of memory cells B – a type of immune system that "remembers" the sequence of certain proteins of the virus. An antibody that blocks the receptor binding site thus prevents the virus from entering the cells and reproduces it in large quantities and is injected into patients as a treatment or treatment.

9.10.3 THE RISK OF STROKE IS HIGHER IN SMOKERS IN COVID-19

Recent reviews have suggested that smoking may increase the severity of COVID-19. Smoking and vaping cause damage to the blood-brain barrier and also increase the risk of blood clots thus increasing the risk of stroke in COVID-19. the nervous system in the brain. Therefore, it has led researchers to review the evidence of how this activity affects the emotional symptoms of people with COVID-19.

9.10.4 OXFORD COVID-19 VACCINE SHOWS REAL PROMISE

Oxford recently published the result of a potential candidate in The Lancet. In this study, it is evident that Oxford tests using adenovirus are safe and promote an important immune response in study volunteers. Pigs were able to produce antibodies to SARS-CoV-2, in addition to showing T-cell responses in further research, which will be reviewed by peers. Therefore, it led to a second booster shot with an improved antibody response. The side effects seen were common but usually mild which included fatigue, headache, pain at the injection site, and flu-like symptoms that could not be treated with paracetamol.

TABLE 9.3 Different Drug Candidates Showing Efficacy in Treatment for COVID-19.

Sr no.	Drug name	Possible mechanism	Country of origin	Status
1.	Umifenovir	Prevent the entry of the virus into human cells	Russia, China	Drug has a good safety profile clinical trials are underway to assess its effectiveness in patients from India
2.	Favilavir	Broad-spectrum inhibitor of viral m – RNA	China	Reported to have efficacy in Covid patients with less side effects in a scientific trial of 70 patients. Approved in China for treating coronavirus
3.	Camostat Mesylate	Blocking the SARS-CoV-2 binding and entry through ACE2	German	Considered for off-label treatment of SARS-CoV-2-infected patients
4.	Ifenprodil	It is a N-methyl-d-aspartate (NDMA) receptor glutamate receptor antagonist	South Korea and Japan	A parenteral and long-acting orally administered product is in production to start medical trials for COVID -19
5.	Rintatolimod	The toll-like receptor 3 (TLR-3) agonist	Japan	Trials are underway to use Rintatolimod has shown a possible action in Covid patients reported by the National Institute of Infectious Diseases (NIID) in Japan and the University of Tokyo
6.	Gimsilumab - a human monoclonal antibody	GM-CSF which is a pro-inflammatory cytokine observed in high levels in the blood serum of COVID-19 infected patients	Riovant Science – New York	Reduce damage to lung and reduce the mortality rate in COVID-19 patients
7.	OyaGen's OYA1	Inhibits SARS-CoV-2 from replicating	United States	Antiviral effectiveness verses coronavirus in laboratory essays, and reported to be more useful than chlorpromazine HCl in inhibiting SARS-CoV-2 from replicating in cell culture

9.11 CONCLUSION

SARS-CoV-2 is a novel and highly contagious virus, and there is no direct treatment for COVID-19 so far, and it has quickly become a pandemic. It should be noted that if no practical action is taken and if drugs, vaccines, and patient follow-up methods are not widely developed or effective, occasional social isolation may continue until 2022. At that time, COVID-19 may have affected 90% of the. world's population and killed over 40 million people. Therefore, it is wise to continue with preventive measures and public health measures until appropriate and effective treatment is available. Combined therapies with some of the above-mentioned medications or supplements, combined with a healthy diet to protect the immune system, and adherence to standards will eventually work against COVID-19. Recent literature findings indicate that there is a recovery rate of more than 65% in the case of COVID Patients. Many Pharma companies, institutions, universities of various countries are in the process of developing and introducing the first vaccine to treat COVID-19. Many companies have developed vaccines in various stages of clinical trials and the public is looking for a positive outcome such as getting a COVID-19 vaccine to end the epidemic.

KEYWORDS

- **COVID-19**
- **CORONA**
- **virus**
- **immunity**
- **WHO**

REFERENCES

Adnan Shereen, M.; Khan, S.; Kazmi, A.; Bashir, N.; Siddique, R. COVID-19 Infection: Origin, Transmission, and Characteristics of Human Coronaviruses. *J. Adv. Res.* **2020,** *24*, 91–98.

Agostini, M. L.; Andres, E. L.; Sims, A. C.; et a Coronavirus Susceptibility to the Antiviral Remdesivir (GS-5734) Is Mediated by the Viral Polymerase and the Proofreading Exoribonuclease. *Mbio* **2018,** *9*, e00221–00218.

Alimian, M.; Pournajafian, A.; Kholdebarin, A.; Ghodraty, M.; Rokhtabnak, F.; Yazdkhasti, P. Analgesic Effects of Paracetamol and Morphine after Elective Laparotomy Surgeries. *Anesthesiol. Pain Med.* **2014,** *4* (2), e12912.

Alzghari, S. K.; Acuna, V. S. Supportive Treatment with Tocilizumab for COVID-19: A Systematic Review. *J. Clin. Virol.* **2020,** *127*, 104380. https://doi.org/10.1016/j.jcv.2020.104380

Amir, M.; Mehrdad, H.; Farhad, S. D.; Reza, R.; Hassan, N. A Narrative Literature Review on Traditional Medicine Options for Treatment of Corona Virus Disease 2019 (COVID-19). *Complement. Ther. Clin. Pract.* **2020,** *40*. https://doi.org/10.1016/j.ctcp.2020.101214

Anderson, R. M.; Fraser, C.; Ghani, A. C.; Donnelly, C. A.; Riley, S.; Ferguson, N. M.; et al. Epidemiology, Transmission Dynamics and Control of SARS: The 2002–2003 Epidemic. *Philos. Trans. R Soc. B Lond. B Biol. Sci.* **2004,** *359* (1447), 1091–1105.

Antinori, S.; Bonazzetti, C.; Gubertini, G.; et al. Tocilizumab for Cytokine Storm Syndrome in COVID-19 Pneumonia: An Increased Risk for Candidemia? Autoimmun. Rev. **2020,** *19* (7), 102564. https://doi.org/10.1016/j.autrev.2020.102564

Arabi, Y. M.; Al-Enezi, F.; Longuere, K. S.; et al. Feasibility of a Randomized Controlled Trial to Assess Treatment of Middle East Respiratory Syndrome Coronavirus (MERS-CoV) Infection in Saudi Arabia: A Survey of Physicians. BMC Anesthesiol. **2016,** *16* (1), 36.

Barratt-Due, A.; Thorgersen, E. B.; Egge, K.; et al. Combined Inhibition of Complement (C5) and CD14 Markedly Attenuates Inflammation, Thrombogenicity, and Hemodynamic Changes in Porcine Sepsis. *J. Immunol.* **2013,** *191* (2), 819–827.

Ben-Zvi, I.; Kivity, S.; Langevitz, P.; Shoenfeld, Y. Hydroxychloroquine: From Malaria to Autoimmunity. *Clin. Rev. Allergy Immunol.* **2012,** *42*, 145–153.

Bijker, E. M.; Bastiaens, G. J. H.; Teirlinck, A. C. Protection Against Malaria After Immunization by Chloroquine Prophylaxis and Sporozoites is Mediated by Preerythrocytic Immunity. *Proc. Natl. Acad. Sci. USA* **2013,** *110*, 7862–7867.

Borner, C.; Hollt, V.; Kraus, J. Mechanisms of the Inhibition of Nuclear Factor Kappab by Morphine in Neuronal Cells. *Mol. Pharmacol.* **2012,** *81* (4), 587–597.

Cao, Y.; et al. Ruxolitinib in Treatment of Severe Coronavirus Disease 2019 (COVID-19): A Multicenter, Single-Blind, Randomized Controlled Trial. *J. Allergy Clin. Immunol.* **2020,** *146* (1), 137–146.

Cao, B.; Wang, Y.; Wen, D. A Trial of Lopinavir–Ritonavir in Adults Hospitalized with Severe COVID-19. *N. Engl. J. Med.* **2020,** *382*,1787–1799.

Chen, J.; Jiang, Q.; Xia, X.; Liu, K.; Yu, Z.; Tao, W.; et al. Individual Variation of the SARS CoV2 Receptor ACE2 Gene Expression and Regulation. Aging Cell Advance [Online] (2020). https://doi.org/10.1111/acel.13168.

Chen, Z.; Li, L.; Cheng, J.; et al.. Clinical Features of COVID-19-Related Liver Functional Abnormality. Clin. Gastroenterol. Hepatol. **2020,** *18*, 1561–1566.

Chen, M.; Tong, R.; Bian, Y.; Shu, Y.; et al. Evidence-Based Rapid Review on Possibility of Treatment of Novel Pneumonia with Subcutaneous interferon-α. Her. Med. **2020,** *39*, 483–488.

Cheng, C. Y.; Lee, Y. L.; Chen, C. P. Lopinavir/Ritonavir did not Shorten the Duration of SARS CoV-2 Shedding in Patients with Mild Pneumonia in Taiwan. *J. Microbiol. Immunol. Infect.* **2020**. https://doi.org/10.1016/j.jmii.2020.03.032.

Cheng, Y.; Wong, R.; Soo, Y. O.; et al. Use of Convalescent Plasma Therapy in SARS Patients in Hong Kong. *Eur. J. Clin. Microbiol. Infect. Dis.* **2005,** *24* (1), 44–46.

Chu, C. M.; Cheng, V. C. C.; Hung, I. F. N.; et al. Role of Lopinavir/Ritonavir in the Treatment of SARS: Initial Virological and Clinical Findings. *Thorax* **2004,** *59*, 252–256.

Colafella, K. M. M.; Uijl, E.; Danser, J. Interference with the Renin-Angiotensin System (ras): Classical Inhibitors and Novel Approaches. In *Reference Module in Biomedical Sciences: Encyclopedia of Endocrine Diseases*; Elsevier, 2018. https://doi.org/ 10.1016/B978-0-12-801238-3.65341-2.

Corman, V. M.; Landt, O.; Kaiser, M.; Molenkamp, R.; Meijer, A.; Chu, D. K.; et al. Detection of 2019 Novel Coronavirus (2019-nCoV) by Real-Time RT-PCR. *Euro Surveill* **2020,** *25* (3). https://doi.org/10.2807/1560-7917.ES.2020.25.3.2000045

Corona Virus, [Online] 2020. https://www.cdc.gov/coronavirus/types.html

Corona Virus, [Online] 2020. http://www.emro.who.int/health-topics/corona-virus/about-COVID-19.html. (Accessed 1 June, 2020).

Corona Virus Types, [Online] 2020. https://www.healthline.com/health/coronavirus-types#types

Cvetkovi, R. S.; Goa, K. L. Lopinavir/Ritonavir: A Review of its Use in the Management of HIV Infection. *Drugs* **2003,** *63*, 769–802.

Delvecchio, R.; Higa, L. M.; Pezzuto, P.; et al. Chloroquine, an Endocytosis Blocking Agent, Inhibits Zika Virus Infection in Different Cell Models. *Viruses* **2016,** *8*, 322.

Deng, L.; Li, C.; Zeng, Q.; et al. Arbidol Combined with LPV/r Versus LPV/r Alone Against Corona Virus Disease 2019: A Retrospective Cohort Study. J. Infect. **2020,** *81* (1), e1–e5. https://doi.org/10.1016/j.jinf.2020.03.002.

Ekstr€om, M.; Dahlander, B. Palliation in Patients with Severe COVID-19. *Lakartidningen* **2020,** *117*, F3PM.

England N, Improvement N. Primary Care and Community Respiratory Resource Pack for use During COVID-19.

Fan, Y.; Zhao, K.; Shi, Z-L.; Zhou, P. Bat Coronaviruses in China. *Viruses* **2019,** *11* (3), 210.

Feldmann, M. Development of Anti-TNF Therapy for Rheumatoid Arthritis. Nat. Rev. Immunol. **2002,** *2*, 364–371.

Fiore, C.; Eisenhut, M.; Krausse, R.; Ragazzi, E.; et al. Antiviral Effects of Glycyrrhiza Species. *Phytother. Res.* **2008,** *22*, 141–148.

Fu, B.; Xu, X.; Wei, H. Why Tocilizumab Could be an Effective Treatment for Severe COVID-19? *J. Transl. Med.* **2020,** *18*, 164.

Furuta, Y.; Gowen, B. B.; Takahashi, K. et al. Favipiravir (T-705), A Novel Viral RNA Polymerase Inhibitor. Antivir. Res. **2013,** *100*, 446–454.

Furuta, Y.; Takahashi, K.; Shiraki, K.; et al. T-705 (Favipiravir) and Related Compounds: Novel Broad-Spectrum Inhibitors of RNA Viral Infections. *Antivir. Res.* **2009,** *82*, 95–102.

Gautret, P.; Lagier, J-C.; Parola, P.; et al. Hydroxychloroquine and Azithromycin as a Treatment of COVID-19: Results of an Open-Label Non-Randomized Clinical Trial. *Int. J. Antimicrob. Agents* **2020**. https://doi.org/10.1101/2020.03.16.20037135.

Gordon, C. J.; Tchesnokov, E. P.; Feng, J. Y.; Porter, D. P.; Gotte, M. The Antiviral Compound 1 Remdesivir Potently Inhibits RNA-Dependent RNA Polymerase from Middle East Respiratory Syndrome Coronavirus. *J. Biol. Chem.* **2020,** *295*, 4773–4779.

Greig, A.; Bouillant, A. Binding Effects of Concanavalin A on a Coronavirus. *Can. J. Comp. Med.* **1977,** *41* (1), 122.

Gu, H.; Xie, Z.; Li, T.; Zhang, S.; Lai, C.; Zhu, P.; et al. Angiotensin-Converting Enzyme 2. Inhibits Lung Injury Induced by Respiratory Syncytial Virus. *Sci. Rep.* **2016,** *6*, 19840. https://doi.org/10.1038/srep19840

Guan, W.-J.; Ni, Z.-Y.; Hu, Y.; Liang, W.-H.; Ou, C.-Q.; He, J.-X.; et al. Clinical Characteristics of Coronavirus Disease 2019 in China. *N. Engl. J. Med.* **2020,** *82* (18), 1708–1720. https://doi.org/10.1056/NEJMoa2002032

Guo, Y.-R.; Cao, Q.-D.; Hong, Z.-S.; Tan, Y.-Y.; Chen, S.-D.; Jin, H.-J.; et al. The Origin, Transmission and Clinical Therapies on Coronavirus Disease 2019 (COVID-19) Outbreak–An Update on the Status. *Mil. Med. Res.* **2020,** *7* (1), 1–10.

Guo, J.; Huang, Z.; Lin, L.; Lv, J. Coronavirus Disease 2019 (COVID-19) and Cardiovascular Disease: A Viewpoint on the Potential Influence of Angiotensin-Converting Enzyme Inhibitors/Angiotensin Receptor Blockers on Onset and Severity of Severe Acute Respiratory Syndrome Coronavirus 2 Infection. *J. Am. Heart Assoc.* **2020,** *9* (7), e016219.

Hanaei, S.; Rezaei, N. COVID-19: Developing from an Outbreak to a Pandemic. *Arch. Med. Res.* 2020. https://doi.org/10.1016/j.arcmed.2020.04.021

Haschke, M.; Schuster, M.; Poglitsch, M.; Loibner, H.; Salzberg, M.; Bruggisser, M.; et al. Pharmacokinetics and Pharmacodynamics of Recombinant Human Angiotensin-Converting Enzyme 2 in Healthy Human Subjects. *Clin. Pharmacokinet.* **2013,** *52* (9), 783–792.

Hendaus, M. A. Remdesivir in the Treatment of Coronavirus Disease 2019 (COVID-19): A Simplified Summary. *J. Biomol. Struct. Dyn.* 2020, 1–6. https://doi.org/10.1080/07391102.2020.1767691

Ho, T.-Y.; Wu, S.-L.; Chen, J.-C.; et al. Emodin Blocks the SARS Coronavirus Spike Protein and Angiotensin-Converting Enzyme 2 Interaction. *Antivir. Res.* **2007,** *74* (2), 92–101.

Hoffmann, M.; Kleine-Weber, H.; Schroeder, S.; Krüger, N.; Herrler, T.; Erichsen, S.; et al. SARS-CoV-2 Cell Entry Depends on ACE2 and TMPRSS2 and is Blocked by a Clinically Proven Protease Inhibitor. *Cell Vol.* **2020,** *181* (2), 271–280.

Holshue, M. L.; DeBolt, C.; Lindquist, S.; et al. First Case of 2019 Novel Coronavirus in the United States. *N. Engl. J. Med.* **2020,** *382*, 929–936.

Hutchinson, M. et al.; Haemophagocytic lymphohisticytosis—an Under Recognized Hyperinflammatory Syndrome. *Rheumatology* **2019,** *58* (Suppl 6), vi23–vi30.

Jacobs, J.; et al. Case Report of a SARS-CoV-2 Infection in a Patient with Ulcerative Colitis on Tofacitinib. *Inflamm. Bowel Dis.* **2020,** *26* (7), e64.

Kadam, R. U.; Wilson, I. A. Structural Basis of Influenza Virus Fusion Inhibition by the Antiviral Drug Arbidol. *Proc. Natl. Acad. Sci. USA* **2017,** *114*, 206–214.

Kaplan, M. M. Ed.; The Use of Methotrexate, Colchicine, and Other Immunomodulatory Drugs in the Treatment of Primary Biliary Cirrhosis. *Semin. Liver Dis.* **1997.**

Kelleni, M. T. Nitazoxanide/Azithromycin Combination for COVID-19: A Suggested New Protocol for Early Management. *Pharmacol. Res.* **2020,** *157*. https://doi.org/10.1016/j.phrs.2020.104874

Keyaerts, E.; Vijgen, L.; Maes, P.; Neyts, J.; Van Ranst, M. In Vitro Inhibition of Severe Acute Respiratory Syndrome Coronavirus by Chloroquine. *Biochem. Biophys. Res. Commun.* **2004,** *323* (1), 264–268.

Khambholja, K.; Asudani, D. Potential Repurposing of Favipiravir in COVID-19 Outbreak Based on Current Evidence. *Travel. Med. Infect. Dis.* **2020**. http://dx.doi.org/ 10.1002/jmv.25798.

Khan, A.; Benthin, C.; Zeno, B.; Albertson, T. E.; Boyd, J.; Christie, J. D.; et al. A Pilot Clinical Trial of Recombinant Human Angiotensin-Converting Enzyme 2 in Acute Respiratory Distress Syndrome. *Crit. Care* **2017,** *21* (1), 234.

Kim, H. Y.; Eo, E. Y.; Park, H.; et al. Medicinal Herbal Extracts of Sophorae Radix, Acanthopanacis Cortex, Sanguisorbae Radix and Torilis Fructus Inhibit Coronavirus Replication in Vitro. *Antiviral. Therap.* **2010,** *15*, 697–709.

Koch, B.; Schult-Dietrich, P.; Büttner, S.; et al. Lectin Affinity Plasmapheresis for Middle East Respiratory Syndrome-Coronavirus and Marburg Virus Glycoprotein Elimination. *Blood Purif.* **2018,** *46* (2), 126–33.

Kuba, K.; Imai, Y.; Rao, S.; Gao, H.; Guo, F.; Guan, B.; et al. A Crucial Role of Angiotensin Converting Enzyme 2 (Ace2) in Sars Coronavirus-Induced Lung Injury. *Nat. Med.* **2005,** *11* (8), 875–879.

La Rosée, P.; et al. Recommendations for the Management of Hemophagocytic Lymphohistiocytosis in Adults. *Blood* **2019,** *133* (23), 2465–2477.

Lam, T. T.-Y.; Shum, M. H.-H.; Zhu, H.-C.; Tong, Y.-G.; Ni, X.-B.; Liao, Y.-S.; et al. Identification of 2019-nCoV Related Coronaviruses in Malayan Pangolins in Southern China. *BioRxiv* **2020**. https://doi.org/10.1101/2020.02.13.945485

Latest Coronavirus News [Online]. https://www.medicalnewstoday.com/coronavirus

Leng, Z.; Zhu, R.; Hou, W.; et al. Transplantation of ACE2- Mesenchymal Stem Cells Improves the Outcome of Patients with COVID-19 Pneumonia. *Aging Dis.* **2020,** *11* (2), 216–28.

Li, Y. C.; Bai, W. Z.; Hashikawa, T. The Neuroinvasive Potential of SARS-CoV2 may be at Least Partially Responsible for the Respiratory Failure of COVID-19 Patients. *J. Med. Virol.* **2020,** *2* (6), 552–555.

Li, S.-Y.; Chen, C.; Zhang, H.-Q.; et al. Identification of Natural Compounds with Antiviral Activities Against SARS-Associated Coronavirus. *Antivir. Res.* **2005,** *67* (1), 18–23.

Li, Q.; Guan, X.; Wu, P.; et al. Early Transmission Dynamics in Wuhan, China, of Novel Coronavirus-Infected Pneumonia. *N. Engl. J. Med.* **2020,** *382*, s1199s–1207.

Li, Z. J.; Teng, B. X.; Luo, J.; et al. Clinical Application of Therapeutic Plasma Exchange in the Three Gorges Area. *Transfus. Apher. Sci.* **2010,** *43* (3), 305–308.

Li, Z.; Yi, Y.; Luo, X.; Xiong, N.; Liu, Y.; Li, S.; et al. Development and Clinical Application of a Rapid IgM-IgG Combined Antibody Test for SARS-CoV-2 Infection Diagnosis. *J. Med. Virol.* **2020**. https://doi.org/10.1002/jmv.25727

Lin, L. T.; Hsu, W. C.; Lin, C. C. Antiviral Natural Products and Herbal Medicines. *J. Tradit. Complement. Med.* **2014,** *4*, 24–35.

Liu, S. Y.; Sanchez, D. J.; Cheng, G. New Developments in the Induction and Antiviral Effectors of Type I Interferon. *Curr. Opin. Immunol.* **2011,** *23*, 57–64.

Luo, M. C.; Wang, W. F.; Yin, W. F.; et al. Clinical Efficacy and Mechanism of Lymphoplasma Exchange in the Treatment of Guillain-Barre Syndrome. Cell Mol. Biol. **2017,** *63* (10), 106–115.

Mair-Jenkins, J.; Saavedra-Campos, M.; Baillie, J. K.; et al. The Effectiveness of Convalescent Plasma and Hyperimmune Immunoglobulin for the Treatment of Severe Acute Respiratory Infections of Viral Etiology: A Systematic Review and Exploratory Meta-Analysis. *J. Infect. Dis.* **2015,** *211* (1), 80–90.

Marano, G.; Vaglio, S.; Pupella, S.; et al. Convalescent Plasma: New Evidence for an Old Therapeutic Tool? *Blood Transfus.* **2016,** *14* (2), 152–157.

Mizui, T.; Yamashina, S.; Tanida, I.; et al. Inhibition of Hepatitis C Virus Replication by Chloroquine Targeting Virus-Associated Autophagy. *J. Gastroenterol.* **2010,** *45,* 195–203.

Mohamed, K.; Rodríguez-Román, E.; Rahmani, F.; Zhang, H.; Ivanovska, M.; Makka, S. A. et al. Borderless Collaboration is Needed for COVID-19: A Disease that Knows no Borders. *Infect. Control Hosp. Epidemiol.* **2020,** 1–2. https://doi.org/10.1017/ice.2020.162

Momtazmanesh, S.; Ochs, H. D.; Uddin, L. Q.; Perc, M.; Routes, J. M.; Nuno Vieira, D.; et al. All Together to Fight Novel Coronavirus Disease (COVID-19). *Am. J. Trop. Med. Hyg.* **2020,** *102* (6), 1181–1183.

Montoya, M.; Schiavoni, G.; Mattei, F.; et al. Type I Interferons Produced by Dendritic Cells Promote Their Phenotypic and Functional Activation. *Blood* **2002,** *99*, 263–3271.

Newton, A. H.; Cardani, A.; Braciale, T. J. The Host Immune Response in Respiratory Virus Infection: Balancing Virus Clearance and Immunopathology. *Semin. Immunopathol.* **2016,** *38*, 471–482.

Oestereich, L.; Luedtke, A.; Wurr, S.; et al. Successful Treatment of Advanced Ebola Virus Infection with T-705 (Favipiravir) in a Small Animal Model. *Antivir. Res.* **2014,** *105* (24),17–21.

Omrani, A. S.; Saad, M. M.; Baig, K. Ribavirin and Interferon Alfa-2a for Severe Middle East Respiratory Syndrome Coronavirus Infection: A Retrospective Cohort Study. *Lancet Infect. Dis.* **2014,** *14*, 1090–1095.

Paraskevis, D.; Kostaki, E. C.; Magiorkinis, G.; Panayiotakopoulos, G.; Sourvinos, G.; Tsiodras, S. Full-Genome Evolutionary Analysis of the Novel Corona Virus (2019-nCoV) Rejects the Hypothesis of Emergence as a Result of a Recent Recombination Event. *Infect. Genet. Evol.* **2020,** *79*. https://doi.org/10.1016/j.meegid.2020.104212

Parry, J. China Coronavirus: Cases Surge as Official Admits Human to Human Transmission. *BMJ* **2020,** *368*, m236. https://doi.org/10.1136/bmj.m236

Patanjali Coronil Medicine [Online]. https://www.timesnownews.com/health/article/COVID-19-drug-patanjali-to-launch-ayurvedic-medicine-coronil-to-treat-coronavirus-infection-today/610441)

Pécheur, E.-I.; Lavillette, D.; Alcaras, F.; Molle, J.; et al. Biochemical Mechanism of Hepatitis C Virus Inhibition by the Broad-Spectrum Antiviral Arbidol. *Biochemistry* **2007,** *46*, 6050–6059.

Peng, Q. Y.; Wang, X. T.; Zhang, L. N. Findings of Lung Ultrasonography of Novel Corona Virus Pneumonia During the 2019–2020 Epidemic. *Intensive Care Med.* **2020,** *46* (5), 849–850.

Prompetchara, E.; Ketloy, C.; Palaga, T. Immune Responses in COVID-19 and Potential Vaccines: Lessons Learned from SARS and MERS Epidemic. Asian Pac. J. Allergy Immunol. **2020,** *38* (1), 1–9.

Qualitative Detection of Nucleic Acid from Severe Acute Respiratory Syndrome Coronavirus 2 (SARS-CoV-2) in Nasopharyngeal Swabs (NPS) from Individuals Suspected of COVID-19 by Their Healthcare Provider. Emergency use of this Test is Limited to Authorized. US Food Drug Adm n.d.

Riou, J.; Althaus, C. L. Pattern of Early Human-to-Human Transmission of Wuhan 2019 Novel Coronavirus (2019-nCoV), December 2019 to January 2020. *Euro Surveill.* **2020,** *25* (4). https://doi.org/10.2807/1560-7917.ES.2020.25.4.2000058

Rocha-Pereira, J.; Jochmans, D.; Dallmeier, K. Favipiravir (T-705) Inhibits in Vitro Norovirus Replication. *Biochem. Biophys. Res. Commun.* **2012,** *424*, 777–780.

Roskoski, R. Jr. Janus Kinase (JAK) Inhibitors in the Treatment of Inflammatory and Neoplastic Diseases. *Pharmacol. Res.* **2016,** *111*, 784–803.

Sabino-Silva, R.; Jardim, A. C.; Siqueira, W. L. Coronavirus COVID-19 Impacts to Dentistry and Potential Salivary Diagnosis. *Clin. Oral Invest.* **2020,** *24* (4), 1619–1621. DOI: 10.1007/s00784-020-03248-x.

Santosh, T. S.; Parmar, R.; Anand, H.; Srikanth, K.; Saritha, M. A Review of Salivary Diagnostics and its Potential Implication in Detection of COVID-19. *Cureus* **2020,** *12* (4), 7708.

Scheinecker, C.; Smolen, J.; Yasothan, U.; Stoll, J.; Kirkpatrick, P. *Tocilizumab. Nat. Rev. Drug Discov.* **2009,** *8*, 273–274.

Schultz. K. R.; Gilman, A. L. The Lysosomotropic Amines, Chloroquine and Hydroxychloroquine: A Potentially Novel Therapy for Graft-Versus-Host Disease. *Leuk. Lymphoma* **1997,** *24*, 201–210.

Sharma, S.; Kumar, V.; Chawla, A.; Logani, A. Rapid Detection of SARS-CoV-2 in Saliva: Can an Endodontist Take the Lead in Point-of-Care COVID-19 Testing? *Int. Endodontic. J.* **2020,** *53* (7), 1017–1019.

Sivakumaran, P.; Vo, A. A.; Villicana, R.; et al. Therapeutic Plasma Exchange for Desensitization Prior to Transplantation in ABO-Incompatible Renal Allografts. *J. Clin. Apher.* **2009,** *24* (4), 155–160.

Strunk, J. L.; Temesgen, H.; Andersen, H.; Packalen, P. Correlation of Chest CT and RTPCR Testing in Coronavirus Disease. *Radiology* **2014,** *80*, 1–8. https://doi.org/10.1148/radiol.2020200642

Sun, D.; Li, H.; Lu, X.-X.; Xiao, H.; Ren, J.; Zhang, F.-R.; et al. Clinical Features of Severe Pediatric Patients with Coronavirus Disease 2019 in Wuhan: A Single Center's Observational Study. *World J. Pediatr.* **2020,** *16* (3), 251–259.

Tchesnokov, E.; Feng, J.; Porter, D.; Götte, M. Mechanism of Inhibition of Ebola Virus RNA-Dependent RNA Polymerase by Remdesivir. *Viruses* **2019,** *11* (4), 326. http://dx.doi.org/10.3390/v11040326.

Tiwari, B. K.; Khosa, R. Hepatoprotective and Antioxidant Effect of Sphaeranthus Indicus Against Acetaminophen-Induced Hepatotoxicity in Rats. *J. Pharmaceut. Sci. Res.* **2009,** *1* (2), 26–30.

Toniati, P.; Piv, S.; Cattalini, M. Tocilizumab for the Treatment of Severe COVID-19 Pneumonia with Hyperinflammatory Syndrome and Acute Respiratory Failure: A Single

Center Study 17 of 100 Patients in Brescia, Italy. *Autoimmun. Rev.* **2020,** *19* (7), 102568. https://doi.org/10.1016/j.autrev.2020.102568

Tsang, K.; Zhong, N. S. SARS: Pharmacotherapy. *Respirology* **2003,** *8* (Suppl), S25–S30.

Usage of Homeopathy to Prevent Corona Virus [Online]. https://www.thailandmedical.news/news/india-slammed-forproposing-usage-of-homeopathy-to-prevent-coronavirus

Vaccine Development and Therapeutic Strategies [Online]. https://indiabioscience.org/columns/general-science/COVID-19-vaccine-development-and-therapeutic-strategies

Vankadari, N. Arbidol: A Potential Antiviral Drug for the Treatment of SARS-CoV-2 by Blocking the Trimerization of Viral Spike Glycoprotein. *Int. J. Antimicrob. Agents* **2020**. https://doi.org/10.1016/j.ijantimicag.2020.105998.

Vimalanathan, S.; Ignacimuthu, S.; Hudson, J. Medicinal Plants of Tamil Nadu (Southern India) are a Rich Source of Antiviral Activities. *Pharmaceut. Biol.* **2009,** *47* (5), 422–429.

Wan, S.; Yi, Q.; Fan, S.; Lv, J.; Zhang, X.; Guo, L.; et al. Characteristics of Lymphocyte Subsets and Cytokines in Peripheral Blood of 123 Hospitalized Patients with 2019 Novel Coronavirus Pneumonia (ncp). *MedRxiv* **2020**. https://doi.org/10.1101/2020.02.10.20021832

Wang, X.; Cao, R.; Zhang, H.; et al. The Anti-influenza Virus Drug, Arbidol is an Efficient Inhibitor of SARS-CoV-2 in Vitro. *Cell Discov.* **2020b,** *6*, 28. https://doi.org/10.1038/s41421-020-0169-8

Wang, C.; Horby, P. W.; Hayden, F. G.; Gao, G. F. A Novel Coronavirus Outbreak of Global Health Concern. *Lancet* **2020,** *395* (10223), 470–473.

Wang, W.; Xu, Y.; Gao, R.; Lu, R.; Han, K.; Wu, G.; et al. Detection of SARS-CoV-2 in Different Types of Clinical Specimens. *J. Am. Med. Assoc.* **2020,** *323* (18), 1843–1844. http://doi.org/10.1001/jama.2020.3786.

Wang, Y.; Zhang, D.; Du, G. Remdesivir in Adults with Severe COVID-19: A Randomised, Double-Blind, Placebo-Controlled, Multicentre Trial. *Lancet* **2020c,** *395*, 1569–1578.

WHO. "Solidarity" Clinical Trial for COVID-19 Treatments April 21, 2020 [Online]. https://www.who.int/emergencies/diseases/novel-coronavirus-2019/global-research-on-novel-coronavirus-2019-ncov/solidarity-clinical-trialfor-COVID-19-treatments.

Wu, C.; Chen, X.; Cai, Y.; Zhou, X.; Xu, S.; Huang, H.; et al. Risk Factors Associated with Acute Respiratory Distress Syndrome and Death in Patients with Coronavirus Disease 2019 Pneumonia in Wuhan, China. *JAMA Intern. Med.* **2020,** *180* (7), 1–11.

Wu, F.; Zhao, S.; Yu, B.; Chen, Y.-M.; Wang, W.; Song, Z.-G.; et al. A New Coronavirus Associated with Human Respiratory Disease in China. *Nature* **2020,** *579* (7798), 265–269. https://doi.org/10.1038/s41586-020-2008-3.

Xu, R.; Cui, B.; Duan, X.; Zhang, P.; Zhou, X.; Yuan, Q. Saliva: Potential Diagnostic Value and Transmission of SARS-CoV-2. *Int. J. Oral Sci.* **2020,** *12* (1), 1–6.

Xudong, X.; Junzhu, C.; Xingxiang, W.; Furong, Z.; Yanrong, L. Age- and Gender Related Difference of ACE2 Expression in Rat Lung. *Life Sci.* **2006,** *78* (19), 2166–2171.

Yan, Y.; Shen, X.; Cao, Y.; Zhang, J.; Wang, Y.; Cheng, Y. Discovery of Anti-2019-ncov Agents from 38 Chinese Patent Drugs Toward Respiratory Diseases via Docking Screening. *Preprints* **2020**. https://doi.org/10.20944/preprints202002.0254.v2.

Yan, R.; Zhang, Y.; Guo, Y.; Xia, L.; Zhou, Q. Structural Basis for the Recognition of the 2019-nCoV by Human ACE2. *BioRxiv* **2020,** *367* (6485), 1444–1448.

Yin, Y.; Wunderink, R. G. MERS, SARS and Other Coronaviruses as Causes of Pneumonia. *Respirology* **2018,** *23* (2), 130–137.

Yu, Y.-B. The Extracts of Solanum nigrum L. for Inhibitory Effects on HIV-1 and its Essential Enzyme. *Kor. J. Orient Med.* **2004,** *10* (1), 119–126.

Zhang, K. Is Traditional Chinese Medicine Useful in the Treatment of COVID-19? *Am. J. Emerg. Med.* **2020**. https://doi.org/10.1016/j.ajem.2020.03.046. In press.

Zhang, H.; Baker, A. Recombinant Human ace2: Acing Out Angiotensin II in ARDS Therapy; Springer, 2017; vol 21, p 305. https://doi.org/10.1186/s13054-017-1882-z

Zhou, P.; Yang, X.-L.; Wang, X.-G.; Hu, B.; Zhang, L.; Zhang, W.; et al. Discovery of a Novel Coronavirus Associated with the Recent Pneumonia Outbreak in Humans and its Potential Bat Origin. *BioRxiv* **2020**. https://doi.org/10.1101/2020.01.22.914952

Zhou, B. P.; Zhong, N. S.; Guan, Y. Treatment with Convalescent Plasma for Influenza (H5N 1) Infection. *N. Engl. J. Med.* **2007,** *357* (14), 1450–1451.

Ziai, S.; Heidari, M. Inhibitory Effects of Germinal Angiotensin Converting Enzyme by Medicinal Plants Used in Iranian Traditional Medicine as Antihypertensive. *J. Kerman Univ. Med. Sci.* **2015,** *16* (2), 134–144.

Zimmerman, P.; Curtis, N. Coronavirus Infections in Children Including COVID-19: An Overview of the Epidemiology, Clinical Features, Diagnosis, Treatment and Prevention Options in Children. *Pediatr. Infect. Dis. J.* **2020,** *39* (5), 355–368.

Zou, Z.; Yan, Y.; Shu, Y.; Gao, R.; Sun, Y.; Li, X.; et al. Angiotensin-Converting Enzyme 2 Protects from Lethal Avian Influenza a h5n1 Infections. *Nat. Commun.* **2014,** *5*, 3594. https://doi.org/10.1038/ncomms4594

CHAPTER 10

Advances in the Traditional System of Medicine for COVID-19

ANUPAM SRIVASTAVA[1], ANAMIKA[2], RITESH TIWARI[3], and AJAY KUMAR SHUKLA[4]

[1]*Department of Kayachikitsa, Chandra Shekhar Singh Ayurved Sansthan, Kaushambi, Uttar Pradesh, India*

[2]*Department of Kaumarbhritya, State Ayurvedic College and Hospital, Lucknow, Uttar Pradesh, India*

[3]*Department of Pharmaceutical Chemistry, Chandra Shekhar Singh College of Pharmacy, Kaushambi, Uttar Pradesh, India*

[4]*Institute of Pharmacy, Dr. Ram Manohar Lohia Avadh University Ayodhya, Faizabad, Uttar Pradesh, India*

ABSTRACT

Coronaviruses have come as a drastic disease outbreak since from last two decades, like severe acute respiratory syndrome (SARS) in 2002 and the all Middle East respiratory syndromes (MERS) in 2012. At present, a novel coronavirus has emerged in late 2019 from the Wuhan City, Hubei Province, China and causing the Coronavirus Disease. The first case was identified on December 12, 2019. On February 11, 2020, World Health Organization (WHO) announced this current viral disease due to coronavirus as "COVID-19," caused by the SARS-CoV type 2. This pandemic disease directly impact peoples' lives at all aspects such as physical, mental, social, and economic wellbeing. Many researchers are doing work on all over the world for the appropriate treatment of this

COVID-19 and Immunomodulation with Special Emphasis on Nutraceutical and Herbal Formulation.
Rajesh K. Kesharwani & Raj K. Keservani (Eds)

disease, but till date no correct cure for this disease could be found. Still vaccine trials for the disease are underway in almost many countries; a few countries have got success so far. The virus still remains a mystery to clinicians and researchers. Reinfection with this virus has also been revealed. In such a situation, the world is also focusing towards alternative medicine for the cure of this disease. Ayurveda is a better option in terms of choice medicine. It is one of the ancient traditional medical systems in the world. It has been developed thousands of years ago in India. In Ayurveda, complete description has been specified about the treatment, prevention, and curative aspects of the disease. However, no disease by the name of COVID-19 is described in the classics of Ayurveda, but diseases with similar symptoms of COVID-19 are described in detail in Ayurvedic lexicons. Based on comparative study of symptoms, it is possible to recognize the probable pathogenesis and treatment of this pandemic.

10.1 INTRODUCTION

In the last years, all over the world SARS (severe acute respiratory syndrome) and MERS (Middle East respiratory syndrome) diseases had come in 2002 and 2012, respectively. Currently a new novel coronavirus has emerged from Wuhan City of China in late 2019 and is continuously ongoing pandemic in many countries throughout the world (Rodriguez-Morales et al., 2020). Coronaviruses belong to the seven members of the family Coronaviridae (subfamily Coronavirinae) (Zhu et al., 2020). Nearly six viruses other than the coronavirus also have infected humans but remain related to mild upper respiratory tract diseases (Wei et al., 2020). These are HCoV-229E, HCoV-NL63, HCoV-OC43, HCoV-HKU1, SARS-CoV, and MERS-CoV (Wei et al., 2020). Coronavirus is an RNA virus that has many hosts. Symptoms range from general cold to more severe respiratory ailments. Recently, the SARS CoV caused havoc in China and gradually infected most of the world population. Despite many efforts, this disease has not been controlled. First, WHO named it 2019 novel coronavirus and then it was later renamed as COVID-19 on February 11, 2020 (https://www.who.int/docs/default-source/coronaviruse/situationreports). In-addition, SARS-CoV-2 is related to member of the order Nidovirales, family Coronaviridae, and subfamily Orthocoronavirinae. It is further subdivided into four genera, namely, Alpha, Beta, Gamma, and Delta coronavirus (Chen et al., 2020). The genera Alpha and Beta coronavirus originate from bats, while the Gamma and Delta coronavirus have evolved from birds and swine gene pools (Li et al., 2020).

10.2 EPIDEMIOLOGY

Initially, the epicenter of COVID-19 was Wuhan city of China. COVID-19 disease first case was recognized on December 12, 2019. Gradually, this disease started spreading in China. When the cases and careers spread to all countries through international flights, gradually many countries of the world became infected with it. According to WHO reports, the disease spread to 203 countries in April 2020 and about 896,450 people were infected with this virus. Gradually this figure kept increasing and by September 2020 more than 30.4 million have been infected. More than 950K patients have died and more than 10 million patients still exist as active cases (https://covid19.who.int/). In the initial phase, this disease had more impact in China. Slowly the virus spread out through all Europe and Italy, and Spain was the most affected. The greatest numbers of infected cases in present scenario are in America and India.

TABLE 10.1 Worldwide Cases.

Worldwide cases by WHO		
Countries	**Confirmed cases**	**Deaths**
America	15,215,110	521,872
South-East Asia	5,871,987	99,001
Europe	5,079,896	228,669
Eastern Mediterranean	2,182,798	56,884
Africa	1,136,235	24,514
Western Pacific	568,943	12,480

Source: World Health Organization.

10.3 THE VIRUS (SARS-COV-2)

Coronaviruses are RNA viruses having wide range of natural hosts (Li et al., 2020; Weiss and Leibowitz, 2011). In the beginning, WHO named this emerging virus as a 2019-novel coronavirus (2019-nCoV) and was later renamed as COVID-19. COVID-19 virus has been recognized as "severe acute respiratory syndrome coronavirus 2" (SARS-CoV-2) by the International Committee on Taxonomy of Viruses (ICTV). The novel coronavirus was identified by scientist within 28 days of the outbreak. Coronaviruses possess an unsegmented, single-stranded (ss) positive-sense RNA genome of 29.891 kb long, with a G + C content of 38%, enclosed by a 5'-cap and 3'-poly-A tail (Fehr and Perlman, 2015; Chan et al., 2020). Coronaviruses having four major structural parts like as proteins, namely, Spike (S), Membrane (M), Envelope (E), and Nucleocapsid (N) (Kuldeep et al., 2019).

10.4 CLINICAL PRESENTATIONS

The clinical researchers' reports represented that COVID-19 causes asymptomatic symptom stage to pathological features like fever, cough, sore throat, and clinical conditions related to severe respiratory failure that requires mechanical ventilation and intensive care unit (ICU). COVID-19 also causes systemic symptoms like sepsis, septic shock, and multiple organ dysfunction syndromes (Lupia et al., 2020). Most of the patients show asymptomatic infections but their frequency is unknown. The key clinical pathophysiological symptoms are fever, cough, dyspnea, headache, sore throat, rhinorrhea, etc. A number of other related clinical symptoms are loss of feeling of smell and taste; and include features of gastrointestinal tract like nausea, vomiting, and diarrhea, etc. in a lesser extent. Pneumonia disease comes to be the most severe manifestation of infection. It is having primary symptoms like COVID-19 disease, and bilateral infiltrates on chest imaging (Yang et al., 2020). COVID-19 disease spread out through the respiratory droplets. It is the key route. In addition, it can also be transmitted through person-to-person contacts by asymptomatic carriers also (Francesco et al., 2020).

10.5 TREATMENT

There is no specific antiviral treatment protocol recommended for COVID-19. The treatment of COVID-19 disease is symptomatic and oxygen treatment chiefly used as the major intervention for patients having severe infection. Sometimes at emergency cases such as respiratory failure the mechanical ventilation may be used, while hemodynamic support facility is necessary for managing septic shock (Yang et al., 2020). For asymptomatic cases, the Home isolation management is suitable where need to check properly evaluation of body temperature, blood pressure, oxygen volume, and respiratory symptoms. Treatment and management of such patients need to focus on prevention of disease transmission from person to person and monitoring for clinical presentations for early hospitalization if required. The time duration of home isolation is uncertain, and incubation time around 14 days approximately without symptoms such as fever, dyspnea, and others are considered adequate to end home isolation (Francesco et al., 2020). Remdesivir drug is approved as novel nucleotide analogue. The researchers have found activity against SARS-CoV-2 and related coronaviruses in animal studies (Wang et al., 2020). Chloroquine and hydroxychloroquine have also shown antiviral effect in vitro and inhibition activity against numerous proinflammatory cytokines such as IL-1 and IL-6 (Francesco et al., 2020). Tocilizumab drug is a recombinant humanized monoclonal antibody. It is used for the treatment and prevention of COVID-19 cases and elevated IL-6 levels (Biggioggero et al., 2018). Tocilizumab drug binds to the interleukin-6 (IL-6) receptor and inhibits it from functioning. Lopinavir–ritonavir is used for HIV infection, but it also has some therapeutic action against SARS-CoV-2 infection (Lim et al., 2020).

10.6 TRADITIONAL SYSTEM OF MEDICINE AND COVID-19

"Health for all" declaration by the WHO is mainly contributed by the Traditional Systems of Medicine (TSM) across the globe. Its importance for the healthcare needs from the past, in the present, and the future are well recognized. The ancient therapeutic systems such as Ayurveda, Siddha, and Unani are the three important Traditional Systems of India, which are now called Indian Systems of Medicine (ISM). Among these three systems, Ayurveda is one of the oldest and the most commonly practiced system in India. It has a very strong conceptual base and has been practiced since a very long time. It takes into consideration all the aspects of health including physical, mental, spiritual, and social components. According to the principle of Ayurveda, good health depends upon the balance of three factors. These three factors are dosha or humor, agni (related to digestive fire), dhatu (related to seven body tissues: lymph, blood, muscle, adipose tissue, bone, bone marrow, and semen), and proper functioning of mala (related to feces, urine, and other waste products) (Shastri et al., 1982). According to the World Health Organization's (WHO) concept of good health, it is a state of complete physical, mental, and social well-being and not merely an absence of disease or illness. It is in close proximity to the definition of good health mentioned in Ayurvedic lexicon (Park, 1983). Considering the modern parameters, COVID-19 can be considered as Aupasargika Roga (Communicable disease) in Ayurveda. This Aupsargika Sankramaka Roga (Communicable Infectious disease) primarily affects the person in which Vyadhikshamatva (immune strength) is compromised in comparison to healthy individuals (Agnivesa, Charaka Samhita).

10.7 AYURVEDIC VIEW OF COVID-19

According to the principles of Ayurveda, no disease can occur without dosha (humor) involvement and also, the diseases that are not mentioned in the Ayurvedic classics. That type of diseases can be treated on the basis of dosha and other pathological factors. As per the modern concept, virus spread easily from person to person through close contact, respiratory droplets released by coughing or sneezing of an infected person, and touching a surface with the virus over hand on it and after touching his or her mouth, nose or eyes. The same is also elaborated in Ayurvedic classics as the concept of gatrasansparsh (bodily contamination) under the Aupsargika Sankramaka Roga. Thus, we can classify COVID-19 under the Aupsargika Sankramaka Roga (Communicable Infectious disease) which is initially represented as a kapha-vaata sansargaja jwara, having association of pitta (Shri et al., 1980) and later on it acquires the status of sannipata jwara (Charakacharya, Charak Samhita).

10.8 AYURVEDIC VIEW OF SAMPRAPTI (PATHOGENESIS) OF COVID-19 INFECTION

As per the concept of Ayurveda, the COVID-19 infection's complication increases may be due to the growth and aggravation of Kapha and Vata dosha followed by Pitta within the Pranavahasrotasa (respiratory system); later on, other channels carrying nutrients, blood, and gastrointestinal tract, etc. The Dushya are initially rasa and rakta (blood) followed by the involvement of all other dhatus in the advanced stages. Due to less functioning of bio-fire (mandagni in abdomen), there is a decrease in digestive process which leads to development of Ama (undigested and improperly processed outcome of digestion and metabolism) causing the obstruction in the pranavahasrotasa which bring abnormality in the Kapha–Vata dosha to a greater extent. These pathophysiological symptoms are like fever, cough, myalgia, fatigue, headache, cough production, dysentery, depression, shortness of breath/dyspnea, and respiratory suffering, etc.; if it is not treated, it will lead to the manifestation of complications like severe pneumonia, septic shock, acute respiratory distress syndrome (ARDS), and multiorgan failure problems, resulting in death (Proposed guidelines by BHU).

10.9 AYURVEDIC APPROACH TOWARDS THE TREATMENT AND MANAGEMENT OF COVID-19

10.9.1 PREVENTIVE MEASURES

Prevention is always the best option to diminish the spread of COVID-19 disease. It is considering the lack of efficient treatment. At the moment, there are few vaccines available all over the world and the best prevention is to avoid contact to the virus (Adhikari et al., 2020).

10.9.2 PERSONAL HYGIENE

Personal hygiene must follow hands wash method. In addition, hands should be washed with soap and water properly for at least 20 s or rubbed with 75% ethyl alcohol-based sanitizer. It kills viruses that may be attached to hands. Spitting by an infected person may contain and spread the virus. So, spitting in public place should be avoided. Contact with hands like shaking and physical touch should be avoided to stop spreading of virus. Frequent touching of own body parts like eyes, nose, and mouth with hands should be avoided because it may transfer virus inside the body (Centers for Disease Control and Prevention). Practice of covering of mouth and nose with handkerchief or with bent elbow should be encouraged. Moreover, while a person without respiratory symptoms is not necessary to wear a medical mask when in public. Those people who are showing respiratory symptoms are advised to use medical masks both in healthcare and homecare settings (Hopman et al., 2020). People should use gloves whenever necessary. People should be advised to maintain physical distancing of minimum 3 ft (World Health Organization Coronavirus Disease) and not to go to crowded places like malls, religious place, markets, etc. Travelling may be avoided until necessary. Work from home culture may be encouraged in present scenario. If anyone has symptoms like fever, cough, difficulty in respiration, etc., then those persons should consult a physician immediately and all the instructions given by doctor should be followed.

10.9.3 DIET

According to individuals' digestive power, diet should be light and easily digestible. The food taken should be fresh and warm. For prevention purpose, lukewarm liquids with some medicinal herbs like shunthi, pippali, marich, dalchini, etc. should be used frequently as a regular drink but not in excess amount. Green vegetables like Patola (*Tricosanthes dioica* Roxb.), Karvellaka (*Momordica charantia* Linn.), Vaastuka (*Chenopodium album* L.), Lashuna (*Allium sativum* L.), Jivanti (*Leptadenia reticulata* Retz.), Shigru (*Moringa oleifera* Lam), Tanduliyak (*Amaranthus spinosus* L.), etc. should be preferred in daily diet (Vaidya Lakshmipati Shastri, Jwara Chikitsa, Yoga Ratnakara). In the fruits, person can use Draksha (*Vitis vinifera* L.), Kapittha (*Feronia limonia* Linn.), Dadima (*Punica granatum* Linn), etc. Food which is heavy to digest and cold in nature or chilled food should be restricted along with over consumption of sweets. Spicy, oily, fried or fermented food should be avoided along with alcohol drinking and beverages too (Govindadasa et al., 2005).

10.9.4 LIFESTYLE MODIFICATION

A healthy lifestyle should be encouraged. Contact with friends and relatives through calls, social media, emails, etc. should be maintained frequently. Adequate sleep of 7–8 h at night should be encouraged and avoided at day time. Also encourage reading books, listening to music (classical or instrumental) or any other creative work. Smoking must be avoided. Exercise and meditation (Dhyaan), daily practice of different Yogasana and Pranayama for at least 30 min, as advised by the Ministry of AYUSH, should be encouraged. Daily and seasonal regimen (Dincharya and Ritucharya) under the supervision of Ayurvedic Physician is always to be encouraged. Self-medication should not be practiced and if medicines are necessary, drug must be used under supervision.

10.9.5 SINGLE DRUGS FOR IMMUNITY ENHANCEMENT

1. Guduchi (*Tinospora cordifolia*)—3–6 gm twice a day in the powder form with lukewarm water or 500–1000 mg of aqueous

extract of Guduchi twice a day or 20 mL twice a day in the form of decoction.

2. Amlaki (*Embilica officinalis*)—fresh Amla fruit powder 3–6 gm twice a day with lukewarm water.
3. Haridra (*Curcuma longa*)—frequent gargling with haldi powder and little warm water used with a pinch of salt or half teaspoon mixed with one glass milk at bed time.
4. Tulsi (*Ocimum sanctum*)—frequent sipping of lukewarm water processed with leaves of Tulsi is advised.

10.9.6 FORMULATIONS FOR IMMUNITY ENHANCEMENT

1. Chyawanprash Avaleha—10–12 gm per day.
2. Draksh Avaleha—10–12 gm per day.
3. Indukantamritam—10–12 gm two times in a day before food.
4. Haridra Khanda—3–5 gm with honey or little warm water.

10.10 MANAGEMENT OF ASYMPTOMATIC PATIENTS

Population that has no symptoms and is home-quarantined may have some symptoms of stress and anxiety. In this critical situation, there is a need for the patient's proper counseling. Health workers should be given information related to the disease and its prevention. Their diet should be healthy and balanced. They should be aware of proper sanitization and should be motivated to exercise according to the nature and physical force. To increase the body's immunity, the following should be consumed.

1. Cow milk, ghee or medicated ghee.
2. Boiled lukewarm water medicated with Yavani (*Trachyspermum ammi* Linn.), Lavanga (*Syzygium aromaticum* Linn.), Sunthi (*Zingiber officinale* Roxb.), Dalchini (*Cinnamomum zeylanicum* Breyn), Pippali (*Piper longum* Linn.), and Tulasi (*Ocimum sanctum* Linn.), etc.
3. Single drug like Guduchi (*Tinospora cordifolia*), Tulsi (*Ocimum sanctum* Linn.), Haridra (*Curcuma longa* Linn.), Manjistha (*Rubia cordifolia* Linn.), Amalaki (*Emblica officinalis* Gaertn.), Ashwagandha (*Withania somnifera* Linn.), Yashtimadhu (*Glycyrrhiza glabra* Linn.), Draksha (*Vitis vinifera* Linn.), Kharjura (*Phoenix sylvestris* Roxb.), etc.

4. Formulations like Giloy ghanvati or Sanshamani Vati (SYS-Jvaradhikara, pg 183), Chyavanprasha (CSChiS-1/1/62–74), Amalaki Rasayana (BR-Rasayana Prakarana, 73/25), etc.

10.11 MANAGEMENT OF MILD SYMPTOMS

For the mild features of symptoms like fever, cough, sore throat, nasal congestion, malaise, and headache following drugs can be used (Guidelines for Ayurveda practitioners).

10.11.1 VATI PREPARATIONS

1. Mahasudarshan Ghanvati for mild fever and headache.
2. Sanjeevani Vati for mild fever and headache.
3. Samshamni Vati for mild fever and headache.
4. Vyoshadivati/Yashtimadhu Ghanvati (Lozenges) for cough.
5. Lavangadi Vati for shortness of breath.
6. Kutajaghan Vati for diarrhea.

10.11.2 CHURNA PREPARATIONS

1. Talishadi Churna + Yastimadhu Churna for cough.
2. Sitopaladi Churna for dry cough and sore throat.
3. Sudarshan Churna for mild fever and headache.
4. Haridra Khanda for allergic features.

10.11.3 KWATH PREPARATIONS

1. Chaturthaka Jvaraharakwatha (Giloya stem either dry or wet 5 gm + Amalaki Dry 5 gm + Nagarmotha 5 gm boiled with 200 mL of water and evaporated to reduce it upto 100 mL)—10 gm boiled in one glass of water, reduced to half BD empty stomach for mild fever.
2. Rasnasaptaka Kwatha for Myalgia—10 gm boiled with one glass of water, reduced to half BD empty stomach.
3. Gojihwadi Kwatha for common cold.
4. Shirishadi Kwath for allergic features.

10.11.4 AVALEHA PREPARATION

1. Chitrak Haritaki Avaleha for common cold.
2. Mridvik Avaleha used for the treatment of dry cough and sore throat.
3. Vasavaleha for shortness of breath.
4. Draksh Avaleha for shortness of breath.

10.11.5 ASAVARISHTA

1. Amritarishta for mild fever.
2. Ashwagandharishta for malaise and bodyache.
3. Balarishta for malaise and bodyache.
4. Dashmularishta for cough.

10.11.6 RASA AUSHADHI

1. Naradiya Lakshmivilasa Rasa for common cold.
2. Tribhuvan kirti Rasa for fever.
3. Shwasakuthara Rasa used for the treatment of shortness of breath.
4. Sameerapannaga Rasa for dry cough and sore throat.
5. Mallasindur Rasa used for the treatment of dry cough and sore throat.
6. Vatavidhwansan Rasa for malaise and bodyache.
7. Soot Shekhar Rasa for allergic features.
8. Rasaraj Rasa for immunity boosting.

10.11.7 BHASMA

1. Godanti bhasma for mild fever and headache.
2. Guduchi satva for mild fever and headache.
3. Swarna bhasma for immunity boosting.
4. Abhrak bhasma for immunity boosting.

10.11.8 KSHAR

1. Yavakshar for shortness of breath.
2. Apamarga kshar for shortness of breath.

10.11.9 OTHERS

Pratimarsha Nasya 2 drops BD with

1. Anu Taila.
2. Shadbindu Taila.
3. Sarshapa Taila.

10.12 MANAGEMENT OF SEVERE FEATURES

For more severe features like moderate to high fever, productive cough, moderate to high dyspnea, etc. following medicines should be taken.

10.12.1 VATI PREPARATIONS

1. Mahasudarshan Ghanvati for moderate to high fever.
2. Bilwadi Gutika for moderate to high fever.

10.12.2 CHURNA PREPARATIONS

1. Talishadi Churna for productive cough.
2. Trikatu Churna for productive cough.
3. Shringyadi Churna for productive cough.

10.12.3 KWATH PREPARATIONS

1. Ashtadashaanga Kwatha for moderate/high fever.
2. Parijatapatra Kwath for moderate/high fever.
3. Dashmoola Kwath for moderate to severe dyspnea.
4. Palashmuladi Kwath for moderate to severe dyspnea.
5. Pushkarmula Kwath for moderate to severe dyspnea.

10.12.4 AVALEHA PREPARATION

1. Vyaghri Haritaki Avaleha for productive cough and dyspnea.
2. Kantakari Avaleha for productive cough and dyspnea.
3. Agastya Haritaki Avaleha used for the treatment of modest to severe dyspnea.
4. Draksh Avaleha for shortness of breath.

10.12.5 ASAVARISHTA

1. Amritarishta for moderate to high fever.

10.12.6 RASA AUSHADHI

1. Putapakwa Vishama Jwarantaka Lauha for moderate to high fever.
2. Vasant malti rasa for moderate to high fever.
3. Mritunjaya rasa for moderate to high fever.
4. Mallachandrodaya rasa for moderate to high fever and productive cough.
5. Laghumalini Vasant rasa for moderate to high fever and dyspnea.
6. Mallasindur rasa for moderate to severe dyspnea.
7. AYUSH 64 for moderate to high fever.
8. Shwas Kasa Chintamani rasa for moderate to severe dyspnea.
9. Chandramrit rasa for moderate to severe dyspnea.
10. Shringabhra rasa for moderate to severe dyspnea.
11. Rasa sindur and makardhwaja for immunity boosting.

10.12.7 BHASMA

1. Abhrak bhasma for moderate to high fever.
2. Guduchi satva for moderate to high fever.
3. Tankan bhasma for productive cough.
4. Shuddhanavasadar for productive cough.
5. Shankha bhasma for moderate to severe dyspnea.
6. Swarna bhasma for immunity boosting.

10.12.8 FOR PNEUMONIA (SHWASAPRADHANAKASA)

1. Sanjeevani Vati—125 mg three times in a day (TDS), Gorochanadi Vati—125 mg three times in a day (TDS), with little warm water.
2. Somasav/Pushkaramoolasava—10–20 mL with equal quantity of water two times in a day (BD).
3. Talisadi (4 g) + Madhuyashti churna (2 gm) + Sameerapannaga rasa (125 mg)—twice in a day with honey or little warm water.

4. Pushkaramoolasava—15–20 mL in BD/TDS with same amount of water
5. Agastya Haritaki/Vyaghri Haritaki/Chitraka Haritaki Avaleha—10–12 gm two times in a day (BD) after food with water.
6. Kanthakari Avaleha—10–12 gm BD after food.
7. Dashamoolakatutrayadi Kashaya—20–30 mL three times in a day (TDS) with lukewarm water before food.
8. Vasakasava—15–20 mL three times in a day (TDS) with lukewarm water after food.
9. Bharangyadi Kwatha—30–40 mL two times in a day (BD) with lukewarm water before food.
10. Chandramrita rasa—250 mg two times in a day (BD) with lukewarm water or honey or tamboolaswarasa or vasa swarasa or ardraka swarasa.

10.13 CONCLUSION

COVID-19 has drastic effects as a pandemic disease for which no definitive treatment has yet been discovered in the contemporary science. The process of research is going on continuously and efforts are also being made to discover vaccines. In such circumstances, the attention of scientists around the world is also focusing towards alternative medicines. This is the time when we can put our ancient medical science in front of the world and give the entire world a direction for the proper management of this pandemic. Ayurveda is a complete and comprehensive science of living beings in which the patient is treated as a whole, not only the disease. Based on this principle, Ayurveda is a better alternative choice for the treatment and management of COVID-19 disease without any harmful effects, economic, safer, and a better way of life emphasizing on immunity too.

KEYWORDS

- **Ayurveda**
- **COVID-19**
- **traditional system of medicine**
- **WHO**

REFERENCES

Adhikari, S. P.; Meng, S.; Wu, Y. J.; Mao, Y. P.; Ye, R. X.; Wang, Q. Z.; Sun, C.; Sylvia, S.; Rozelle, S.; Raat, H.; et al. Epidemiology, Causes, Clinical Manifestation and Diagnosis, Prevention and Control of Coronavirus Disease (COVID-19) During the Early Outbreak Period: A Scoping Review. *Infect. Dis. Poverty* **2020,** *9*, 29.

Agnivesa. *Charaka Samhita*, Sutra Sthana 28/07, ed. 18; Shastri, R. D. ed.; Chaukhamba Bharti Academy: Varanasi, 1992; p 571.

Biggioggero, M.; Crotti, C.; Becciolini, A.; Favalli, E. G. Tocilizumab in the Treatment of Rheumatoid Arthritis: An Evidence-Based Review and Patient Selection. *Drug Des. Dev. Ther.* **2018,** *13*, 57–70.

Centers for Disease Control and Prevention 2019 Novel Coronavirus, Wuhan, China. [Online] 2020. https://www.cdc.gov/coronavirus/2019-ncov/prevent-getting sick/prevention. html (accessed on 13 April 2020).

Chan, J. F.; Kok, K. H.; Zhu, Z.; Chu, H.; To, K. K.; Yuan, S.; Yuen, K. Y. Genomic Characterization of the 2019 Novel Human-Pathogenic Coronavirus Isolated from a Patient with Atypical Pneumonia after Visiting Wuhan. *Emerg. Microbes Infect.* **2020,** *9* (1), 221–236. DOI: 10.1080/22221751.2020.1719902.

Chen, Y.; Liu, Q.; Guo, D. Emerging Coronaviruses: Genome Structure, Replication, and Pathogenesis. *J. Med. Virol.* **2020,** 92 (4), 418–423. DOI: 10.1002/jmv.25681.

Charak Acharya. Charak Samhita; Commentary by Sashtri, K., Goraknath, C., 13th ed.; Chaukambha Bharti Academy: Varanasi, India, 1986; ChikitsaSthan 3/103.

Dhama, K.; Khan, S.; Tiwari, R.; Rodriguez, A. J.; et al. Coronavirus Disease 2019 - COVID-19, Preprints (www.preprints.org) | NOT PEER-REVIEWED | Posted: 13 April 2020. DOI: 10.20944/preprints 202003.0001.v2.

Di Gennaro, F.; et al. Coronavirus Diseases (COVID-19) Current Status and Future Perspectives: A Narrative Review. *Int. J. Environ. Res. Public Health* **2020,** *17*, 2690. DOI: 10.3390/ijerph17082690.

Dutta, S. A. *Sushrut Samhita*, 8th ed.; Chowkhembha Sanskrit Samsthan: Varanasi, 1982; p 64 (or Chap. 15, Verse 48).

Fehr, A. R.; Perlman, S. Coronaviruses: An Overview of Their Replication and Pathogenesis. *Methods Mol. Biol.* **2015,** *1282*, 1–23. DOI: 10.1007/978-1-4939-2438-7_1.

Govindadasa. Jwara Adhikara. In *Bhaishajya Ratnavali*, 18th ed.; Chowkambha Samskrita Samstana: Varanasi, 2005.

Guidelines for Ayurveda Pracitioners for Covid 19. Draft Version 3.1 Dated 08/04/2020.

Gupta, Shri A. D. *AstangaHrdya*, Chaukhamba Sanskrit Sansthana: Varanasi, India, 1980; NidanaSthana, 2/25.

Hopman, J.; Allegranzi, B.; Mehtar, S. Managing COVID-19 in Low- and Middle-Income Countries. *JAMA* **2020.**

https://covid19.who.int/WHO Coronavirus Disease (COVID-19) Dashboard, Data last updated: 2020/9/18, 4:01pm CEST.

Li, G.; Fan, Y.; Lai, Y.; Han, T.; Li, Z.; Zhou, P.; Pan, P.; Wang, W.; Hu, D.; Liu, X.; Zhang, Q.; Wu, J. Coronavirus infections and immune responses. *J. Med. Virol.* **2020,** *92* (4), 424–432 DOI: 10.1002/jmv.25685.

Lim, J.; Jeon, S.; Shin, H. Y. The Author's Response: Case of the Index Patient who Caused Tertiary Transmission of Coronavirus Disease 2019 in Korea: The Application of Lopinavir/Ritonavir for the Treatment of COVID-19 Pneumonia Monitored by Quantitative RT-PCR. *J. Korean Med. Sci.* **2020,** 35.

Lupia, T.; Scabini, S.; Mornese Pinna, S.; Di Perri, G.; De Rosa, F. G.; Corcione, S. 2019 Novel Coronavirus (2019-nCoV) Outbreak: A New Challenge. *J. Glob. Antimicrob. Resist.* **2020,** *21*, 22–27.

Park, G. E. *Textbook of Preventive and Social Medicine*, 9th ed.; M/F Banarasi Das Bhanot: Jabalpur, India, 1983; p 12.

Pneumonia in China, 2019. *N. Engl. J. Med.* 10.1056/NEJMoa2001017. DOI: 10.1056/NEJMoa2001017.

Proposed Guidelines for the Management of COVID-19 (To be used by Ayurvedic Practitioners) Faculty of Ayurveda, Institute of Medical Sciences, Banaras Hindu University: Varanasi, 2020.

Rodriguez-Morales, A. J.; Bonilla-Aldana, D. K.; Balbin-Ramon, G. J.; Rabaan, A. A.; Sah, R.; Paniz-Mondolfi, A.; Pagliano, P.; Esposito, S. History is Repeating Itself: Probable Zoonotic Spillover as the Cause of the 2019 Novel Coronavirus Epidemic. *Infez. Med.* **2020,** *28* (1), 3–5.

Wang, H.; Wang, S.; Yu, K. COVID-19 Infection Epidemic: The Medical Management Strategies in Heilongjiang Province, China. *Crit. Care* **2020,** *24*, 107.

Wei, X.; Li, X.; Cui, J. Evolutionary Perspectives on Novel Coronaviruses Identified in Pneumonia Cases in China. Natl. Sci. Rev. **2020**. DOI: 10.1093/nsr/nwaa009.

Weiss, S. R.; Leibowitz, J. L. Coronavirus Pathogenesis. *Adv. Virus Res.* **2011,** *81*, 85–164. DOI:
10.1016/B978-0-12-385885-6.00009-2.

WHO 2020. World Health Organization. Coronavirus Disease 2019 (COVID-19) Situation Report. *Situation Report – 33* [Online], February 22, 2020. https://www.who.int/docs/default-source/coronaviruse/situationreports/20200222-sitrep-33-COVID-19.pdf (accessed September 10, 2020).

WHO 2020. World Health Organization. Coronavirus Disease 2019 (COVID-19) situation report. *Situation Report – 33* [Online]. https://www.who.int/docs/default-source/coronaviruse/situationreports/20200222-sitrep-33 COVID-19.pdf

World Health Organization Coronavirus Disease (COVID-19) Advice for the Public [Online]. https://www.who.int/emergencies/diseases/novel-coronavirus-2019/advice-for-public (accessed Aug 23, 2020).

Yang, Y.; Peng, F.; Wang, R.; Guan, K.; Jiang, T.; Xu, G.; Sun, J.; Chang, C. The Deadly Coronaviruses: The 2003 SARS Pandemic and the 2020 Novel Coronavirus Epidemic in China. *J. Autoimmun.* **2020**.

Zhu, N.; Zhang, D.; Wang, W.; Li, X.; Yang, B.; Song, J.; Zhao, X.; Huang, B.; Shi, W.; Lu, R.; Niu, P.; Zhan, F.; Ma, X.; Wang, D.; Xu, W.; Wu, G.; Gao, G. F.; Tan, W.; China Novel Coronavirus Investigating and Research Team. A Novel Coronavirus from Patients with Vaidya Lakshmipati Shastri. Jwara Chikitsa. In *Yoga Ratnakara*, Ed. 2018; Chaukhamba Prakashan: Varanasi, pp 251–253.

BIBLIOGRAPHY

1. Ayurvedic Formulary of India
2. Ashtang Hridayam Uttarasthana
3. Bhavprakasha Nighantu
4. Bhavprakasha Nighantu uttarardha
5. Bhaishajya Ratnavali
6. Charaka Samhita Chikitsa Sthana
7. Charadatta
8. Rasamrita
9. Rasendra Sara Sangraha
10. Rasa Tarangini
11. Rasa Tantra Saar & Siddha Prayoga Samghraha
12. Siddha Bheshaja Manimala
13. Sharangdhara Samhita Madhyama Khand
14. Siddha yoga Samgraha
15. Yoga Ratnakara

Index

D

P

R

S

T

9781774913178